Varney's Pocket Midwife

SECOND EDITION

Jan M. Kriebs, CNM, MSN, FACNM
Assistant Professor
Department of Obstetrics, Gynecology,
and Reproductive Sciences
University of Maryland School of Medicine
Baltimore, Maryland

Carolyn L. Gegor, CNM, MS, RDMS
Nurse Midwifery Education Program
Georgetown University
School of Nursing and Health Studies
Washington, D.C.

JONES AND BARTLETT PUBLISHERS
Sudbury, Massachusetts
BOSTON   TORONTO   LONDON   SINGAPORE

World Headquarters
Jones and Bartlett Publishers
40 Tall Pine Drive
Sudbury, MA 01776
978-443-5000
info@jbpub.com
www.jbpub.com

Jones and Bartlett Publishers Canada
6339 Ormindale Way
Mississauga, ON L5V 1J2
Canada

Jones and Bartlett Publishers
International
Barb House, Barb Mews
London W6 7PA
United Kingdom

Jones and Bartlett's books and products are available through most bookstores
and online booksellers. To contact Jones and Bartlett Publishers directly, call
800-832-0034, fax 978-443-8000, or visit our website www.jbpub.com.

Substantial discounts on bulk quantities of Jones and Bartlett's publications are
available to corporations, professional associations, and other qualified organiza-
tions. For details and specific discount information, contact the special sales
department at Jones and Bartlett via the above contact information or send an
email to specialsales@jbpub.com.

Production Credits
Acquisitions Editor: Kevin Sullivan
Associate Editor: Amy Sibley
Production Director: Amy Rose
Associate Production Editor: Carolyn F. Rogers
Marketing Manager: Emily Ekle
Manufacturing and Inventory Coordinator: Amy Bacus
Composition: ATLIS Graphics
Cover Design: Anne Spencer
Text Design: Paw Print Media
Printing and Binding: Malloy, Inc.
Cover Printing: Malloy, Inc.

Library of Congress Cataloging-in-Publication Data

Kriebs, Jan M.
    Varney's pocket midwife.—2nd ed. / Jan M. Kriebs, Carolyn L. Gegor.
        p. ; cm.
    Rev. ed. of: Varney's pocket midwife / Helen Varney, Jan M. Kriebs, Carolyn
L. Gegor. 1998.
    Includes bibliographical references and index.
    ISBN 0-7637-2671-0 (pbk.)
    1. Midwifery. 2. Gynecologic nursing. 3. Maternity nursing.
    [DNLM: 1. Midwifery—Handbooks. 2. Nurse Midwives—Handbooks.
WY 49 K92v 2004] I. Title: Pocket midwife. II. Gegor, Carolyn L.
III. Varney, Helen. Varney's pocket midwife. IV. Title.
    RG950.V37 2004 Suppl.
    618.2—dc22
                                                                    20044013103
6048
Printed in the United States of America
15 14 13 12 11   10 9 8 7 6 5 4 3

Table of Contents

Appendix A

Appendix B

Introduction

The first edition of the *Pocket Midwife* grew out of our desire to supplement the personal collections of reminders that almost all of us as midwives carry through our clinical lives. In this second edition we have again planned to create a quick resource and guidebook. This is not a complete reference source—it is a mental refresher. Nor is it intended to replace those very personal creations of the medication dose you just cannot remember at midnight, or the lab results you always reverse in your head. We do hope that this guide will provide students and practicing midwives alike a background to which such personal data can be added.

Varney's Midwifery, for which this is a clinical companion, contains a wealth of detail and description that does not fit into anyone's pocket. Some important, even essential, topics are not included here, because if you do not know them when the need arises, you either do not have time to look them up, or you need more detail than we can provide. Each section of the *Pocket Midwife* cites the relevant chapters of the text, and other useful references as well. In particular, Web sites that offer easy and up-to-date access to information are included in relevant sections.

Although the title page bears two names, there are others whose advice and support have been invaluable. Chief among these is Jenifer Fahey, CNM, whose expert review has improved the product you hold in your hands. Our excellent contributing authors for the fourth edition of *Varney's Midwifery* were the original developers of much of the material on which we have relied. The midwives at Maryland Women's Health—Rachel Payne Lovett, Jennifer Kaye, and Courtney Marshall—have each shared ideas, suggestions, and material. Our thanks also to Linda Sparks, our administrative assistant, for efforts "above and beyond." The editorial staff at Jones and Bartlett are also major contributors to the completion of this book.

Finally, we acknowledge the hard work and leadership of Helen Varney, whose determination to create and maintain an American midwifery textbook has provided the foundation on which we stand. Although Helen has officially "retired" from the book, she contributed an historical timeline to help us all remember the midwives and others who have worked for better care for mothers and babies, and to support the modern practice of midwifery. No one knows our history better than Helen, and few have done as much to make our future happen.

The Profession of Midwifery

Documents of the American College of Nurse-Midwives (ACNM)

The ACNM, as the professional organization for CNMs and CMs, creates and publishes many documents to support the education and practice of midwives in the United States. Included here are several of those most significant for practicing midwives, accurate as of May 15, 2004, and used by permission of the American College of Nurse-Midwives.

Standards for the Practice of Midwifery

Midwifery practice as conducted by Certified Nurse-Midwives (CNMs) and Certified Midwives (CMs) is the independent management of women's health care, focusing particularly on pregnancy, childbirth, the postpartum period, care of the newborn, and the family planning and gynecologic needs of women. The CNM and CM practice within a health care system that provides for consultation, collaborative management, or referral, as indicated by the health status of the client. CNMs and CMs practice in accord with the *Standards for the Practice of Midwifery*, as defined by the American College of Nurse-Midwives (ACNM).

STANDARD I: *Midwifery care is provided by qualified practitioners.*

The midwife:

1. Is certified by the ACNM designated certifying agent
2. Shows evidence of continuing competency as required by the ACNM designated certifying agent
3. Is in compliance with the legal requirements of the jurisdiction where the midwifery practice occurs

STANDARD II: *Midwifery care occurs in a safe environment within the context of the family, community, and a system of health care.*

The midwife:

1. Demonstrates knowledge of and utilizes federal and state regulations that apply to the practice environment and infection control
2. Demonstrates a safe mechanism for obtaining medical consultation, collaboration, and referral
3. Uses community services as needed
4. Demonstrates knowledge of the medical, psychosocial, economic, cultural, and family factors that affect care
5. Demonstrates appropriate techniques for emergency management including arrangements for emergency transportation
6. Promotes involvement of support persons in the practice setting

STANDARD III: Midwifery care supports individual rights and self-determination within boundaries of safety.

The midwife:

1. Practices in accord with the Philosophy and the Code of Ethics of the American College of Nurse-Midwives
2. Provides clients with a description of the scope of midwifery services and information regarding the client's rights and responsibilities
3. Provides clients with information regarding, and/or referral to, other providers and services when requested or when care required is not within the midwife's scope of practice
4. Provides clients with information regarding health care decisions and the state of the science regarding these choices to allow for informed decision-making

STANDARD IV: Midwifery care is composed of knowledge, skills, and judgments that foster the delivery of safe, satisfying, and culturally competent care.

The midwife:

1. Collects and assesses client care data, develops and implements an individualized plan of management, and evaluates outcome of care
2. Demonstrates the clinical skills and judgments described in the ACNM *Core Competencies for Basic Midwifery Practice*
3. Practices in accord with the ACNM *Standards for the Practice of Midwifery*

4. Practices in accord with service/practice guidelines that meet the requirements of the particular institution or practice setting

STANDARD V: Midwifery care is based upon knowledge, skills, and judgments which are reflected in written practice guidelines.

The midwife:

1. Describes the parameters of service for independent and collaborative midwifery management and transfer of care when needed
2. Establishes practice guidelines for each specialty area which may include, but is not limited to, primary health care of women, care of the childbearing family, and newborn care
3. Includes the following information in each specialty area:
   a. Client selection criteria
   b. Parameters and methods for assessing health status
   c. Parameters for risk assessment
   d. Parameters for consultation, collaboration, and referral
   e. Appropriate interventions including treatment, medication, and/or devices

STANDARD VI: Midwifery care is documented in a format that is accessible and complete.

The midwife:

1. Uses records that facilitate communication of information to clients, consultants, and institutions
2. Provides prompt and complete documentation of evaluation, course of management, and outcome of care

3. Promotes a documentation system that provides for confidentiality and transmittability of health records
4. Maintains confidentiality in verbal and written communications

STANDARD VII: Midwifery care is evaluated according to an established program for quality management that includes a plan to identify and resolve problems.

The midwife:

1. Participates in a program of quality management for the evaluation of practice within the setting in which it occurs
2. Provides for a systematic collection of practice data as part of a program of quality management
3. Seeks consultation to review problems, including peer review of care
4. Acts to resolve problems identified

STANDARD VIII: Midwifery practice may be expanded beyond the ACNM Core Competencies to incorporate new procedures that improve care for women and their families.

The midwife:

1. Identifies the need for a new procedure taking into consideration consumer demand, standards for safe practice, and availability of other qualified personnel
2. Ensures that there are no institutional, state, or federal statutes, regulations, or bylaws that would constrain the midwife from incorporation of the procedure into practice

3. Demonstrates knowledge and competency, including:
   a. Knowledge of risks, benefits, and client selection criteria
   b. Process for acquisition of required skills
   c. Identification and management of complications
   d. Process to evaluate outcomes and maintain competency
4. Identifies a mechanism for obtaining medical consultation, collaboration, and referral related to this procedure
5. Reports the incorporation of this procedure to the ACNM

Source: ACNM Division of Standards and Practice. Approved: ACNM Board of Directors, March 8, 2003.

Hallmarks of Midwifery

The art and science of midwifery are characterized by these hallmarks:

1. Recognition of pregnancy, birth, and menopause as normal physiologic and developmental processes
2. Advocacy of non-intervention in the absence of complications
3. Incorporation of scientific evidence into clinical practice
4. Promotion of family-centered care
5. Empowerment of women as partners in health care
6. Facilitation of healthy family and interpersonal relationships
7. Promotion of continuity of care
8. Health promotion, disease prevention, and health education
9. Promotion of a public health care perspective
10. Care to vulnerable populations

11. Advocacy for informed choice, shared decision making, and the right to self-determination
12. Cultural competence
13. Familiarity with common complementary and alternative therapies
14. Skillful communication, guidance, and counseling
15. Therapeutic value of human presence
16. Collaboration with other members of the health care team

Source: ACNM Core Competencies for Basic Midwifery Practice.

A Framework for Midwifery Clinical Management

The midwifery management process includes:

1. Systematically compiling and updating a complete and relevant database for the comprehensive assessment of each client's health, including a thorough health history and physical examination
2. Identifying problems and formulating diagnoses based upon interpretation of the database
3. Identifying health care needs/problems in collaboration with the client
4. Providing information and support to enable clients to make informed decisions and to assume primary responsibility for their own health
5. Developing a comprehensive plan of care with the client
6. Assuming primary responsibility for the implementation of individualized plans
7. Obtaining consultation, planning, and implementing collaborative management; referral or transferring the care of the client as appropriate
8. Initiating management of specific complications, emergencies, and deviations from normal

9. Evaluating, with the client, the effectiveness of care and modifying the plan of care as appropriate.

Source: ACNM Core Competencies for Basic Midwifery Practice.

References

American College of Nurse Midwives Web site. Available at: http://www.acnm.org. Accessed June 14, 2004.

Varney, H., Kriebs, J. M., & Gegor, C. L. (2003) Chapter 1. In *Varney's midwifery*, (4th ed.) Sudbury, MA: Jones and Bartlett Publishers.

SECTION 2

Basic Tools for Patient Care

Characteristics of the Culturally Competent Practitioner

Just as it is important to utilize a management framework to provide care that is skillful, as well as respectful of the woman, it is equally important to recognize and respect cultural differences that affect how one gives or receives health care.

Table 2-1 Practitioners and Cultural Awareness

Practitioners who are culturally competent:

- Move from cultural unawareness to an awareness and sensitivity of their own cultural heritage
- Recognize their own values and biases and are aware of how they might affect clients from other cultures
- Demonstrate comfort with cultural differences that exist between themselves and clients
- Know specifics about the particular cultural groups with which they are working
- Understand the historical events that may have caused harm to a particular cultural group
- Respect and are aware of the unique needs of clients from diverse communities
- Understand the importance of diversity within, as well as between, cultures

- Endeavor to learn more about cultural communities through client interactions, participation in cultural diversity dynamics, and consultations with community experts
- Make a continuous effort to understand a client's point of view
- Demonstrate flexibility and tolerance of ambiguity, and are nonjudgmental
- Maintain a sense of humor and an open mind
- Demonstrate a willingness to relinquish control in clinical encounters, to risk failure, and to look within for the source of frustration, anger, and resistance
- Acknowledge that the process is as important as the product

Source: Randall-David, E. *Culturally Competent HIV Counseling and Education.* Rockville, MD: DHHS Maternal and Child Health Bureau, 1994.

Components of a Complete History

Demographic/identifying information
    Age, ethnicity, education, contact information
Chief complaint
    Always recorded, even "Annual examination"
History of present illness (HPI)
    Current symptoms related to chief complaint, or
    "noncontributory" if no physical complaint at
    well-woman examination

Medical history	Social history
Surgical history	Family history
Menstrual history	Gynecologic history
Obstetric history	Sexual history
	Contraceptive history

The medical, surgical, family, and social histories are sometimes identified by the acronym PFSH.

Choose an order in which to ask the history that moves through the questions in an organized fashion and from least intimate to most. Establish a pattern that is consistent regardless of type or complexity of visit.

Phrasing Sociosexual Questions

Respect for women and respect for culture are both essential to best care. Another aspect of competent care is awareness of and respect for the varieties of sexual experience. One key issue occurs when the clinician assumes that all women are practicing heterosexuals. The following questions can be used to decrease the risk of discouraging some women from providing a complete history or seeking needed care.

SECTION 2

Table 2-2   Questions to Ensure a Complete Sexual History

With whom do you live? (alone / friend / partner / husband / children / pets / other)

Who is your emergency contact?

Do you currently have a sexual partner? Have you ever had a sexual partner?

Is your current sexual partner female / male / both / transgender / none?

Have your sexual partner(s) in the past been male / female / both / transgender?

Do you have a need for birth control at this time?

Have you ever used contraception?

What methods have you used?

Are you currently using any birth-control method?

Do you identify yourself as being heterosexual / lesbian / bisexual / transgender / celibate / other?

Do you experience orgasm?

Does your sexual activity include vaginal entry?

Do you have pain with vaginal entry?

Are you aware of safer sex practices?

Do you use safer sex practices? If yes, please list the methods you are currently using.

Have you ever had sex without your consent?

Source: Adapted from Carroll, NM. Providing gynecological and obstetric care for lesbians. *Contemp Rev Obstet Gynecol.* March 2000; Table 1, 76.

Review of Systems

Current or recent symptoms and signs relating to any body system relevant to the current examination, whether or not they appeared as part of the chief complaint or HPI

Components of the Physical Examination

> Constitutional
> Vital signs, height, and weight
> General appearance
> Skin and Hair
> Head / eyes / ears / nose / mouth and throat

Neck	Genitourinary
Heart	Musculoskeletal
Lungs	Vascular
Breast	Neurologic
Abdomen	Lymphatic

- If performing a single-system primary-care examination in well-woman gynecology, at least seven items from that system must be noted on the examination, which can include the breasts, axillary and inguinal lymphatics, bladder, and urethra as well as the reproductive system. A complete abdominal examination should also be included.

Anatomy of the Pelvis and Perineum

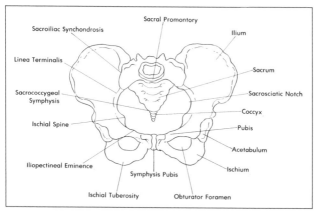

Figure 2-1   Bones of the pelvis.

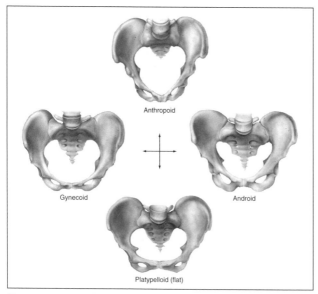

Figure 2-2   Four basic pelvic types. Caldwell-Moloy classification.

Table 2-3 Muscles of the Perineum

Muscles	Boundaries	Function
Bulbocavernosus	There are two bulbocavernosus muscles, one on either side of the vaginal orifice; posteriorly they attach to the central tendinous point of the perineum and the inferior fascia of the urogenital diaphragm; anteriorly they insert into the corpora cavernosa clitoridis; laterally they surround the orifice of the vagina, covering the vestibular bulbs and Bartholin's glands on either side.	Known as the sphincter vaginae, their contraction reduces the size of the vaginal orifice; the anterior muscle fibers contribute to clitoral erection.
Ischiocavernosus	There are two ischiocavernosus muscles, one on either lateral boundary of the perineum; posteriorly they arise from the inner surface of the ischial tuberosities; anteriorly they cover and insert into the sides and posterior surface of the crus clitoridis; laterally they extend from the clitoris to the ischial tuberosities along the ischial ramus, from which they derive some of their fibers.	Maintain clitoral erection
Superficial transverse perineal (transversus perinei superficialis)	There are two superficial transverse perineal muscles, which generally follow the transverse diameter of the pelvic outlet; they arise from the inner and anterior surface of the ischial tuberosity of the superior ramus of the ischium by a small tendon; they insert into the central tendinous point of the perineum.	Fix the location of the central tendinous point of the perineum
Deep transverse perineal (transversus perinei profundus)	There are two deep transverse perineal muscles, which are broader than the superficial transverse perineal muscles; they arise from the inferior ramus of the ischium; they insert into the sides of the vagina.	Help to fix the vagina

Sphincter of the membranous urethra muscles (sphincter urethrae membranaceae)	There are two sphincters of the membranous urethra muscles, consisting of external and innermost fibers; they arise from the margin of the inferior ramus of the pubis on either side; they cross the space of the pubic arch, pass around all sides and encircle the urethra, and unite with the muscle fibers from the other side by blending with them.	Urethral sphincter
External anal sphincter (sphincter ani externus)	The external anal sphincter consists of two strata of fibers (superficial and deep), which together form one flat plane of muscular fibers; it arises from the anococcygeal body, which is a tendinous band extending from the tip of the coccyx to the posterior margin of the anus; it passes around, encircles, and surrounds the anal canal; it inserts in the central tendinous point of the perineum.	Anal sphincter; helps to fix the location of the central tendinous point of the perineum
Central tendinous point of the perineum	A fibromuscular structure in the midline between the vagina and the anus and at the base of the urogenital diaphragm; the tissue is fibrous because it is the point of fusion of both the superior and inferior fascia of the urogenital diaphragm and the external perineal fascia and Colles' fascia; it has muscular fibers because it is a common point of attachment for a number of muscles whose fibers blend together into the central tendinous point of the perineum, among them the bulbocavernosus, superficial transverse perineal, some fibers of the deep transverse perineal, external anal sphincter, and the levator ani-pubococcygeus.	Common point of attachment for a number of layers of fascia and muscles

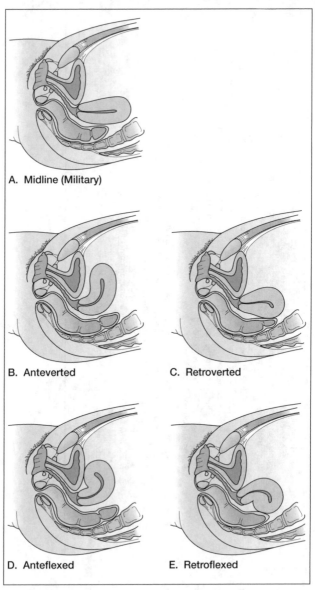

Figure 2-3 Positions of the uterus.

Anatomy of the Breast

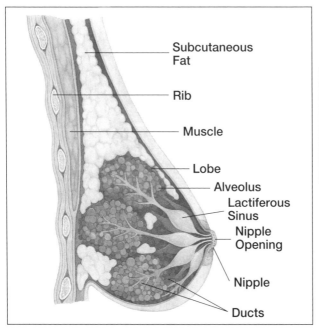

Figure 2-4 Side view of lactating breast.

Source: Walker, M.L. *Core Curriculum for Lactation Consultant Practice.* (2002). Sudbury, MA: Jones and Bartlett Publishers.

Complete Breast Examination

Utilize relevant components of the PFSH to reinforce assessment of changes in breast appearance, tissue, and shape. These include:

- Age
- Previous mammography/breast sonography
- Previous breast disease, masses
- Menstrual cycle, menarche, and menopause

- Pregnancies and breastfeeding
- Use of hormonal products
- Surgery of the reproductive system, e.g., oophorectomy
- Use of alcohol and tobacco

Relevant items in an HPI include:

- Nipple discharge
- Breast pain or tenderness
- Changes in breast shape, appearance
- New masses

Clinical breast examination:

- Inspection both erect and supine
- Palpation of both breasts in an organized pattern including the area from the clavicle to the mammary ridge, and under the axilla
- Assessment of supraclavicular and axillary lymph nodes
- Assessment of any accessory breast tissue, such as supernumerary nipples

Abnormalities requiring further assessment and physician consultation:

- Asymmetry of breast contour—mass, indentation, or shrinking
- Retraction of breast tissue
- Nipple deviation or retraction (does not include inverted nipples)
- Edema, *peau d'orange* skin changes
- Firmness or thickening of breast tissue
- Dilated subcutaneous veins not associated with pregnancy and lactation
- Heat or erythema, particularly if localized
- Ulcerations or lesions

- Palpable lymph nodes
- Nipple erosion, ulceration, thickening; erythema not associated with breastfeeding or breast sex play
- Nipple discharge or crusting
- Localized granular nodularity
- Masses within the breast tissue

Complete Pelvic Examination

Consider relevant items from the patient history as guides for particular observations during the examination.

- Age
- Menarche, menstrual age
- Menstrual cycle
- Perimenopausal symptoms
- Sexually transmitted infections, recurrent vaginal infections
- Use of contraceptive or other hormonal products
- Obstetric experience
- Gynecologic surgery

Review of systems:

- Assessment of gastrointestinal complaints
- Urinary problems
- Vaginal discharge
- Abdominal or pelvic pain
- Vaginal odor
- Lesions

The pelvic examination can be considered to include the entire genitourinary tract. Thus it can include:

- Bladder and urethra
- External genitalia
- Bartholin's and Skene's glands

- Vagina
- Cervix
- Uterus
- Adnexa
- Anus and perirectal area

Inspection of visible components is followed by speculum examination and bimanual evaluation. Rectovaginal examination is included as needed for adequate assessment of the uterus.

The Normal Menstrual Cycle

The normal menstrual cycle is regular in pattern and duration, ranging from 25 to 35 days in length, and up to seven days duration.

Normal Laboratory Values

Estrogen (as estradiol)

Follicular phase	60–200 pg/ml
Midcycle peak	150–750 pg/ml
Luteal phase	30–450 pg/ml
Perimenopause	≤ 20 pg/ml

Progesterone

Follicular phase	< 50 ng/dl
Luteal phase	200–2500 ng/dl
Postmenopausal	< 40 ng/dl

Luteinizing hormone

Follicular phase	1–12 IU/liter
Ovulatory peak	16–104 IU/liter
Luteal phase	1–12 IU/liter
Postmenopausal	14–66 IU/liter

Follicle-stimulating hormone

Follicular phase	1–9 IU/liter
Ovulatory peak	6–26 IU/liter
Luteal phase	1–9 IU/liter
Postmenopause	20–180 IU/liter
Prolactin	0–25 ng/dl, or < 25 µg/liter
Testosterone	<1 ng/ml, < 3.5 nmol/liter (SI units)

Source: Tietze, Pagnana.

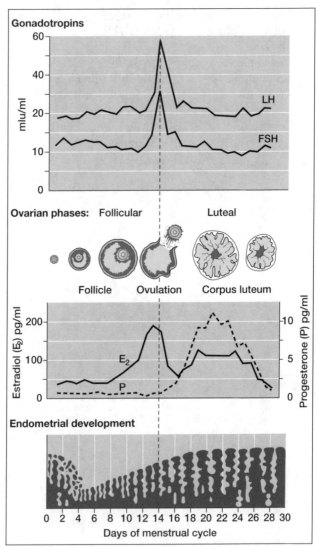

Figure 2-5   Events of the menstrual cycle, incorporating pituitary, ovarian, and uterine function.

Standard (Universal) Precautions

*Gloving, Gowning, Masking and Other Protective
Barriers as Part of Universal Precautions*

All health care workers should routinely use appropriate
barrier precautions to prevent skin and mucous membrane exposure during contact with any patient's blood or
body fluids that require universal precautions.

Gloves should be worn:

- For touching blood and body fluids requiring
  universal precautions, mucous membranes, or
  nonintact skin of all patients
- For handling items or surfaces soiled with blood
  or body fluids to which universal precautions
  apply

Gloves should be changed after contact with each
patient. Hands and other skin surfaces should be washed
immediately or as soon as patient safety permits if contaminated with blood or body fluids requiring universal
precautions. Hands should be washed immediately after
gloves are removed. Gloves should reduce the incidence
of blood contamination of hands during phlebotomy, but
they cannot prevent penetrating injuries caused by needles or other sharp instruments. Institutions that determine that routine gloving for all phlebotomies is not
necessary should periodically reevaluate their policy.
Gloves should always be available to health care workers
who wish to use them for phlebotomy. In addition, the
following general guidelines apply:

1. Use gloves for performing phlebotomy when the
   health care worker has cuts, scratches, or other
   breaks in his or her skin.
2. Use gloves in situations in which the health care
   worker judges that hand contamination with blood

may occur, e.g., when performing phlebotomy on an uncooperative patient.

3. Use gloves for performing finger and heel sticks on infants and children.

4. Use gloves when persons are receiving training in phlebotomy.

Masks and protective eyewear or face shields should be worn by health care workers to prevent exposure of mucous membranes of the mouth, nose, and eyes during procedures that are likely to generate droplets of blood or body fluids requiring universal precautions. Gowns or aprons should be worn during procedures that are likely to generate splashes of blood or body fluids requiring universal precautions.

All health care workers should take precautions to prevent injuries caused by needles, scalpels, and other sharp instruments or devices during procedures; when cleaning used instruments; during disposal of used needles; and when handling sharp instruments after procedures. To prevent needlestick injuries, needles should not be recapped by hand, purposely bent or broken by hand, removed from disposable syringes, or otherwise manipulated by hand. After they are used, disposable syringes and needles, scalpel blades, and other sharp items should be placed in puncture-resistant containers for disposal. The puncture-resistant containers should be located as close as practical to the use area. All reusable needles should be placed in a puncture-resistant container for transport to the reprocessing area.

General infection control practices should further minimize the already minute risk for salivary transmission of HIV. These infection control practices include the use of gloves for digital examination of mucous membranes and endotracheal suctioning, hand washing after exposure to saliva, and minimizing the need for emergency mouth-to-mouth resuscitation by making mouth-pieces and other ventilation devices available for use in areas where the need for resuscitation is predictable.

Although universal precautions do not apply to human breast milk, gloves can be worn by health care workers in situations where exposures to breast milk might be frequent, e.g., in breast milk banking.

Source: Adapted from the universal precautions page. Centers for Disease Control and Prevention. Available at: http://www.cdc.gov/ncidod/hip/Blood/UNIVERSA.HTM. Accessed March 1, 2004.

Information regarding workplace exposure to bloodborne infections can be found in the following document: Centers for Disease Control and Prevention. Updated US Public Health Service guidelines for the management of occupational exposures to HBV, HCV, and HIV and recommendations for post-exposure prophylaxis. *Morb Mortal Wkly Rep.* Jun 29 2001, 50(RR11):1-42.

Assessment for Intimate Partner Violence (IPV)

This topic includes physical, psychological, and sexual abuse. One in four American women experience physical assaults or rape during their lifetime. More than 1% are abused each year.

Risk factors include:

- Alcohol use
- Partner's unemployment or substance abuse
- Witnessing or experiencing IPV as a child (increases both risk of adult abuse and of becoming an abuser)
- Partner's lack of communication skills
- Partner depression, aggression, poor self-esteem

Clinical presentation is often nonspecific and may include headaches, dyspareunia, worsening PMS, depression or anxiety, irritable bowel syndrome, substance abuse, or other symptoms. Patients may offer inconsistent explanations for recurrent injuries. Frequent falls, bruises at different stages of healing, central distribution of injuries, or facial injuries may suggest IPV. Often an overprotective or antagonistic significant other is present.

It is important that there be some private space and time during the visit to question the woman about possible IPV injuries. Asking directly about whether she is safe at home, whether she is afraid of her partner, and whether anyone in her home has tried to injure, strike, or hurt her, can open the way for her to bring up current abuse. If one asks about prior abuse, responses may reflect childhood trauma or sexual events, and offer an opportunity to inquire about ongoing mental health needs.

Mnemonic for Intimate Partner Violence Screening:

Remember to ask.
Ask directly.
Document findings.
Assess safety.
Review options and refer.

Used by permission of Glass R. H., Curtis M. G., Hopkins M. P., eds. (1999). *Glass's Office Gynecology* (5th ed.). Baltimore, MD: Lippincott Williams and Wilkins.

A resource for IPV information is the Intimate Partner Violence fact sheet available from the Centers for Disease Control and Prevention.

Documenting the history and the physical examination related to violence is as essential as any component of the visit. Remember that one of the hallmarks of abuse is loss of self-esteem by the victim. Thus, it may take several attempts before the woman can leave the setting in which she has been abused. The U.S. Preventive Services Task Force Guideline on screening for domestic violence states that there is not enough evidence to recommend for or against routine screening.

References

Carroll, N. M. (2000). Providing gynecological and obstetric care for lesbians. *Contemp Rev Obstet Gynecol.* March, 75–79.

Centers for Disease Control and Prevention. Updated U.S. Public Health Service guidelines for the management of occupational exposures to HBV, HCV, and HIV and recommendations for post-exposure prophylaxis. *Morb Mortal Wkly Rep.* Jun 29 2001; 50(RR11):1–42.

Deska, K., Pagana, T. J. (2002). *Mosby's diagnostic and laboratory test reference* (6th ed.). St. Louis: C.V. Mosby.

Glass, R. H., Curtis, M. G., Hopkins, M. P. (Eds.). (1999). *Glass's office gynecology* (5th ed.). Baltimore, MD: Lippincott Williams & Wilkins.

Intimate partner violence fact sheet. Available at: http://www.cdc. gov/ncipc/factsheets/ipvfacts.htm. Accessed March 17, 2004.

Pagnana, K. D. & Pagnana, T. J. (2002). *Mosby's manual of diagnostic and laboratory tests* (2nd ed.). St. Louis: Mosby, Inc.

Randall-David, E. (1994). *Culturally competent HIV counseling and education.* Rockville, MD: DHHS Maternal and Child Health Bureau.

Report of the U.S. Preventive Services Task Force. (1996). *Guide to clinical preventive services* (2nd ed.). Baltimore, MD: Lippincott Williams & Wilkins.

Tietze, N. W. (1995). *Clinical guide to laboratory tests* (3rd ed.). Philadelphia: WB Saunders.

Walker, M. L. (2002). *Core curriculum for lactation consultant practice.* Sudbury, MA: Jones and Bartlett Publishers.

Universal precautions Web site. Available at: http://www. cdc.gov/ncidod/hip/Blood/UNIVERSA.HTM. Accessed March 1, 2004.

Varney, H., Kriebs, J. M., & Gegor, C. L. (2003). *Varney's midwifery* (4th ed.). Sudbury, MA: Jones and Bartlett Publishers. Chapters 2, 3, 11, 45, 52, 61, 79.

SECTION 2

SECTION 3

Lifestyle: Nutrition, Exercise, and Substance Abuse

Proper nutrition is key to healthy human growth and development, and to lifelong well-being. Four of the leading causes of death among American women are affected by diet: coronary heart disease, certain cancers, stroke, and diabetes. The promotion of good nutrition for all women is essential to the provision of primary care.

Food Pyramids

The U.S. Department of Health and Human Services released new general dietary guidelines in 2000. The areas included were: (1) aiming for fitness by working towards a healthy weight and being physically active every day; (2) building on the food pyramid to make healthy food choices and keeping food safe to eat; (3) choosing a sensible diet with low saturated fats and cholesterol, moderate total fat intake, moderating sugars in the diet, decreasing the use of salt, and moderating alcohol intake.

While not a perfect summary of good nutrition, the food pyramid is an easy tool to use when explaining the components of a healthy diet to women.

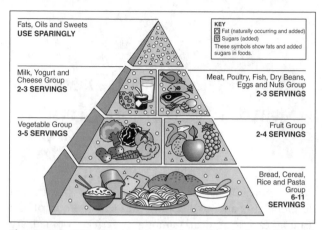

Figure 3-1 U.S. Department of Agriculture's Food Pyramid. *Source:* USDA and the U.S. Department of Health and Human Services, 1992.

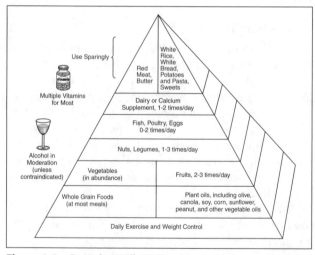

Figure 3-2 Dr. Walter Willett's Food Pyramid. *Source:* Reprinted with permission of Simon & Schuster Source, a division of Simon & Schuster Adult Publishing, from *Eat, Drink, and Be Healthy* by Walter C. Willett, M.D. Copyright © 2001 by the President and Fellows of Harvard College.

What Counts as One Serving
(approximate values for estimating intake)

Breads, cereals, rice, pasta
    1 slice bread
    $\frac{1}{2}$ cup cooked rice or pasta
    $\frac{1}{2}$ cup cooked cereal
    1 ounce dry cereal

Vegetables
    $\frac{1}{2}$ cup chopped raw or cooked vegetables
    1 cup leafy vegetables

Fruits
    1 piece of most fruits
    1 wedge of melon
    $\frac{3}{4}$ cup juice
    $\frac{1}{2}$ cup canned fruit

Milk, yogurt, cheese
    1 cup fresh milk or yogurt
    $1\frac{1}{2}$ to 2 ounces cheese

Meat, poultry, fish, eggs, dried beans, nuts
    $2\frac{1}{2}$ to 3 ounces cooked lean meat, poultry, meat
    1 egg is equivalent to 1 ounce of meat
    2 tablespoons peanut butter

*Some vegetable proteins require combination with other foods to provide complete proteins.

SECTION 3

Table 3-1   Food Sources of Protein

Food	Quantity	Amount of Protein (grams)
Complete Proteins		
Lentils	1 cup (cooked)	30
Beef, chuck, roasted	3 oz	28
Pork, center loin	3 oz	27
Turkey	3 oz	27
Chicken breast	3 oz	26
Flounder	3 oz	25
Tuna, canned	3 oz	24
Beef, lean ground	3 oz	22
Scallops	3 oz	16
Cottage cheese	$\frac{1}{2}$ cup	15
Ham	3 oz	15
Eggs	2 large	12
Shrimp	3 oz	11
Yogurt	1 cup	8
Milk, any type	8 oz	8
Cheddar cheese	1 oz	7
Incomplete Proteins		
Tofu	$\frac{1}{2}$ cup	10
Green peas	1 cup	9
Peanut butter	2 tbsp	8
Egg noodles	1 cup	7
Brown rice	1 cup	5
White rice	1 cup	4
Bread, whole wheat	1 slice	3

Recommended Values and Common Sources for Nutrients

Table 3-2 Daily Values

Daily Values (DVs) are made up of two sets of dietary guidelines:

1. Daily Reference Values (DRVs)—guidelines for intake of the following nutrients:
   - Fat (including saturated fat)*
     No more than 30% of total daily calories; saturated fat should comprise no more than 10% of daily calories**
   - Cholesterol
     No more than 300 mg per day
   - Carbohydrates*
     60% of daily calories
   - Protein*
     10% of daily calories (for adults and children over the age of 4)
   - Fiber*
     11.5 g per 1000 daily calories
   - Sodium
     No more than 2400 mg per day
   - Potassium
     No more than 3500 mg per day
2. Recommended Daily Intakes (RDIs)—guidelines for intake of certain essential vitamins and minerals (independent of total caloric intake):
   - Vitamin A: 5000 International Units (IU)
   - Vitamin C: 60 mg
   - Thiamin (vitamin B1): 1.5 mg
   - Riboflavin (vitamin B2): 1.7 mg
   - Niacin (vitamin B3): 20 mg
   - Calcium: 1000 mg (1.0 g)
   - Iron: 18 mg
   - Vitamin D
   - Vitamin E: 30 IU

- Vitamin B6: 2.0 mg
- Folic acid: 0.4 mg (400 mcg)
- Vitamin B12: 6 mcg
- Phosphorus: 1000 mg (1.0 g)
- Iodine: 150 mcg
- Magnesium: 400 mg
- Zinc: 15 mg
- Copper: 2 mg
- Biotin: 0.3 mg (300 mcg)
- Pantothenic acid: 10 mg

*These DRVs depend upon total caloric intake. Please refer to Table 6-2, *Varney's Midwifery,* 4th edition, on calculating DRVs based on caloric intake.

**The National Cholesterol Program of the National Institutes of Health (NIH) now considers 7% to be the cutoff for the maximum number of calories that should come from saturated fat.

Source: Institute of Medicine Food and Nutrition Board.

Table 3-3 Vitamins Categorized by Solubility

Fat-Soluble Vitamins
- Vitamin A
- Vitamin D
- Vitamin E
- Vitamin K

Water-Soluble Vitamins
- Vitamin C
- B vitamins

Thiamin (B1)
Riboflavin (B2)
Niacin (B3)
Vitamin B6
Pantothenic acid
Vitamin B12
Biotin
Folic acid (folate)

Essential Minerals
- Calcium
- Chloride
- Chromium
- Copper
- Fluoride
- Iodine
- Iron
- Magnesium
- Manganese
- Molybdenum
- Phosphorus
- Potassium
- Selenium
- Sodium
- Zinc

Table 3-4 Dietary Reference Intakes for Selected Vitamins and Minerals for Nonpregnant, Nonlactating Women

Vitamin	RDA/Adequate Intake for Women		Food Sources
A[1] Given in retinal activity equivalents (RAEs)	9–13 y 14–70 y >70 y	600 mcg/day 900 mcg/day 900 mcg/day	Liver, dairy products, egg yolks, fish, carrots, green leafy vegetables, pumpkins, sweet potatoes
D (calciferol)[2] 1 mcg calciferol = 40 IU vitamin D	9–50 y 50–70 y >70 y	5 mcg/day 900 mcg/day 15 mcg/day	Fortified dairy products and cereals, fish liver oils, egg yolks
E[3]	9–13 y 14–70 y >70 y	11 mg/day 15 mg/day 15 mg/day	Vegetable oils, unprocessed cereal grains, nuts, fruits, vegetables, meats, wheat germ
K[4]	9–13 y 14–18 y 19–70 y >70 y	60 mcg/day 75 mcg/day 90 mcg/day 90 mcg/day	Green leafy vegetables, brussels sprouts, cabbage, plant oils, margarine
C (ascorbic acid)[5]	9–13 y 14–18 y 19–70 y >70 y	45 mg/day 65 mg/day 75 mg/day 75 mg/day	Citrus fruits, tomatoes, potatoes, broccoli, brussels sprouts, spinach
B₆	9–13 y 14–18 y 19–50 y	1.0 mg/day 1.2 mg/day 1.3 mg/day	Fortified cereals, whole grain breads, organ meats, meat, poultry, legumes

Vitamin	RDA/Adequate Intake for Women		Food Sources
B[12] (cobalamin)[6]	50–70 y	1.5 mg/day	Fortified cereals, meat, fish, shellfish, poultry, dairy products
	>70 y	1.5 mg/day	
	9–13 y	1.8 mcg/day	
	14–70 y	2.4 mcg/day	
	>70 y	2.4 mcg/day	
Folate (folic acid)[7]	9–13 y	300 mcg/day	Enriched cereals, green leafy vegetables, enriched whole grain bread, fortified foods
	14–70 y	400 mcg/day	
	>70 y	400 mcg/day	
Mineral			
Calcium[8]	9–18 y	1300 mg/day	Milk, cheese, yogurt, corn tortillas, calcium-set tofu, kale, broccoli
	19–50 y	1000 mg/day	
	50–70 y	1200 mg/day	
	>70 y	1200 mg/day	
Iron[9]	9–13 y	5 mg/day	Fortified dairy products and cereals, fish liver oils, egg yolks
	14–18 y	10 mg/day	
	19–50 y	15 mg/day	
	50–70 y	8 mg/day	
	>70 y	8 mg/day	
Iodine[10]	9–13 y	120 mcg/day	Processed food, iodized salt
	14–70 y	150 mcg/day	
	>70 y	150 mcg/day	

Zinc[11]	9–13 y	8 mg/day	Fortified cereals, red meats, certain seafood
	14–18 y	9 mg/day	
	19–70 y	8 mg/day	
	>70 y	8 mg/day	

[1]Individuals with high alcohol intake are especially susceptible to adverse effects of excess.

[2]Patients on glucocorticoid therapy may need additional vitamin D.

[3]Patients on anticoagulants need to be monitored when taking vitamin E supplements.

[4]Patients on anticoagulant therapy should monitor vitamin K intake.

[5]Smokers and nonsmokers regularly exposed to smoke may require additional vitamin C.

[6]Patients older than 50 may need to supplement dietary sources of vitamin B_{12}:

[7]Maternal folate intake is inversely related to the risk of neural tube defects in the fetus.

[8]Amenorrheic women have reduced net calcium absorption.

[9]Recommended intake assumes 75% of iron is from heme iron sources. Those consuming vegetarian diets may need up to twice the suggested iron intake than someone consuming a nonvegetarian diet.

[10]Individuals with autoimmune thyroid disease, previous iodine deficiency, or nodular goiter are distinctly susceptible to the adverse effects of excess iodine.

[11]Zinc absorption is lower for those consuming vegetarian diets than for those eating nonvegetarian diets.

Sources: National Academy of Sciences. Dietary Reference Intakes for Calcium, Phosphorous, Magnesium, Vitamin D, and Fluoride, 1997; Dietary Reference Intakes for Thiamin, Riboflavin, Niacin, Vitamin B6, Folate, Vitamin B12, Pantothenic Acid, Biotin, and Choline, 1998; Dietary Reference Intakes for Vitamin C, Vitamin E, Selenium and Carotenoids, 2000; and Dietary Reference Intakes for Vitamin A, Vitamin K, Arsenic, Boron, Chromium, Copper, Iodine, Iron, Manganese, Molybdenum, Nickel, Silicon, Vanadium, and Zinc, 2001. Washington, DC: National Academy Press.

Table 3-5 Function of Selected Vitamins and Minerals

Vitamin	Function	Adverse Effects of Excessive Consumption
A Given in retinal activity equivalents (RAEs)	Required for normal vision, gene expression, reproduction, embryonic development, and immune function	Teratological effects and liver toxicity (from preformed vitamin A only)
D (calciferol) 1 mcg calciferol = 40 IU vitamin D	Maintains serum calcium and phosphorus (important for bone formation and maintenance)	Hypercalcemia, GI distress, anorexia, headache, nausea, vomiting, metallic taste in mouth
E	Major function appears to be as a nonspecific chain-breaking antioxidant	None reported from vitamin E naturally occurring in foods but hemorrhagic toxicity possible from excess intake of vitamin E in supplements
K	Coenzyme during the synthesis of many proteins involved in blood clotting and bone metabolism	None identified
C (ascorbic acid)	Cofactors for reactions requiring reduced copper or iron metalloenzyme and as a protective antioxidant	GI disturbances, kidney stones, excess iron absorption
B_6	Coenzyme in the metabolism of amino acids and glycogen	No adverse effects from vitamin B_6 in food. Sensory neuropathy has occurred from high intakes from supplement forms.

B$_{12}$ (cobalamin)	Coenzyme in nucleic acid metabolism; prevents megaloblastic anemia	None identified
Folate (folic acid)	Coenzyme in nucleic acid metabolism; prevents megaloblastic anemia	Masks neurological complications in people with vitamin B$_{12}$ deficiency.
Mineral		
Calcium	Essential role in blood clotting, muscle contraction, nerve transmission, and bone and tooth formation	Kidney stones, hypercalcemia, renal insufficiency
Iron	Used to make hemoglobin, which transports oxygen to all body tissues	Gastrointestinal distress
Iodine	Component of thyroid hormones	Elevated thyroid stimulating hormone (TSH concentration)
Zinc	Component of multiple enzymes and proteins; involved in the regulation of gene expression	Reduced copper status

Sources: National Academy of Sciences. Dietary Reference Intakes for Calcium, Phosphorous, Magnesium, Vitamin D, and Fluoride, 1997; Dietary Reference Intakes for Thiamin, Riboflavin, Niacin, Vitamin B6, Folate, Vitamin B12, Pantothenic Acid, Biotin, and Choline, 1998; Dietary Reference Intakes for Vitamin C, Vitamin E, Selenium and Carotenoids, 2000; and Dietary Reference Intakes for Vitamin A, Vitamin K, Arsenic, Boron, Chromium, Copper, Iodine, Iron, Manganese, Molybdenum, Nickel, Silicon, Vanadium, and Zinc, 2001. Washington, DC: National Academy Press.

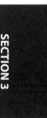

SECTION 3

Table 3-6   Food Sources of Heme Iron

Food	Quantity	Amount of Iron (mg)
Clams	3 oz	24
Oysters	3 oz	11
Chicken liver, cooked	3 oz	7
Beef liver, cooked	3 oz	6
Mussels	3 oz	6
Beef, chuck, braised	3 oz	3
Beef, tenderloin, roasted	3 oz	3
Turkey, dark meat, roasted	3 oz	2
Beef, eye of round, roasted	3 oz	2
Turkey, light meat, roasted	3 oz	1
Tuna, fresh bluefin, cooked, dry heat	3 oz	1
Chicken, leg, meat only, roasted	3 oz	1
Crab, cooked, moist heat	1 cup	1
Chicken, breast, roasted	3 oz	1
Halibut, cooked, dry heat	3 oz	0.9
Pork, loin, meat only, broiled	3 oz	0.8
Tuna, white, canned in water	3 oz	0.8

Table 3-7   Food Sources of Nonheme Iron

Food	Quantity	Amount of Iron (mg)
Ready-to-eat cereal, 100% fortified	$\frac{3}{4}$ cup	18.0
Ready-to-eat cereal, 50% fortified	$\frac{3}{4}$ cup	9.0
Soybeans, mature, cooked, boiled	1 cup	8

Lentils, cooked, boiled	1 cup	6
Molasses, blackstrap	2 tbsp	6
Kidney beans, cooked, boiled	1 cup	5
Pinto beans, cooked, boiled	1 cup	5
Lima beans, cooked, boiled	1 cup	4
Navy beans, cooked, boiled	1 cup	4
Black beans, cooked, boiled	1 cup	4
Oatmeal, instant, fortified	$\frac{1}{2}$ cup	4
Prunes, dried	6 oz	4
Prune juice	8 oz	3
Spinach, cooked, boiled	$\frac{1}{2}$ cup	3
Tofu, firm	$\frac{1}{2}$ cup	2
Black-eyed peas, cooked, boiled	1 cup	2
Spinach, frozen, cooked, boiled	$\frac{1}{2}$ cup	1
Whole wheat bread	1 slice	1
White bread, enriched	1 slice	1

SECTION 3

Table 3-8 Oral Iron Preparations

Preparation	Typical Dose	Elemental Iron/Dose
Ferrous sulfate	325 mg tid	65 mg
Ferrous sulfate exsiccated (Feosol)	200 mg tid	65 mg
Ferrous gluconate	325 mg tid	36 mg
Ferrous fumarate (Hemocyte)	325 mg bid	106 mg

Table 3-9   Tips to Increase Absorption of Iron

1. Take iron supplements between meals or 30 minutes before meals.
2. Avoid calcium ingestion with iron (milk, antacid, prenatal supplements).
3. Take with vitamin C (orange juice, vitamin C supplement).
4. Cook foods in a minimal amount of water, for the shortest possible time.
5. Eat meat, poultry, and fish—foods in which iron is absorbed and utilized more readily than the iron in other foods.
6. Eat a wide variety of foods.

Table 3-10   Folic Acid
RDA: 400 mcg before and during pregnancy

Food	Quantity	Folic Acid (mcg)
Meats		
Liver	$3\frac{1}{2}$ oz	220
Egg	1	22
Ground beef	3 oz	8
Turkey	3 oz	6
Chicken	3 oz	5
Ham	3 oz	5
Fish and shellfish		
Oysters, raw	1 c	25
Crabmeat	1 c	21
Scallops	6	15
Haddock	3 oz	14
Salmon	$3\frac{1}{2}$ oz	14
Cod	$3\frac{1}{2}$ oz	10
Shrimp	$3\frac{1}{2}$ oz	5

Fruit and fruit juices

Orange juice	8 oz	100
Grapefruit juice	8 oz	52
Cantaloupe	1 cup	48
Orange	1 med	45
Strawberries	1 cup	26
Banana	1 med	22
Pineapple, fresh	1 c	16
Grapefruit	$\frac{1}{2}$ med	15
Pear	1 med	12

Vegetables

Asparagus	$\frac{1}{2}$ c	108
Romaine lettuce	1 c	76
Broccoli	$\frac{1}{2}$ c	65
Spinach	$\frac{1}{2}$ c	54
Peas	$\frac{1}{2}$ c	51
Brussels sprouts	$\frac{1}{2}$ c	47
Tomatoes, canned	1 c	35
Iceberg lettuce	1 c	31
Baked potato	1 med	22

Legumes

Navy beans	1 c	225
Chickpeas, canned	1 c	160
Kidney beans, canned	1 c	126
Baked beans	1 c	61

Nuts

Almonds	1 oz	88
Peanuts	1 oz	24
Cashews	1 oz	20
Walnuts	1 oz	19
Pistachios	1 oz	17
Pecans	1 oz	12

Food	Quantity	Folic Acid (mcg)
Bread and grain products		
Oatmeals, instant and fortified	$\frac{3}{4}$ c	150
Wheat germ	$\frac{1}{4}$ c	100
Bran muffin	1	19
Whole wheat bread	1 slice	16
Macaroni	1 c	10
White bread	1 slice	10
Rice, brown or white	1 c	8
Milk and milk products		
Cottage cheese	1 c	28
Yogurt	1 c	25
Milk	1 c	13
Cheddar cheese	1 oz	5
Ice cream	1 c	3
American cheese	1 oz	2
Other		
Brewer's yeast	1 tbsp	313
Cereals		

Many cereals are fortified with folacin. Check labels because amounts vary.

Table 3-11   Food Sources of Calcium

Food	Quantity	Amount of Calcium (mg)
Ricotta cheese	1 cup	669
Sardines	$3\frac{1}{2}$ oz	437
Yogurt, low-fat plain	1 cup	415
Yogurt, low-fat fruit varieties	1 cup	350
Collard greens	1 cup	357

Milk, low-fat 1%	8 oz	300
Tums E-X	1 tab	300
Milk, whole	8 oz	288
Spinach, cooked	1 cup	278
Molasses, blackstrap	2 tbsp	274
Tofu, firm made with calcium sulfate	4 oz	250-265
Cheese, Swiss	1 oz	272
Cheese, provolone	1 oz	214
Cheese, cheddar	1 oz	204
Cheese, mozzarella	1 oz	185
Sesame seeds	2 tbsp	176
Ice cream, vanilla, 16% fat	1 cup	151
Salmon, canned with bones	3 oz	133
Cheese, American	1 oz	124
Tofu, regular made with calcium sulfate	4 oz	120-392
Tofu made with nijare	4 oz	80-146
Cottage cheese	4 oz	70
Hummus	$\frac{1}{2}$ cup	62
Almonds, blanched	1 oz	50
Chickpeas	$\frac{1}{2}$ cup	40
Broccoli	$\frac{1}{2}$ cup	36

Table 3-12 Amount of Elemental Calcium in Common Supplements

Calcium carbonate	40%
Calcium citrate	24%
Calcium lactate	14%
Calcium gluconate	9%

At 40% elemental calcium, a 500-mg tablet yields 200 mg of calcium.

SECTION 3

Table 3-13 Body Mass Index (BMI) Chart

Height (inches)

BMI	58	59	60	61	62	63	64	65	66	67	68	69	70	71	72	BMI	
19	91	94	97	100	104	107	110	114	118	121	125	128	132	136	140	**19**	
20	96	99	102	106	109	113	116	120	124	127	131	135	139	143	147	**20**	Normal
21	100	104	107	111	115	118	122	126	130	134	138	142	146	150	154	**21**	
22	105	109	112	116	120	124	128	132	136	140	144	149	153	157	162	**22**	
23	110	114	118	122	126	130	134	138	142	146	151	155	160	165	169	**23**	
24	115	119	123	127	131	135	140	144	148	153	158	162	167	172	177	**24**	
25	119	124	128	132	136	141	145	150	155	159	164	169	174	179	184	**25**	
26	124	128	133	137	142	146	151	156	161	166	171	176	181	186	191	**26**	Overweight
27	129	133	138	143	147	152	157	162	167	172	177	182	188	193	199	**27**	

Obese

28	29	30	31	32	33	34	35	36	37	38	39	40
134	138	143	148	153	158	162	167	172	177	181	186	191
138	143	148	153	158	163	168	173	178	183	188	193	198
143	148	153	158	163	168	174	179	184	189	194	199	204
148	153	158	164	169	174	180	185	190	195	201	206	211
153	158	164	169	175	180	186	191	196	202	207	213	218
158	163	169	175	180	186	191	197	203	208	214	220	225
163	169	174	180	186	192	197	204	209	215	221	227	232
168	174	180	186	192	198	204	210	216	222	228	234	240
173	179	186	192	198	204	210	216	223	229	235	241	247
178	185	191	198	204	211	217	223	230	236	242	249	255
184	190	197	203	210	216	223	230	236	243	249	256	262
189	196	203	209	216	223	230	236	243	250	257	263	270
195	202	209	216	222	229	236	243	250	257	264	271	278
200	208	215	222	229	236	243	250	257	265	272	279	286
206	213	221	228	235	242	250	258	265	272	279	287	294

Table 3-14 Body Mass Index Calculations

$\dfrac{\text{Weight in kilograms}}{(\text{Height in meters})^2}$	$\dfrac{\text{Weight in pounds} \times 703}{(\text{Height in inches})^2}$

Table 3-15 Classifications for Body Mass Index (BMI)

BMI

Underweight	$<18.5 \text{ kg/m}^2$
Normal weight	$18.5\text{-}24.9 \text{ kg/m}^2$
Overweight	$25\text{-}29.9 \text{ kg/m}^2$
Obesity (Class 1)	$30\text{-}34.9 \text{ kg/m}^2$
Obesity (Class 2)	$35\text{-}39.9 \text{ kg/m}^2$
Extreme obesity (Class 3)	$\geq 40 \text{ kg/m}^2$

Source: From National Institutes of Health—National Heart, Lung, and Blood Institute. *The Practical Guide to Identification, Evaluation, and Treatment of Overweight and Obesity in Adults,* 2000.

Table 3-16 General Guidelines for Caloric Intake for Moderately Active Females

- 11 to 18 years of age: 2200 calories/day
- 19 to 24 years of age: 2100 calories/day
- 25 to 50 years of age: 2000 calories/day
- 51 years of age or older: 1900 calories/day
- Pregnant women (second and third trimesters): Add 300 calories/day
- Nursing mothers: Add 500 calories/day

Table 3-17 Factors Affecting Necessary Caloric Intake

- Body size
- Age
- Height
- Weight
- Activity level/Base Metabolic Rate (BMR)
- Pregnancy status
- Lactation status

Table 3-18 Guideline Questions for a Nutritional Assessment

Measure weight, height, and blood pressure and calculate BMI. Ask the following:

1. Are you currently taking any medications or undergoing treatment for any health problem?
2. Do you smoke? If so, how much do you smoke in one day?
3. Do you drink alcohol at all? If so, how much do you drink in one day? In one week?
4. Do you use any street drugs?
5. Do you exercise? If so, how often and for how long? What type of exercise?
6. How many meals do you eat in one day?
7. How often do you snack during the day?
8. How many times do you eat out during one week? (Include all carry-out and fast food.)
9. How many glasses of fluid do you drink in one day? How many glasses of water do you drink in one day?
10. Are you allergic to any foods? If so, what happens when you eat this particular food?
11. Are you on a diet? If so, what kind of diet? How long have you been on it and with what results?

SECTION 3

12. Do you take any of the following:
     *   Multivitamins
     *   Calcium supplement
     *   Iron supplement
     *   Folic acid supplement
     *   Diet pills
     *   Laxatives
     *   Power drinks/diet drinks (such as Ensure, Slimfast, etc.)
13. Which of the following terms would you use to describe your current weight?
     *   High
     *   Just right
     *   Low
14. Do you or a first-degree family member (mother, father, brothers, or sisters) suffer from any of the following medical conditions?
     *   Hypertension (high blood pressure)
     *   Diabetes (high blood sugar)
     *   Heart disease
     *   Kidney disease
     *   Liver disease
     *   Anemia, sickle cell disease
     *   Immune disorder such as lupus or HIV infection
     *   Cancer
     *   Crohn's disease, irritable bowel syndrome, ulcerative colitis

Ask patient to conduct a three-day diet/exercise recall by doing the following:

1. Write down everything you eat AND drink in one day including all snacks (no matter how small).
2. Write down any physical activity beyond your activities of daily living (for example, include a half-hour walk but do not include housework or walking done during your job).

Table 3-19 Signs and Symptoms of Eating Disorders

Anorexia	Bulimia
Severe weight loss, emaciation	Near normal weight in most cases
Acceptance of appearance as normal	Dizziness
Poor sleep habits	Fainting
Cold intolerance	Increased thirst
Constipation	Muscle cramps
Anemia (mild)	Constipation
Restlessness/sleep disturbance	Tooth damage, loss of enamel
Pale, dry skin	Reflux esophagitis
Loss of scalp and pubic hair and/or lanugo	Petachiae in and around eyes
Brittle, dry nails	
Tooth disease/decay	

SECTION 3

Exercise

Both how one begins exercise and how effectively one exercises are dependent on many factors. The U.S. Department of Health and Human Services Office of Women's Health has several guidelines for women in various age groups and with certain health conditions. The following recommendations are tips to help encourage someone to begin exercising.

- Choose an activity that's fun.
- Change your activities so you don't get bored.
- Doing housework may not be fun, but it does get you moving! So do gardening, yardwork, and walk the dog.
- If you can't set aside one block of time, do short activities during the day, such as three 10-minute walks.

- Create opportunities for activity, such as parking your car farther away, taking the stairs instead of the elevator, or walking down the hall to talk to a co-worker instead of using e-mail.
- Don't let the cold weather keep you on the couch! You can still find activities to do in the winter like exercising to a workout video or joining a sports league. Or get a head start on your spring cleaning by choosing active indoor chores like window washing or reorganizing closets.
- Use different jogging, walking, or biking paths to vary your routine.
- Exercise with a friend or family member.
- If you have children, make time to play with them outside. Set a positive example!
- Turn activities into social occasions—have dinner after you and a friend work out.
- Read books or magazines to inspire you.
- Set specific, short-term goals, and reward yourself when you achieve them.
- Don't feel badly if you don't notice body changes right away.
- Make your activity a regular part of your day, so it becomes a habit.
- Build a community group to form walking clubs, build walking trails, start exercise classes, and organize special events to promote physical activity.

Some women need a physical evaluation before beginning to exercise. Among these are women who:

- Have heart disease or had a stroke or are at high risk for them
- Have diabetes or are at high risk for it

- Are obese (body mass index of 30 or greater)
- Have an injury (such as a knee injury)
- Are older than age 50
- Are pregnant

Source: The physical activity (exercise) page. *National Women's Health Information Center*. Available at: http://www.4woman.gov/faq/exercise. htm#5. Accessed April 4, 2004.

Kegel Exercises

1. Help the woman identify her pubococcygeus muscle by having her tighten her vaginal muscles around your finger during a bimanual examination.
2. Instruct her that her abdominal, hip, or leg muscles should not move during this exercise.
3. To help the woman identify the correct muscle movement at home suggest she contract the same muscles used when "trying to stop the flow of urine" or "trying not to pass gas." She can only recognize these sensations if she has some tone in the muscles.
4. Slow Kegel exercises are done by slowly and steadily tightening the muscle and holding for 5-10 seconds, then slowly releasing. These can be done in sets of 10, three to five times a day. Alternatively, instructions to perform the exercise 50 times daily can be given.
5. Rapid tightening and release of the muscle can be taught as a second exercise.

SECTION 3

Substance Abuse

Just as proper nutrition and regular exercise improve or maintain health, the immoderate use of legal substances such as caffeine can cause health problems. Tobacco and excessive alcohol use, as well as illicit drugs, can damage one's health. Even legal medications can have potential for abuse. This is true regardless of whether the woman is using her own prescription or using someone else's medications. It is the clinician's responsibility to screen for substance abuse, and to counsel women appropriately.

Table 3-20   Caffeine Content of Common Foods and Beverages

Food	Estimated Caffeine (mg)	Serving Size
Brewed coffee	180-250	10 oz
Instant coffee	70-320	10 oz
Decaffeinated coffee	2-12	10 oz
Tea	50-250	10 oz
Coca Cola (caffeinated)	46	12 oz (1 can)
Mountain Dew soft drink	54	12 oz (1 can)
Red Bull energy drink	80	8.3 oz
Chocolate bar	1-35	1 oz

Source: Hanson, G. R., Venturelli, P. J., and Fleckenstein, A. E. (2002). *Drugs and Society* (7th ed.). Sudbury, MA: Jones and Bartlett Publishers.

Tobacco Cessation

"More people die annually in the United States from tobacco-related illnesses than all deaths due to alcohol, cocaine, heroin, AIDS, suicides, homicides, fires, airplane and car crashes, . . . drowning, and the death penalty combined" (*Varney's Midwifery*, 4th edition, p. 321).

Table 3-21 Results of Evidence-Based Systematic Reviews of Various Methods Used for Tobacco Cessation

Evidence of Effectiveness*

Antidepressants: bupropion (Zyban, Wellbutrin), nortriptyline (Sensaval)

Clonidine: Catapres

Community interventions for youth

Group therapy

Individual counseling

Nicotine replacement therapy (NRT)

Self-help groups

Insufficient Evidence of Effectiveness†

Aversion therapy

Anxiolytics: diazepam or Valium; meprobamate or Equanil, Meprospan and Miltown; metoprolol or Toprol; and oxprenol or Trasicor

Exercise

Mecamylamine or Inversine (nicotine antagonist/antihypertensive)

Opiate antagonist: naloxone or Narcan

Telephone counseling

No Evidence of Effectiveness

Acupuncture

Hypnosis

Lobeline (partial nicotine agonist)

*Degree of effectiveness is not the same for each intervention, but all demonstrate some effectiveness.

†Usually too few studies available.

Substance Abuse Screening

There are several scoring tools designed to provide a rapid screen for substance abuse. They are primarily developed for alcohol abuse, and are not as clearly useful in screening for other substance abuse.

Table 3-22   The TWEAK Questionnaire for Alcohol Use

T   Tolerance (2 points)   How many drinks can you hold? (Cutoff: Four or more is a conservative cutoff for use with women compared to six or more for men)

W   Worried (2 points)   Have close friends or relatives worried or complained about your drinking in the past year?

E   Eye Openers (1 point)   Do you sometimes take a drink in the morning when you first get up?

A   Amnesia (1 point)   Has a friend or family member ever told you about things you said or did while you were drinking that you could not remember?

K   Cut down (1 point)   Do you sometimes feel the need to cut down on your drinking?

Note: A total of 2 to 3 points may indicate an alcohol abuse problem.

Source: Chan, A. K., Pristach, E. A., Welte, J. W., et al. (1993). The TWEAK test in screening for alcoholism/heavy drinking in three populations. *Alcoholism: Clinical and Experimental Research* 6:1188-1192. Used by permission.

Table 3-23 Substances of Abuse, Maternal Overdose, and Fetal/Neonatal Effects

Substance of Abuse	Maternal Overdose/Withdrawal	Fetal/Neonatal Effects
Alcohol	*Overdose*: Unusual behavior, depression, amnesia, hypotension *Withdrawal*: Agitation, tremors	Microcephaly, growth retardation, mental retardation, craniofacial abnormalities, abortion Growth restriction occurs both before and after birth Nutritional deficiencies, smoking and polypharmacy confound data The fetus of a woman who ingests six drinks per day is at a 40% risk of developing some features of FAS, but the threshold is still unknown
Anticholinergics Atropine Belladonna Scopolamine	*Overdose*: Pupils dilated and fixed, increased heart rate and temperature, amnesia, vagueness *Withdrawal*: None	None noted
Cannabis Marijuana THC Hashish	*Overdose*: Infected conjunctiva with normal pupils, decreased blood pressure when standing, increased heart rate, time and space disoriented *Withdrawal*: None	Some subtle behavioral alterations noted but no anomalies or growth delay
CNS sedatives Barbiturates Chlordiazepoxide Diazepam Flurazepam Glutethimide Meprobamate	*Overdose*: Normal pupils, decreased, shocky blood pressure, depressed respiration, depressed tendon reflexes, coma, ataxia, slurring, convulsions *Withdrawal*: Tremulousness, insomnia, chronic blink reflex, agitation, toxic psychosis	No anomalies Limp baby

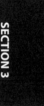

SECTION 3

Substance of Abuse	Maternal Overdose/Withdrawal	Fetal/Neonatal Effects
CNS stimulants	*Overdose:* Dilated and reactive pupils, shallow respirations, increased blood pressure, hyperactive reflexes, cardiac arrhythmias, dry mouth, tremors, sensorium hyperacute	Questionable increased rate of abortion, hyperactivity in utero, depression of interactive behavior, controversy about anomalies
Antiobesity		Cocaine has been linked with some bowel atresias and possible
Amphetamines		congenital malformations of heart, limbs, face, and GU tract as well
Cocaine		as growth restriction. Maternal and fetal complications include
Methylphenidate	*Withdrawal:* Muscle aches, abdominal pain, hunger,	sudden death and placental abruption (sixfold increase in
Phenmetrazine	prolonged sleep, possibly suicidal	obstetrical complications)
Methaqualone		
Hallucinogens	*Overdose:* Dilated pupils, increased blood pressure, heart rate and tendon reflexes, flush face, euphoria, anxiety, illusions, hallucinations	Dysmorphic face Behavioral problems
LSD		
Ketamine		
Mescaline	*Withdrawal:* None	
Dimethyltryptamine		
Phencyclidine (PCP)		
Opiates	*Overdose:* Constricted pupils, decreased blood pressure, heart rate and reflexes, hypoactive sensorium	Intrauterine withdrawal with increased fetal activity
Codeine		Neonatal withdrawal
Heroin		Depressed breathing movements
Hydromorphone	*Withdrawal:* Agitation, flulike symptoms, dilated	Methadone usually treatment of choice
Meperidine	pupils, abdominal pain	
Morphine	pupils, abdominal pain	
Opium		
Pentazocine		
Tripelennamine		

Sources: Rayburn, W. F., and Zuspan, F. P. *Drug therapy in obstetrics and gynecology* (1992). St. Louis, MO: Mosby Year Book; American College of Obstetricians and Gynecologists. (1997). Teratology. *ACOG Educational Bulletin, 233,* 1–8; Dunbar, A. E., O'Neil, M., & Marben, L. (1999). *Johns Hopkins Children's Center NICU Guidebook 1999–2000.* Baltimore, MD: Johns Hopkins University.

References

American College of Obstetricians and Gynecologists. (1997). Teratology. *ACOG Educational Bulletin*, 233, 1–8.

Chan, A. K., Pristach, E. A., Welte, J. W., et al. (1993). The TWEAK test in screening for alcoholism/heavy drinking in three populations. *Alcoholism: Clinical and Experimental Research*, 6, 1188–1192.

Dunbar, A. E., O'Neil, M., & Marben, L. (1999). *Johns Hopkins Children's Center NICU Guidebook 1999–2000.* Baltimore, MD: Johns Hopkins University.

Hanson, G. R., Venturelli, P. J., and Fleckenstein, A. E. (2002). *Drugs and society* (7th ed.). Sudbury, MA: Jones and Bartlett Publishers.

National Academy of Sciences. Dietary reference intakes for calcium, phosphorus, magnesium, vitamin D, and fluoride, 1997; Dietary reference intakes for thiamin, riboflavin, niacin, vitamin B6, folate, vitamin B12, pantothenic acid, biotin, and choline, 1998; Dietary reference intakes for vitamin C, vitamin E, selenium, and carotinoids, 2000; Dietary reference intakes for vitamin A, vitamin K, arsenic, boron, chromium, copper, iodine, iron, manganese, molybdenum, nickel, silicon, vanadium, and zinc, 2001. Washington, DC: National Academy Press.

Physical activity (exercise) Web page. *National Women's Health Information Center.* Available at: http://www.4woman.gov/faq/exercise.htm#5. Accessed April 4, 2004.

Rayburn, W. F. and Zuspan, F. P. *Drug therapy in obstetrics and gynecology* (1992). St. Louis, MO: Mosby Year Book.

Varney, H., Kriebs, J. M., & Gegor, C. L. (2003). *Varney's midwifery* (4th ed.). Sudbury, MA: Jones and Bartlett Publishers.

Wang, E. C. (1999). Methadone treatment during pregnancy. *JOGNN*, 28, 6, 615–622.

Willett, W. C. (2001). *Eat drink and be healthy.* New York: Simon and Schuster Source.

SECTION 3

SECTION 4

Primary Care

Definition of Primary Care

"The provision of integrated, accessible, health care services by clinicians who are accountable for addressing a large majority of personal health care needs, developing a sustained partnership with patients, and practicing in the context of family and community."

Source: Donaldson, M. S., et al. (Eds.). *Primary care: America's health in a new era.* Washington, DC: National Academy Press.

Table 4-1 Clinical Preventive Services for Normal-Risk Adults, Recommended by the U.S. Preventive Services Task Force

---

Screening

Blood pressure, height, and weight: Periodically, ages 18–75

Cholesterol: *Men,* every 5 years, ages 35–75
             Women, every 5 years, ages 45–75

Pap smear: Women, every 1–3 years, ages 18–65

Chlamydia: Women, periodically, ages 18–25

Mammography: Women, every 1–2 years, ages 40–75

Sigmoidoscopy: Every 5 years, ages 50–75

And/or fecal occult blood: Yearly, ages 50–75

Alcohol use: Periodically, ages 18–75

Vision, hearing: Periodically, ages 65–75

Immunization

Tetanus-diphtheria (Td): Every 10 years, ages 18–75

Varicella (VZV): Susceptibles only, two doses, ages 18–75

Measles, mumps, rubella (MMR): Women of childbearing age, one dose, ages 18–50

Pneumococcal: One dose, ages 65–75

Influenza: Yearly, ages 65–75

Chemoprevention

Aspirin to prevent cardiovascular events:

Men, periodically, ages 40–75

Women, periodically, ages 50–75

Counseling

Calcium intake: Women, periodically, ages 18–75

Folic acid: Women of childbearing age, ages 18–50

Tobacco cessation, drug and alcohol use, STDs and HIV, nutrition, physical activity, sun exposure, oral health, injury prevention, and polypharmacy: Periodically, ages 18–75

Source: Clinical Preventive Services for Normal-Risk Adults Recommended by the U.S. Preventive Services Task Force. (2002). *Put prevention into practice.* Rockville, MD: Agency for Health Care Quality and Research.

Table 4-2 Recommended Adult Immunization Schedule*

Age group Vaccine	19–49 (years)	50–64 (years)	65 and older
Tetanus, diphtheria (Td) Only one lifetime series needed	1 booster every 10 years	1 booster every 10 years	1 booster every 10 years
Td	Primary series of 2 injections, 4 weeks apart, and 1 injection 6–12 months later if unknown status	Primary series of 2 injections 4 weeks apart, and 1 injection 6–12 months later if unknown status	Primary series of 2 injections 4 weeks apart, and 1 injection 6–12 months later if unknown status
Influenza* Low risk adults under 50 can have intranasal vaccine if desired	1 dose annually for medical risk, health care workers, those in long-term care facilities (workers or residents)	1 dose annually	1 dose annually
Pneumococcal (polysaccharide)	1 dose for those at risk	1 dose	1 revaccination, after 5 years if vaccinated before age 65
Hepatitis B Only one series needed	3 doses at 0, 1–2, 4–6 months For those at risk	3 doses at 0, 1–2, 4–6 months	3 doses at 0, 1–2, 4–6 months

SECTION 4

Age group Vaccine	19–49 (years)	50–64 (years)	65 and older
Hepatitis A Only one lifetime vaccination series	2 doses at 0, 6–12 months for those at risk	2 doses at 0, 6–12 months for those at risk	2 doses at 0, 6–12 months for those at risk
Measles, mumps, rubella (MMR) Only one lifetime vaccination needed	1 dose if history unreliable, 2 doses for those with occupational or other indications	1 dose if history unreliable, 2 doses for those with occupational or other indications	1 dose if history unreliable, 2 doses for those with occupational or other indications
Varicella Only one lifetime series needed	2 doses 0, 4–8 weeks for susceptible persons with no clinical or serologic evidence	2 doses 0, 4–8 weeks for susceptible persons	2 doses 0, 4–8 weeks for susceptible persons
Meningococcal (polysaccharide) Only one lifetime series needed	1 dose at any time for those at risk	1 dose at any time for those at risk	1 dose at any time for those at risk

*See http://www.cdc.gov/nip/ for full information on risk categories.

Causes of Mortality for American Women

Lifestyle and environmental factors may precipitate disease or be directly responsible for death. For example, obesity and limited exercise may lead to heart disease or diabetes; tobacco use increases cancer risks.

Table 4-3 Leading Causes of Death, Women Only

All Races, Females	Percent*
1. Diseases of the heart (heart disease)	29.9
2. Malignant neoplasms (cancer)	21.8
3. Cerebrovascular diseases (stroke)	8.4
4. Chronic lower-respiratory diseases	5.1
5. Diabetes mellitus (diabetes)	3.1
6. Influenza and pneumonia	3.0
7. Alzheimer's disease	2.9
8. Accidents (unintentional injuries)	2.8
9. Nephritis, nephrotic syndrome, and nephrosis (kidney disease)	1.6
10. Septicemia	1.4

*Percent of total deaths due to the cause indicated.

Source: CDC Office of Women's Health. Available at: http://www.cdc.gov/od/spotlight/nwhw/lcod/00all.htm. Accessed April 22, 2004.

Pharmacology

FDA Classification for Drugs in Pregnancy

Table 4-4 FDA Pregnancy Risk Categories for Prescription and Nonprescription Drugs

A Controlled studies in women fail to demonstrate a risk to the fetus in the first trimester (and there is no evidence of a risk in later trimesters), and the possibility of fetal harm appears remote.

B   Either animal reproduction studies have not demonstrated a fetal risk but there are no controlled studies in pregnant women or animal reproduction studies have shown an adverse effect (other than a decrease in fertility) that was not confirmed in controlled studies in women in the first trimester (and there is no evidence of a risk in later trimesters).

C   Either studies in animals have revealed adverse effects on the fetus (teratogenic or embryocidal or other) or there are no controlled studies in women and animals are not available. Drugs should be given only if the potential benefit justifies the potential risk to the fetus.

D   There is positive evidence of human fetal risk, but the benefits from use in pregnant women may be acceptable despite the risk (e.g., if the drug is needed in a life-threatening situation or for a serious disease for which safer drugs cannot be used or are ineffective).

X   Studies in animals or human beings have demonstrated fetal abnormalities or there is evidence of fetal risk based on human experience or both, and the risk of the use of the drug in pregnant women clearly outweighs any possible benefit. The drug is contraindicated in women who are or may become pregnant.

Source: From the *Federal Register,* 44:37434-37467, 1980.

Teratogens

Table 4-5 Medications That Have Moderate to High Teratogenicity

Drug (Class)	Generic (Trade) Names	FDA Pregnancy Category	Trimester When Most Teratogenic	Fetal/Infant Effects
Androgen	Danazol (Danocrine)	X	2nd, 3rd	Virilization of females and ambiguous genitalia
Angiotensin converting enzyme (ACE) inhibitors	Captopril (Capoten) Enalapril (Vasotec)	C	All	Fetal hypotension syndrome, fetal kidney hypoperfusion, anuria, oligohydramnios, pulmonary hypoplasia
Angiotensin II receptor blockers	Candesartan Cilexetil (Atacand) Irbesartan (Avapro)	D	2nd, 3rd	Fetal and neonatal hypotension, skull hypoplasia, anuria, renal failure and death
Antibiotics	Aminoglycosides: Spectinomycin Gentamicin Streptomycin	D	All	8th nerve toxicity, discoloration of teeth, altered bone growth
	Tetracycline	D		Bone and teeth staining
Anticoagulants	Warfarin (Coumadin)	X	All	Hypoplastic nasal bridge (1st trimester) CNS malformations (2nd trimester) Risk of bleeding (3rd trimester)

Drug (Class)	Generic (Trade) Names	FDA Pregnancy Category	Trimester When Most Teratogenic	Fetal/Infant Effects
Anticonvulsant	Carbamazepine	C	1st	Neural tube defects
	Phenytoin	D		Hydantoin syndrome
	Trimethadione	D		
	Valproic acid	D		
Anti-infective	Iodine	D	All	Congenital goiter, transient hypothyroidism
Antineoplastic	Aminopterin	X	1st	Multiple unspecified malformations and low birth weight
	Busulfan	D	1st	
	Cyclophosphamide	D	1st	
	Cytarabine	D	1st	
	Methotrexate	D	All	
	Tamoxifen	D	All	
Antituberculosis therapy	Isoniazid	C	All	Shown to have an embryocidal effect in rats and rabbits when given in pregnancy; no well-controlled studies in pregnant women
	Rifamycin	C	All	CNS abnormalities with chronic use
Antiviral (HIV)	Efavirenz (Sustiva)	C	All	Teratogenic in primate lab animals; no well-controlled human data
Benzodiazepine	Lorazepam (Ativan)	D	3rd	Neonatal dependence with chronic use
	Clonazepam (Klonopin)	C		
	Chlordiazepoxide (Librium)	D		

	Oxazepam (Serax)	D		
	Diazepam (Valium)	D		
Chelating agent	Penicillamine	D	1st	Cutis laxa, other congenital anomalies
Dermatologic preparation	Minoxidil	C	2nd, 3rd	Newborn hirsutism
Hallucinogen	Phencyclidine	X	All	Abnormal neurologic exam, including poor suck reflex and poor feeding
Hypoglycemic agents	Chlorpropamide	C	All	Prolonged neonatal hypoglycemia
Prostaglandin analog	Misoprostol (Cytotec)	X	All	Embryocidal in early pregnancy; may cause preterm labor and birth
Retinoid, systemic	Isotretinoin (Accutane)	X	All	CNS, cardioaortic, ear, and clefting defects; microtia, anotia, thymic aplasia, brachial arch and aortic arch abnormalities; certain congenital heart malformations
Retinoid, topical	Tretinoin (Retin-A)	C	All	Very unlikely to attain therapeutic topical exposure to retinoids
Sedative	Thalidomide	X	1st, 2nd	Phocomelia, limb reduction
Thyroid drugs	Propylthiouracil	D	All	Goiter
	Methimazole	D	All	Aplastic cutis

Source: Adapted from Reynolds, H.D. (1998). Preconception care: An integral part of primary care for women. *J. Nurse-Midwifery, 43*(6), 452.

Classification of Medication Safety During Lactation

L1 Safest—Frequently used and no adverse effects seen in infants: not orally bioavailable: or controlled studies fail to demonstrate risk and there is little chance of harm.

L2 Safer—Has been studied in small numbers of breastfeeding women and no adverse effects seen; or evidence of risk demonstrated to be likely is remote.

L3 Moderately safe—Controlled studies show minimal effect or no controlled study, but possible infant risk. Give if benefit justifies risk.

L4 Possibly hazardous—Positive evidence of risk to infant or milk supply; benefits may make use acceptable, such as with serious illness not otherwise treatable or risk of death.

L5 Contraindicated—Significant, well-documented risk in human infants, or high risk of the medication harming infants. Risk outweighs benefit of continued breast-feeding. Not to be used while breastfeeding. (Hale, 2002)

FDA Classification of Controlled Substances

Table 4-6   FDA Classification of Controlled Substances

Schedule	Interpretation
I	High potential for abuse and no current accepted medical use. Examples are heroin and LSD.
II	High potential for abuse. Use may lead to severe physical or psychological dependence. Examples are opioids, amphetamines, short-acting barbiturates, and preparations containing codeine. Prescriptions must be written in ink or typewritten and signed by the practitioner. Verbal prescriptions must be confirmed in writing within 72 hours and may be given only in a genuine emergency. No renewals are permitted.

Schedule	Interpretation
III	Some potential for abuse. Use may lead to low-to-moderate physical dependence or high psychological dependence. Examples are barbiturates and preparations containing small quantities of codeine. Prescriptions may be oral or written. Up to five renewals are permitted within six months.
IV	Low potential for abuse. Examples include chloral hydrate, phenobarbital, and benzodiazepines. Use may lead to limited physical or psychological dependence. Prescriptions may be oral or written. Up to five renewals are permitted within six months.
V	Subject to state and local regulations. Abuse potential is low; a prescription may not be required. Examples are antitussive and antidiarrheal medications containing limited quantities of opioids.

SECTION 4

Common Medical Problems in Women

Anemia

Table 4-7 Laboratory Values in Common Anemias

Laboratory Test	Iron Deficiency	Vitamin B$_{12}$ Deficiency	Folate Deficiency	Thalassemia	Chronic Disease
RBC	low	high	high	normal	normal
Hemoglobin	low	low	low	low	low
MCV	low	high	high	low	normal-low
MCH	low	high	high	low	low
MCHC	low	normal	normal	low	normal-low
Iron	low	high	high	high	low
TIBC	high	normal	normal	normal	low
Ferritin	low	high	high	high	normal-high

Hypertension

While few midwives will manage hypertension independently, all midwives should be able to correctly assess hypertension and risk of cardiovascular disease, counsel women on the lifestyle modifications that are an essential component of effective blood pressure management, and consult or refer for medication therapy.

Table 4-8 Classification of Blood Pressure

Category	SBP mmHg		DBP mmHg
Normal	<120	and	<80
Prehypertension	120–139	or	80–89
Hypertension Stage 1	140–159	or	90–99
Hypertension Stage 2	≥160	or	≥100

Table 4-9 Blood Pressure Measurement Techniques

Method	Notes
In office	Two readings 5 minutes apart, seated in chair, confirm elevation in opposite arm
Ambulatory BP monitoring	Indicated for evaluation of "white coat" hypertension
Patient self-check	Provides information on response to therapy and may help improve adherence to therapy

SECTION 4

A risk-scoring tool for cardiovascular disease developed by the National Cholesterol Education Program can be found in *JAMA*. 2001;285:2486–2497.

Principles of Lifestyle Modification

- Encourage healthy lifestyles for all individuals.
- Prescribe lifestyle modifications for all patients with prehypertension and hypertension.

Table 4-10   Lifestyle Modification Recommendations

Modification	Recommendation	Average SBP Reduction
Weight reduction	Maintain normal body weight (BMI 18.5–24.9 kg/m^3)	5–20 mm Hg/ 10 kg
DASH eating plan	Adopt a diet rich in fruits, vegetables, and low-fat dairy products with reduced content of saturated and total fat	8–14 mm Hg
Dietary sodium restriction	Reduce dietary sodium intake to ≤100 mmol/ day (2.4 g sodium or 6 g sodium chloride)	2–8 mm Hg
Aerobic physical activity	Regular aerobic physical activity (e.g., brisk walking) at least 30 minutes per day, most days of the week	4–9 mm Hg
Moderation of alcohol consumption	Women: limit to ≤1 drink per day	2–4 mm Hg

Source for hypertension tables: National Heart Lung and Blood Institute. *Seventh Report of the Joint National Committee on Prevention, Detection, Evaluation, and Treatment of High Blood Pressure (JNC 7).* May 2003. Available at: http://nhlbi.nih.gov.

Table 4-11 Classification of LDL, Total, and HDL
Cholesterol (mg/dL)

LDL Cholesterol
<100 Optimal
100–129 Near optimal/above optimal
130–159 Borderline high
160–189 High
>190 Very high
Total Cholesterol
<200 Desirable
200–239 Borderline high
>240 High
HDL Cholesterol
<40 Low
>60 High

Source: National Cholesterol Education Program, *Third Report of the National Cholesterol Education Program (NCEP) on Detection, Evaluation, and Treatment of High Blood Cholesterol in Adults (Adult Treatment Panel III).* National Institutes of Health and National Heart, Lung, and Blood Institute, May 2001. Available at: www.nhlbi.nih.gov/guidelines/index. Accessed on August 2, 2002.

Heart Disease

SECTION 4

Table 4-12 New York Heart Association Classification
of Heart Disease

Class I	Able to maintain normal physical activity levels without pain, shortness of breath, or other symptoms.
Class II	Some limitation of physical activity; will notice symptoms with normal activity levels.
Class III	Physical activity is limited; symptoms occur with even mild activity.
Class IV	Symptoms of congestive heart failure occur even at rest; physical activity is severely limited.

Respiratory Infections
Upper respiratory infections (URI)

- Symptoms include nasal congestion, clear to white discharge, sore throat, muscle aches, headache, cough. Influenza—higher fever
- Symptomatic management—rest, increased humidity, fluids, antipyretics, analgesics, cough suppressants, decongestants
- Ipratropium bromide (Atrovent) nasal spray, 1–2 sprays each nostril 3–4 times daily
- Antihistamines are not effective
- Influenza (not colds)—Rimantidine (Flumantidine) or neuraminidase inhibitors (Tamiflu) used within 48 hours of onset; reduces symptoms by about 24 hours
- Influenza vaccine for those at risk—health care workers, immunocompromised, chronic respiratory conditions, elderly

Sinusitis

- Usually a superimposed bacterial infection, with symptoms of greenish discharge, pain over affected sinus, fever, cough that worsens when reclining
- Symptomatic treatment as above
- Antibiotics for infections not resolving with supportive treatment, or frequent infections. Referral to physician if resistant or with periorbital edema.

Bronchitis

- Limited to infection of trachea and bronchi, usually a viral syndrome in healthy women

- Symptoms/signs include a viral syndrome of fever, malaise, fatigue, sore throat, chest pain, cough (may or may not be productive); lung sounds clear except over bronchi, chest x-ray clear
- Supportive therapy; albuterol inhaler (Proventil, Ventolin) as needed for cough; use 2 puffs every 4–6 hours. Prolonged inhaler dependence or more frequent use indicates need for physician referral.
- Antibiotics only for symptoms of bacterial infection such as productive colored sputum on coughing, chronic or recurrent disease

Community-Acquired Pneumonia

- Predisposing factors include chronic cough, repeated viral infections, smoking.
- Bacteria cause two thirds of community acquired disease.
- Symptoms: abrupt onset of fever, cough, chest pain, shortness of breath, sweats and chills, generalized aches, headache, fatigue
- Signs: rales and wheezing over affected lung fields; decreased air flow with consolidation
- Chest x-ray is diagnostic; sputum for culture is useful.
- Healthy adults under 50 years old, with pulse less than 125 bpm, normal mental status, temperature between 35°C and 40°C, respiratory rate less than 30, DBP less than 90, can be managed outpatient initially and observed for disease progress.
- The midwife should consult to confirm the plan of care.
- Macrolides, quinolones, and doxycycline are the most common antibiotics used initially.

SECTION 4

Table 4-13 Examples of Antibiotics Commonly Used in the Treatment of Respiratory Infections

Class	Dose Range/ Duration	Pregnancy Category
Cephalosporins		
Cefaclor (Ceclor)	250 mg q8h × 10 days	B
Cefixime (Suprax)	400 mg po QD × 10 days	B
Cefuroxime Axetil (Ceftin)	250 mg po q12h × 10 days	B
Cephalexin (Keflex)	250 mg po q6h × 10 days	B
	500 mg po q12h × 10 days	B
Macrolides		
Azithromycin (Zithromax)	500 mg po × 1, then 250 mg po QD × 4 days	B
Clarithromycin (Biaxin)	250-500 mg po q12h × 10–14 days	C
Penicillins		
Amoxicillin (e.g., Amoxil)	500 mg po q8h × 10 days 500-875 mg q12h × 10 days	B
Amoxicillin/ Clavulanate (Augmentin)	500-875 mg po q12h × 10 days (based on amoxicillin dose)	B
Quinolones		
Ciprofloxacin (Cipro)	500 mg po BID × 10 days	C
Levofloxacin (Levoquin)	500 mg po QD × 10 days	C
Trimethoprim/ sulfamethoxazole (Bactrim)	160/800 mg po BID × 10 days	C

Asthma

Asthma symptoms include chronic airway inflammation associated with spasm, edema, increased mucus production, and hyperresponsiveness to stimuli.

Symptoms in adults include chest tightness, shortness of breath, and wheezing. A dry cough is sometimes present and may be the only complaint.

Table 4-14 Classification of Asthma Severity: Clinical Features Before Treatment

	Days with Symptoms	Nights with Symptoms	PEF or FEV$_1$*	PEF Variability
Step 4 *Severe Persistent*	Continual	Frequent	≤60%	>30%
Step 3 *Moderate Persistent*	Daily	≥5/month	>60%–<80%	>30%
Step 2 *Mild Persistent*	3–6/week	3–4/month	≥80%	20–30%
Step 1 *Mild Intermittent*	≤2/week	≤2/month	≥80%	<20%

*Percent predicted values for forced expiratory volume in 1 second (FEV$_1$) and percent of personal best for peak expiratory flow (PEF) (relevant for children 6 years old or older who can use these devices).

NOTES
• Patients should be assigned to the most severe step in which *any* feature occurs. Clinical features for individual patients may overlap across steps.

- An individual's classification may change over time.
- Patients at any level of severity of chronic asthma can have mild, moderate, or severe exacerbations of asthma. Some patients with intermittent asthma experience severe and life-threatening exacerbations separated by long periods of normal lung function and no symptoms.
- Patients with two or more asthma exacerbations per week (i.e., progressively worsening symptoms that may last hours or days) tend to have moderate-to-severe persistent asthma.

Source: Practical Guide for the Diagnosis and Management of Asthma. NIH Publication No. 97-4053.

Initial Asthma Therapy

- Check for decreased airflow with peak flow meter.
- Counsel for smoking cessation.
- Consult or refer for initial medication regimen. Rescue inhalers alone are not adequate therapy for persistent asthma symptoms.

Abdominal Complaints
Gastroesophageal Reflux Disease (GERD)
Symptoms:

- Heartburn, worse with meals, bending over, lying down
- Wheeze, cough, laryngitis
- Chest pain

Treatment for GERD

- Weight reduction
- High protein, low-fat diet
- Avoidance of triggers
- Remain upright after eating
- Medication with antacids for mild symptoms

- H2 receptor antagonists
- If therapy fails, refer to physician management for treatment including treatment for *H. pylori*, endoscopy, surgical revision.

Table 4-15 Medications for the Management of Gastroesophageal Reflux Disease (GERD)

Medication	Dose	Duration of Therapy	FDA Pregnancy Category
H2 Receptor Antagonists			
Cimetidine (Tagamet)	400 mg po QID or 800 mg po BID	12 weeks	B
Famotidine (Pepcid)	20 mg po BID	6 weeks	B
Nizatidine (Axid)	150 mg po BID	12 weeks	B
Ranitidine (Zantac)	150 mg po BID	12 weeks	B
Proton Pump Inhibitors			
Esomeprazole (Nexium)	20 mg po QD 20 mg po QD	4 weeks maintenance	B
Iansoprazole (Prevacid)	15 mg po QD	8 weeks	B
Omeprazole (Prilosec)	20 mg po QD	4-8 weeks	C

Acute Diarrhea/Gastroenteritis

- Usually infectious
- Refer persistent watery diarrhea lasting more than 2 weeks for physician management.
- Refer patients with unresolved dehydration for physician management.

- Symptoms of infection include:
  - Nausea and vomiting
  - Explosive onset of diarrhea
  - Fever
  - Malaise
  - Increased bowel sounds
  - Tender abdomen without guarding
- Workup includes:
  - Stool sample for bleeding/WBCs
  - Electrolytes if dehydration is suspected
  - Medications such as kaolin/pectin (Kaopectate), diphenoxylate (Lomotil), loperamide (Imodium) to reduce frequency of stools
  - Stool for ova and parasites with persistent diarrhea

Constipation

Causes

- Inadequate dietary fiber
- Inadequate fluid intake
- Iron therapy
- Medications (tricyclics, anticholinergics, calcium channel blockers)
- Misuse of laxatives
- Opiate use
- Stress
- Neurologic dysfunction

Management

- Dietary counseling
- Increased exercise
- Avoidance of straining
- Stop overuse of laxatives and cathartics

- If needed, a bulk-forming laxative can be tried, adding docusate sodium as necessary.
- If none of the above is helpful, referral to a physician is appropriate.

Cholecystitis

Symptoms or signs include:

- Right-upper quadrant pain
- Diffuse discomfort after eating
- Severe, acute abdominal pain, may refer to right shoulder or central back.
- Murphy's sign: inspiratory arrest with deep palpation of the right-upper quadrant
- Palpable mass below the liver
- Leukocytosis, elevated liver functions, elevated bilirubin

Management includes medical referral. The definitive treatment is surgical.

Appendicitis

Symptoms and signs include:

- Anorexia
- Acute right-lower quadrant pain
- Vomiting
- Fever
- Leukocytosis
- Deep tenderness over McBurney's point
- Rovsing's sign: rebound pain with release of pressure on lower-left abdomen

Management is by medical referral. Definitive treatment is surgical.

Diagnosis and Management of Urinary Tract Infections

Diagnosis is by culture; treatment in healthy women can be started based on symptoms of dysuria and increased frequency of voiding. In the office a positive leukocyte esterase on a clean catch urine is adequate for treatment.

Table 4-16 Anti-Infectives Commonly Used in the Treatment of Uncomplicated Urinary Track Infections

Trimethoprim/sulfamethoxazole (Bactrim)	160 mg/800 mg po BID × 3 days*
Nitrofurantoin (Macrodantin)	100 mg po BID × 3 days*
Amoxicillin (Amoxil)	500 mg po TID × 3 days
Cephalexin (Keflex)	500 mg po QID × 3 days
During pregnancy, treat with 7-day therapy at same dose.	

*Avoid use in term pregnancy.

Single-dose therapy is clinically effective, but is associated with an increased recurrence rate. Seven-day therapy can be reserved for pregnant women, the immunocompromised, diabetics, and women whose symptoms were present for several days before seeking treatment.

Assessing CVA Tenderness

Expose the costovertebral angle. Strike gently but firmly with either the ulnar surface of a fist, or with your open hand striking your fist placed on the costovertebral angle.

Pyelonephritis

Symptoms include:

- Flank pain/positive CVAT
- Nausea

- Urinalysis positive for WBCs or pyuria
- Positive urine culture

Referral to a physician is indicated, as pyelonephritis is commonly treated with IV therapy initially. In some cases young, healthy, nonpregnant women can be treated entirely on an outpatient basis. Careful monitoring of progress is required.

Common regimens for the treatment of pyelonephritis last 10-14 days and may include:

Cephalosporins (Rocephin)
Quinolones (Cipro)
Trimethoprim/ sulfamethoxazole (Bactrim)

Diabetic Screening

Characteristics of Type I diabetes:

- Polyuria
- Increased thirst
- Increased hunger, with weight loss
- Fatigue

Characteristics of Type II diabetes:

- As well as the above, which may be present
- Persistent vaginal yeast infections
- Pruritis
- Skin infections
- Blurred vision
- Neuropathy

Criteria for Diagnosis of Diabetes

Table 4-17   Criteria for the Diagnosis of Diabetes Mellitus

1. Symptoms of diabetes plus casual plasma glucose (PG) concentration ≥200 mg/dl (11.1 mmol/l). Casual is defined as any time of day without regard to time since last meals. The classic symptoms of diabetes include polyuria, polydipsia, and unexplained weight loss.

or

2. FPG ≥126 mg/dl (7.0 mmol/l). Fasting is defined as no caloric intake for at least 8 h.

or

3. 2-h PG ≥200 mg/dl (11.1 mmol/l) during an OGTT. The test should be performed as described by WHO, using a glucose load containing the equivalent of 75 g anhydrous glucose dissolved in water.

In the absence of unequivocal hyperglycemia with acute metabolic decompensation, these criteria should be confirmed by repeat testing on a different day. The third measure (OGTT) is not recommended for routine clinical use.

Source: Copyright © 2003 American Diabetes Association. From *Diabetes Care,* Vol. 26, Supplement 1, 2003; S5-S20. Reprinted with permission from The American Diabetes Association.

Diagnosis of diabetes in the midwife's office should be followed by:

- Performance of hemoglobin A_{1C}
- Referral for nutritional counseling
- Referral to a provider experienced in the management of diabetes
- Recommendations of lifestyle modifications including smoking cessation, improved diet, exercise, weight loss

- Consideration of contraceptive needs and pre-conception counseling

Thyroid Disease

Table 4-18   Common Clinical Features of Thyroid Disease: Signs and Symptoms

---

Hyperthyroid
Anxiety, nervousness
Fatigue
Weakness
Increased sweating
Heat intolerance
Diarrhea
Warm, moist skin
Tremor
Irregular menses
Lid lag, stare
Hyperreflexia
Increased appetite with weight loss
Palpitations with angina
Goiter
Ophthalmopathy

Hypothyroid
Fatigue, sleepiness
Lethargy
Muscle weakness
Muscle cramping or pain
Cold intolerance
Constipation
Dry skin, brittle nails, thinning hair
Headaches

Menorrhagia, amenorrhea (late)
Delay in deep tendon reflex relaxation
Depression
Decreased sweating
Edema (non-pitting)
Hoarseness
Pallor
Loss of appetite
Weight gain (occasionally weight loss)
Slowed speech and body movements
Bradycardia
Goiter

Thyroid Hormone Values

Table 4-19 Thyroid Hormone Values

Condition	Thyroid-Stimulating Hormone (TSH)	Free T4	Serum T3
Graves' disease	Absent	Elevated	Elevated
Subclinical hyperthyroid	<0.1 mU/L	Normal	Normal
Hypothyroid	High with primary, low with secondary	Low	Low/normal
Subclinical hypothyroid	Mildly elevated (<10.0 mU/L)	Low/normal	

Clinical Characteristics of the Primary Headache Types

Table 4-20 Clinical Characteristics of the Primary Headache Syndromes

Feature	Migraine without Aura	Migraine with Aura	Tension-Type Headache (Episodic)	Cluster Headache (Episodic)
Prevalence	Common	Uncommon	Common	Rare
Gender	Females>males	Females>males	Females>males	Males>females
Family history	Frequent	Frequent	Frequent	Rare
Age at onset (yr)	10–30	10–30	20–40	20–40
Prodrome	Common	Common	None	None
Aura (visual)	None	Present	None	None
Site of pain	Hemicranial, bilateral	Hemicranial, bilateral	Bilateral, occipital, frontal	Unilateral, frontotemporal periorbital
Charter of pain	Pulsatile	Pulsatile	Aching, tight, squeezing	Boring
Severity of pain	Moderate to severe	Moderate to severe	Mild to moderate	Severe
Onset to peak pain	Minutes to hours	Minutes to hours	Hours	Minutes (rapid)

Feature	Migraine without Aura	Migraine with Aura	Tension-Type Headache (Episodic)	Cluster Headache (Episodic)
Duration of pain	Usually 4–24 hrs	Usually 4–24 hrs	Hours to days	30–90 min
Frequency of attack	Variable, several per month	Variable, several per month	Variable, several per month	Daily during cluster period
Periodicity of attacks	No (exception, menstrual migraine)	No (exception, menstrual migraine)	No	Yes, "like clockwork"
Accompaniments	Nausea, vomiting, photophobia, phonophobia, osmophobia	Nausea, vomiting, photophobia, phonophobia, osmophobia	Nausea on occasion	Ipsilateral nasal congestion, rhinorrhea, conjunctival injection, ptosis, lacrimation
Behavior during headache	Still, quiet	Still, quiet	No change	Pace
Nocturnal attacks of pain	Can occur	Can occur	Very rare	Extremely frequent
Triggering factors	Multiple	Multiple	Stress, elevation	Alcohol, sleep, emotional upset

Source: From *Mayo Clin. Proc.*, 71, 1055–1066 (November) 1996. Available at www.ama-assn.org/spec/migraine/library/readroom/mayoful.htm and used by permission of the publisher.

Management of Headaches
Chronic Tension Headaches:

- Empathy
- Assessment for anxiety/depression disorders
- Relaxation/stress reduction
- NSAIDS, acetaminophen, possibly supplemented with 200 mg caffeine

Migraine:

- Avoidance of dietary triggers
- High dose NSAIDS, 1000 mg acetaminophen as abortive therapy with mild disease
- Caffeine-containing compounds (Caffergot)
- Sumatriptan (Imitrex), naratriptan (Amerge)
- Tricyclic antidepressants
- Use consultation as appropriate to determine medical regimen.
- Ensure adequate contraception as indicated. Some medications (e.g., ergotamines) are contraindicated in pregnancy.

Depression
Major Depression

The DSM-IV criteria for major depression include five or more of the following symptoms, present for a 2-week period and representing a change from prior function. Either of the first two criteria must be present:

1. Depressed mood nearly every day for most of the day either by self-report or observation
2. Diminished or absent pleasure in all or most activities, most of the day, most days
3. Significant weight loss or gain (>5%), or decreased or increased appetite nearly every day

4. Insomnia or hypersomnia
5. Psychomotor agitation or retardation (must be observed by others)
6. Fatigue or loss of energy
7. Feelings of worthlessness, or inappropriate or excessive guilt, possibly delusional
8. Decreased ability to concentrate or think clearly, indecisiveness
9. Recurrent thoughts of death, suicidal ideation, or a suicide plan or attempt

The symptoms must cause significant impairment of life activities or distress, and cannot be accounted for by loss of a loved one or other major life loss.

For more information, see *Varney's Midwifery*, 4th edition, p. 159.

Depression in the postpartum period is diagnosed and treated by the same criteria as at any other time in a woman's life.

Dysthymia

Dysthymia is a more low-grade, chronically depressed state, in which mood is depressed most days, for most of the day, for two or more years. It is associated with at least two of the following characteristics:

1. Changes in appetite
2. Insomnia or hypersomnia
3. Fatigue, decreased energy
4. Low self-esteem
5. Poor concentration, difficulty with decision making
6. Hopeless feelings

Medical conditions may cause symptoms of depression either as part of their own symptoms or because living with that problem has induced depressive feelings.

Examples include hypothyroidism, severe anemia, chronic pain, disabilities as a result of stroke, arthritis, or heart disease.

Therapeutic Options for Depression

Both psychotherapy and medications are important in the management of depression. Behavioral changes need to be incremental, as women with depression are already feeling overwhelmed. Goals need to be set in increments that allow for the positive reinforcement of visible achievements. Apart from crisis intervention, counseling is a long-term process, one which few midwives have the time to provide in the office setting. Maintaining a referral network that includes psychiatric services is essential (see *Varney's Midwifery*, 4th edition, p. 159, for more details).

Table 4-21   Examples of Medications Used in the Treatment of Depression and Related Disorders

Class	Initial Dose	Maximum Dose	FDA Pregnancy Category
Selective Serotonin Reuptake Inhibitors (SSRIs)			
Citalopram (Celexa)	20 mg po QD	60 mg po QD	C
Fluoxetine (Prozac)	20 mg po QAM	90 mg po QAM	C
Paroxetine (Paxil)	20 mg po QD	50 mg po QD	C
Sertraline (Zoloft)	50 mg po QD	200 mg po QD	C

Antidepressants

Venlafaxine (Effexor)	37.5–75 mg po bid	375 mg/day	C
Buproprion (Wellbutrin)	100 mg po bid	450 mg/day	B

Tricyclic Antidepressants

Amitriptyline (Elavil)	50–100 mg po QHS	150 mg/day	C
Imipramine (Tofranil)	75 mg/day	200 mg/day	N

Infectious Diseases

HIV

The human immunodeficiency virus (HIV) is an RNA retrovirus that preferentially attacks T-helper lymphocytes (CD4) cells as well as other cell types. Initial exposure may produce a viral syndrome within the first month, including fever, muscle aches, sore throat, and lymphadenopathy. Rapid viral replication at this time causes a steep drop in the CD4 count and high viral load. As the body mounts an immune response, the viral load subsides and the CD4 cell number increases. The body continues to produce CD4 cells to replace those lost to the virus. This period can last for 10 or more years. Age, race, gender, drug abuse, and viral characteristics affect disease progress. In the later stages of HIV/AIDS, falling CD4 cell counts reach a point at which the body cannot defend itself from common ailments or from diseases that do not normally infect humans (opportunistic infections).

When the final risk determination is made, about two thirds of all women in the United States with HIV/AIDS have been infected sexually.

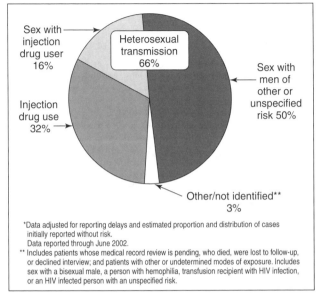

Sex with injection drug user 16%

Heterosexual transmission 66%

Sex with men of other or unspecified risk 50%

Injection drug use 32%

Other/not identified** 3%

*Data adjusted for reporting delays and estimated proportion and distribution of cases initially reported without risk.
Data reported through June 2002.
** Includes patients whose medical record review is pending, who died, were lost to follow-up, or declined interview; and patients with other or undetermined modes of exposure. Includes sex with a bisexual male, a person with hemophilia, transfusion recipient with HIV infection, or an HIV infected person with an unspecified risk.

Figure 4-1   Risk factors for transmission of HIV in women.

Source: From Centers for Disease Control and Prevention. Accessed on February 14, 2003, at http://www.cdc.gov.

SECTION 4

Counseling prior to HIV testing includes a focused discussion of risk reduction, acknowledgment of current efforts the woman is making to reduce her risks, and being specific in discussing her individual risks and her understanding of HIV. This session is also the time when further risk reduction plans can be made and skills reinforced—for example, negotiating condom use.

Table 4-22 Recommendations for When to Test for HIV

---

1. All clients in settings where the population is at increased behavioral or clinical risk of HIV
   a. adolescent and school-based clinics with high STD rates
   b. clinics serving men who have sex with men
   c. correctional facilities including juvenile detention
   d. drug and alcohol programs
   e. freestanding HIV testing sites
   f. homeless shelters
   g. outreach (e.g., needle exchange) programs
   h. STD clinics
   i. TB clinics
2. Individuals in settings with <1% HIV prevalence
   a. clinical signs or symptoms of HIV infection
   b. have diagnoses suggesting increased HIV risk
   c. self-report HIV risks
   d. specifically request the test
3. All clients in settings where the prevalence of HIV is >1%
4. Regardless of any of the above
   a. all pregnant women
   b. all persons with possible occupational exposure
   c. all clients known to be exposed to an HIV positive person sexually or through needle sharing

---

Source: From Revised guidelines for HIV counseling, testing, and referral. (2001). *MMWR, 50,* RR-19. Accessed at http://www.cdc.gov/mmwr/pdf/rr/rr5019.

Table 4-23   Risk Assessment Questions for HIV in Women

How many sexual partners have you had in your lifetime?
This year?

How old were you the first time you were sexually active?

Are your partners men, women, or both?

What have you used to protect yourself from pregnancy?
From sexually transmitted infections?

Have you ever had an abnormal Pap smear or an STD or
hepatitis?

Have you ever used an IV drug or used other drugs like crack?

Have you abused alcohol?

Have you ever shared a needle?

Have any of your partners ever used drugs, shared needles,
been in jail, had an STD, had hepatitis, worked as a prostitute,
or traded sex for drugs/money?

Are you concerned that you have been put at risk for catching
HIV?

Source: From Anderson, J. R. (2001). *A guide to the clinical care of women with HIV.* Accessed at http://www.hab.hvsa.gov/publications/women-care.htm.

Post-test counseling for women whose test results are negative reinforces positive messages about preventing infection and makes sure that women understand the limitations of the test. Frequency of retesting is included.

Counseling the newly diagnosed woman takes time; it often takes more than one visit. Emotional issues take precedence. Have a specific plan to offer her for follow-up and simple, positive messages about living with HIV. Specific topics include:

- Test results interpretation
- Course of HIV, monitoring health

- Referral for medical care and case management
- Notification of partners, disclosure issues
- Issues of confidentiality and discrimination
- Behavior changes to prevent transmission and protect her own health
- Assessment of mental and emotional status

Reading HIV Labs

ELISA/Western Blot: Tests for diagnosis of HIV infection. The ELISA is a nonspecific measure of antibodies which is subject to cross-reaction with other conditions and can result in a false positive if performed without confirmatory testing. The Western Blot measures specific antibody response to HIV infection. Other rapid tests are becoming available, which are also nonspecific. As with the ELISA, they require confirmation with a Western Blot, or with a different nonspecific test using different technology.

Persistent inconclusive results can be caused by autoimmune or collagen vascular diseases, alloantibodies from pregnancy or transfusion, infection with a rare subtype, or HIV-2. True false positives are less than 0.0001 percent in low-prevalence areas.

CD4 count: T-lymphocytes involved in immune response to HIV infection. Normal counts are 500-1500 cells/mm^3. Below 200 cells/mm^3 the diagnosis of AIDS is made based on decreased immune competence. Pregnancy, substance abuse, steroids, and illnesses other than HIV can also suppress CD4 counts.

Viral load: Measure of amount of virus present in the blood of infected persons. The most common test is RNA based. All tests have both a lower and upper limit of accuracy. Ultrasensitive tests can identify the presence of as few as 40 viral particles per milliliter.

Basics of HIV Therapy

Current recommendations for management of HIV include delaying medication therapy until the body's own immune system begins to weaken (around 350 cells/mm^3). The desired response is a drop in viral load to a non-detectable level. Treatment of HIV is a complex issue, and choices made for medications now can affect the usefulness of others as the disease progresses. For this reason, everyone living with HIV should be referred for care to a provider specializing in infectious disease management.

Women living with HIV need to be seen for gynecological examinations and Pap testing every 6 months for 1 year after diagnosis. After that, annual testing is adequate until the CD4 count drops below 500 cells/mm^3 or high-risk HPV is found on the Pap test. Aggressive management of abnormal Pap smears is recommended. HIV is known to increase the likelihood and rapidity of cervical disease progression. The vagina and vulva should also be inspected for lesions that may indicate malignant changes. Contraceptive management includes checking for drug-drug interactions with antiretrovirals, promotion of regular condom use, and education about sexual transmission. Counseling includes STD prevention and disclosure issues. Ten percent of AIDS cases are in persons over 50. Women of all ages need safe-sex counseling to reduce transmission.

The Centers for Disease Control and Prevention regularly updates guidelines for HIV management and therapy. These are found on the Web at http://www.cdc.gov. The midwife whose patient is positive for HIV should review these documents for better understanding of the disease and its management. The U.S. Department of Health Resources and Services

SECTION 4

Administration also publishes *A Guide to the Clinical Care of Women with HIV*.

HIV Therapy in Pregnancy

Counseling during the initial pregnancy visit includes the risks of mother-to-child transmission, management options to reduce that risk, and the importance of regular care.

HIV therapy during pregnancy is continued without interruption for the woman already on antiretrovirals. The one exception is the woman taking efavirenz (Sustiva), who should be advised to stop this medication. She should involve her primary provider in this decision as an alternative medication will need to be provided without a break in therapy. Women not taking medication prior to pregnancy should not begin until organogenesis is complete, or around 12 weeks. The midwife caring for women with HIV must establish a consulting relationship with a primary care provider expert in HIV management to determine pregnancy regimens and alter them as needed.

During pregnancy the CD4 count should be assessed at least every trimester. Viral load testing is done before medication is started, 4 weeks later, and at least once a trimester, plus at 36 weeks. Liver function, metabolic status, and CBC are measured at intervals determined by the medication regimen and patient status.

Risk factors that increase the risk of mother-to-child transmission include:

- Elevated viral load
- Clinical disease progression
- Coinfection with STDs, Hepatitis C, other diseases
- Substance abuse, including smoking

- Multiple sexual partners, unprotected intercourse
- Preterm birth
- Chorioamnionitis
- Invasive fetal monitoring or testing

Decisions regarding route of childbirth are made in discussion with the mother. For women on antiretroviral therapy whose viral load is less than 1000 cells/mm^3 at term, vaginal birth is considered a safe alternative, with the risk of perinatal transmission at 1–2%. Other women should be counseled to consider a cesarean birth, which independently reduces the risk of transmission.

Artificial rupture of the membranes is avoided. Active management of labor can be considered, particularly if the membranes rupture early in labor.

Women whose HIV status is unknown at the start of labor should be offered rapid HIV testing. If the test is positive, a single dose of nevirapine 200 mg po at the onset of active labor and IV AZT should be offered, and neonatal AZT prescribed, pending the results of a confirmatory test. When nevirapine is given in labor, the pediatrician must be informed.

Access the CDC Web site for the most current information on management of HIV in pregnancy.

Table 4-24 Classes of HIV Medication

Nucleoside/Nucleotide Reverse Transcriptase Inhibitors (NRTIs)

Generic Drug Name, Abbreviation (Brand)	FDA Category	Dose
Zidovudine, AZT (Retrovir)	C	300 mg po bid
Lamivudine, 3TC (Epivir)	C	150 mg po bid
Didanosine, ddI (Videx)	B	<60 kg 250 mg po qd or 125 mg po bid (tabs)
		OR 250 mg po qd or 167 mg po bid (powder)
		>60 kg 400 mg po qd or 200 mg po bid (tabs)
		OR 500 mg po qd or 250 mg po bid (powder)
		OR Videx EC 400 mg po qd
Zalcitabine, ddC (Hivid)	C	0.75 mg po tid
Stavudine, d4T (Zerit)	C	<60 kg 30 mg po bid
		>60 kg 40 mg po bid
Abacavir, APV (Ziagen)	C	300 mg po bid
AZT + 3TC (Combivir)	C	300 mg AZT + 150 mg 3TC po bid
AZT + 3TC + ABC (Trizivir)	C	300 mg AZT + 150 mg 3TC + 300 mg ABC po bid
Tenofovir DF (Viread)	B	300 mg po qd

Non-nucleoside Reverse Transcriptase Inhibitors (NNRTIs)

Generic Drug Name, Abbreviation (Brand)	FDA Category	Dose
Nevirapine, NVP (Viramune)	C	200 mg po bid
Delavirdine, DLV (Rescriptor)	C	400 mg po tid
Efavirenz, EFV (Sustiva)	C*	600 mg po qhs

Protease Inhibitors (PIs)

Generic Drug Name, Abbreviation (Brand)	FDA Category	Dose
Saquinavir, SQV, hgc (Invirase)	B	400 mg po bid with RTV
Saquinavir, SQV, sgc (Fortovase)	B	1200 mg po tid
Ritonavir, RTV (Norvir)	B	600 mg po bid
Indinavir, IDV (Crixivan)	C	800 mg po q 8 hours
Nelfinavir, NFV (Viracept)	B	750 mg po tid OR 1250 mg po bid
Amprenavir, APV (Agenerase)	C	1200 mg po bid (caps) OR 1400 mg po (oral solution)
Lopinavir/Ritonavir, LPV/RTV (Kaletra)	C	400 mg LPV + 100 mg RTV po bid

*Not used in pregnancy due to primate studies showing teratogenicity.

Note: Many of these drugs have specific dosing requirements, medication interactions, and/or significant side effects beyond the scope of this reference. Interested readers are referred to www.hivatis.org for current antiretroviral information.

Sources: https://www.hivatis.org; Bartlett, J. G., & Gallant, J. *Medical Management of HIV Infection* (2001-2002 Ed). Baltimore, MD: Johns Hopkins University.

SECTION 4

Tuberculosis

Table 4-25   Risk Factors for Tuberculosis Infection and Progression

---

Overcrowded environment
Immigration from areas where TB is endemic
Nosocomial exposure (e.g., nursing homes)
Evidence of prior TB infection
HIV
Diabetes
Steroid therapy
Immunosuppressive therapy
Head and neck cancers
Renal disease
Malabsorption syndromes
Gastrectomy, intestinal bypass
Malnutrition, low body weight
Alcoholism
Substance abuse

Diagnosis of Tuberculosis

Exposure to tuberculosis (TB) is by droplet or aerosolization. Latent TB is identified by a positive reaction to the PPD test without symptoms and is noninfectious. It occurs in 21–23% of those exposed. Ten percent of healthy women without risk factors will progress to active TB.

To interpret PPD results, read 48–72 hours after administration. Positive results are identified at:

- Induration >15 mm in persons with no risk factors

- Induration >10 mm in
  - Recent immigrants from endemic TB areas
  - Persons with high-risk health conditions
  - Children exposed to those at high risk
  - IV drug abusers
  - Mycobacteriology lab staff
  - Inhabitants and staff of congregate living facilities (jails, nursing homes) and the homeless
- Induration >5 mm in
  - Persons with HIV/AIDS
  - Persons with close exposure to an active TB patient
  - Persons whose CXR suggests prior TB without treatment
  - Those who are immune suppressed

Anergy is the condition in which the reaction decreases or disappears in the presence of exposure. In TB, causes include AIDS, acute viral illness, overwhelming TB, sarcoidosis, live virus vaccines, and immune suppression.

Table 4-26   Signs and Symptoms of Active Tuberculosis

Fever: Initially minimal to moderate temperature elevation occurs daily in the late afternoon or evening, usually accompanied by a feeling of euphoria and well-being; as disease progresses, temperature elevations reach 103°F (39.5°C) or higher.

Night sweats: The daily rise in body temperature reverses at night with accompanying diaphoresis.

Weight loss: Minor weight loss with anorexia occurs early in the disease; increased weight loss, fatigue, and irritability occurs as the disease progresses.

Chronic cough: A cough that is worse in the morning.

Chronic, productive cough: A cough that produces large amounts of purulent, greenish-yellow sputum sometimes accompanied by hemoptysis.

Pleurisy with effusion: This is particularly significant in young childbearing women, as pleurisy in this age group is uncommon.

Spontaneous atelectasis: Especially in a young person, this may be a sign of active tuberculosis.

Crepitant rales: This is heard best on auscultation after the woman coughs.

Table 4-27   Factors That May Cause False-Positive and False-Negative Responses to the Tuberculin Skin Test

False Positive	Nontuberculous mycobacteria
	BCG vaccination
False Negative	Anergy
	Recent TB infection
	Very young age (<6 months old)
	Live-virus vaccination
	Overwhelming TB disease

Source: Centers for Disease Control and Prevention. (2000). *Core curriculum on tuberculosis: What the clinician should know* (4th ed.). Accessed at http://www.cdc.gov/nchstp/tb/pubs/corecurr/default.htm.

Treatment of Latent Tuberculosis

- Screen for HIV, liver disease, contraindications to medications (no.)
- Isoniazid (INH) 300 mg po qd for 9 months
- In pregnancy, add pyridoxine (B6).
- Persons resistant to INH should be referred for management.
- Teach the importance of adherence, risks, and benefits of long-term therapy, side effects.

- The patient should be seen monthly to assess adherence, symptoms of progression, and signs of hepatitis.

Management of tuberculosis is by the consultant physician who should be notified prior to ordering chest x-ray or sputum culture.

Hepatitis

Viral hepatitis is the term which refers to a group of pathogenic viruses, not all related to one another.

Hepatitis A

- Fecal-oral transmission of the hepatitis A virus, occasionally household exposure
- Incubation averages 28 days, most infectious prior to onset of symptoms
- Signs and symptoms include flulike syndrome, rash, muscle and joint pain, jaundice, upper-right quadrant pain, itching, weight loss, enlarged and tender liver, splenomegaly
- Care is palliative.
- Vaccine is available.

Hepatitis B

- Vaccine is available.
- Incubation averages 60–90 days, range 45–180 days
- 50–70% will have subclinical infection without jaundice.
- Chronic infection fewer than 10%
- Nonhepatic symptoms: rash, fever arthralgia, myalgia, arthritis can precede jaundice
- Nausea, vomiting
- Right-upper quadrant pain

- Enlarged, tender liver
- Fever, chills weakness/exhaustion, headache

Risk Factors for Hepatitis B

- Use of contaminated needles for IVDU
- Unsafe sex, multiple sexual partners
- Exposure to blood, semen, saliva, vaginal secretions
- Immigrants from areas where hepatitis B is endemic
- Men who have sex with men (MSM)
- Women intimate with MSM
- Infants born to mothers with hepatitis B
- Hemodialysis patients

Laboratory Values in Hepatitis B

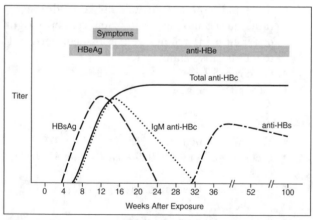

Figure 4-2   Progressive serology changes with acute hepatitis B infections.

Source: From Centers for Disease Control and Prevention. Accessed on February 14, 2003, at: http://www.cdc.gov.

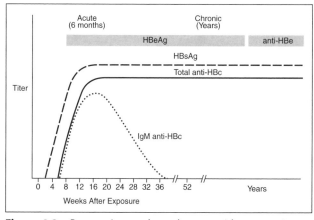

Figure 4-3 Progressive serology changes with progression to chronic hepatitis B infection.

Source: From Centers for Disease Control and Prevention. Accessed on February 14, 2003 at: http://www.cdc.gov.

Table 4-28 Serologic Markers of Hepatitis B Status

Stage of HBV Infection	Hepatitis B Surface Antigen (HbsAg)	Hepatitis B Surface Antibodies (Anti-HBs)	Hepatitis B Core Antibodies (Anti-HBc)	Total IgM (Anti-HBc Detects both IgM and IgG)
Late incubation	+	−	−	±
Acute	+	−	+	+
Chronic	+	− Rarely +	+	−
Recent (<6 months) window	−	±	+	+

Stage of HBV Infection	Hepatitis B Surface Antigen (HbsAg)	Hepatitis B Surface Antibodies (Anti-HBs)	Hepatitis B Core Antibodies (Anti-HBc)	Total IgM (Anti-HBc Detects both IgM and IgG)
Distant (>6 months) resolved	−	+	+	−
Immunized	−	+ with titer >10 mIU/ml	−	−

Hepatitis C

- Transmission is primarily bloodborne, less commonly sexual or perinatal
- Incubation takes an average of 6–7 weeks, range 2–26 weeks
- Acute infection with jaundice fewer than 20%
- Management of acute infection is palliative.
- 85% chronic infection; 5–20% will have cirrhosis.
- Acute infection with recovery: HCV RNA will be positive up to 6 months; anti-HCV will rise after 2–3 months; ALT will spike 4–6 weeks after exposure, peak around 3 months, and be normal around 6 months later
- Progression to chronic infection is reflected in persistent positive HCV-RNA and elevation of ALT

Target Groups for Testing

- IVDU
- Hemodialysis patients
- Recipients of clotting factors before 1987, blood or organ transplants before 1992

- Undiagnosed liver disease
- Infants of infected mothers (test at 12-18 months)
- Health care and public safety workers with known exposure

Management of the Woman with Hepatitis

Table 4-29 Diagnosis of Hepatitis

History

- Blood transfusion or blood products/organs prior to June 1992
- Previous hepatitis or jaundice
- Exposure to someone who has hepatitis or is jaundiced
- Multiple sex partners
- MSM
- Women having sex with MSM
- Intravenous drug use, even one episode, even in the remote past
- Immigration or travel from a country with endemic hepatitis
- Occupation—health care worker or public safety worker, day care worker
- Hemophilia
- History of dialysis

Clinical Signs of Hepatitis

- Anorexia
- Nausea
- Vomiting
- Upper-right quadrant abdominal pain
- Epigastric pain
- Malaise
- Weakness

- Fatigue
- Arthralgia
- Arthritis
- Urticaria
- Myalgia

Physical Examination

- Tender, enlarged liver
- Enlarged spleen
- Jaundice (of sclera or entire body)

Laboratory tests

- Positive hepatitis screening test or identification of specific hepatitis antigens and antibodies
- Elevated liver function tests AST (SGOT), ALT (SGPT), LDH, and bilirubin

---

The treatment of acute hepatitis is palliative. Consultation with or referral to a physician for management is appropriate, depending on the patient's status.

References

American Diabetes Association Web site. Available at: http://www.diabetes.org.

Anderson, J. R. A guide to the clinical care of women with HIV (2001). From http://www.hab.hvsa.gov/publications/womencare.htm.

Bartlett, J. G. & Gallant, J. (2002). *Medical Management of HIV Infection* (2001–2002 ed.). Baltimore, MD: Johns Hopkins University.

Centers for Disease Control and Prevention. (2000). *Core curriculum on tuberculosis: What the clinician should know* (4th ed.). From http://www.cdc.gov/nchstp/tb/pubs/corecurr/default.htm.

Centers for Disease Control and Prevention Web site. Available at: http://www.cdc.gov.

Clinical Preventive Services for Normal-Risk Adults Recommended by the U.S. Preventive Services Task Force. (2002). *Put prevention into practice.* Rockville, MD: Agency for Health Care Quality and Research.

Donaldson, M. S., et al. (Eds.). (1996). *Primary care: America's health in a new era.* Washington, DC: National Academy Press.

Expert Panel on Detection, Evaluation, and Treatment of High Blood Cholesterol in Adults. (2001). Executive summary of the third report of the National Cholesterol Education Program (NCEP) expert panel on detection, evaluation, and treatment of high blood cholesterol in adults (Adult Treatment Panel III). *JAMA, 285,* 2486–2497.

Federal Register (1980), 44, 37434–37467.

Hale, T. W. (2002). *Medications and mother's milk* (10th ed.). Amarillo, TX: Pharmasoft Publishing.

Institute of Medicine, Yordy, K. D., Lohr, K. N., Vanselow, N. A., et al. (Eds.). (1996). *Primary care: America's health in a new era.* Washington, DC: National Academy Press.

Mayo Clinic Proceedings 71, 1055–1066 (1966). Available at: http://www.ama-assn.org/spec/migraine/library/readroom/mayoful.htm.

Miniño, A. M., Arias, E., Kochanek, K. D., Murphy, S. L. & Smith, B. L. (2000). Deaths: Final data for 2000. *National Vital Statistics Reports, 50,* 15, 1–120.

Mokdad, A. H., Marks, J. S., Stroup, D. F., & Gerberding, J. L. (2004). Actual causes of death in the United States, 2000. *JAMA, 291,* 10, 1238–1246.

National High Blood Pressure Education Program. (2003). Seventh report of the Joint National Committee on Prevention, Detection, Evaluation, and Treatment of High Blood Pressure (JNC 7). Washington, DC: National Heart Lung and Blood Institute, National Institutes of Health, Department of Health and Human Services.

National Institutes of Health. (1997). Guidelines for the diagnosis and management of asthma. Expert Panel Report 2. NIH Publication No. 97-4051.

Reynolds, H. D. Preconception care: An integral part of primary care of women (1998). *Journal of Nurse Midwifery, 43*(6), 452.

Revised guidelines for HIV counseling, testing, and referral (2001). *MMWR, 50*, RR-19. From http://www.cdc.gov/mmwr/pdf/rr/rr5019.

Varney, H., Kriebs, J. M., & Gegor, C. L. (2003). *Varney's midwifery* (4th ed.). Sudbury, MA: Jones and Bartlett Publishers.

U.S. Preventive Services Task Force. (1966). *Guide to clinical preventive services*. Baltimore, MD: Lippincott William & Wilkins.

U.S. Department of Health Resources and Services Administration. *A guide to the clinical care of women with HIV*. Available at: http://www.hrsa.gov.

SECTION 5

Reproductive Health

Menstrual Abnormalities

Table 5-1   Common Definitions Referring to
Menstrual Changes

Amenorrhea: Absence of any menses by age 16 (primary),
   or absence of menses in woman who has previously
   menstruated (secondary).

Menorrhagia (Hypermenorrhea): Normal menstrual intervals
   with excessive flow and/or duration.

Metrorrhagia: Menstruation occurring at irregular intervals, or
   incidences of spotting or bleeding between periods.

Menometrorrhagia: Excess/prolonged menses at irregular
   intervals.

Polymenorrhea: Normal menses at more frequent intervals than
   normal (i.e., more frequent periods).

Oligomenorrhea: Normal menses at greater than normal
   intervals (i.e., fewer periods).

Hypomenorrhea: Scant bleeding at normal intervals.

Disorders Associated with Amenorrhea

Table 5-2 Disorders Associated with Amenorrhea

Genital Outflow Track (Uterus and Vagina)	Ovaries	Pituitary Gland	Hypothalamus (CNS)
Asherman's syndrome	Gonadal dysgenesis	Pituitary adenomas	Stress
Müllerian tube anomalies	Polycystic ovaries	Empty sella syndrome	Weight loss, eating disorders
Androgen insensitivity syndrome (testicular feminization)	Turner syndrome		Strenuous exercise
	Mosaicism		Posthormone use for birth control
	Premature ovarian shutdown		
	Side effects from radiation and/or chemotherapy		

Evaluation and Management of Amenorrhea

Taking these steps in order provides an orderly approach to assessment. At any point in the workup when the midwife feels it is appropriate, or when the practice guidelines require it, physician consultation and, possibly, referral are warranted.

1. Rule out pregnancy.
2. Consider normal variations of perimenopause.
3. Verify contraceptive method and possible endometrial suppression.
4. Evaluate general health, nutrition, medication/herbal use, exercise, weight gain or loss, emotional status.
5. Check TSH and prolactin.
6. Progesterone challenge:
   - Medroxyprogesterone acetate (Provera) 5–10 mg po qd × 5-10 days

   OR
   - Progesterone capsules 400 mg po qhs × 10 days
7. Estrogen challenge:
   - Estradiol (Estrace) 4.0 mg qd × 21 days

   OR
   - Conjugated equine estrogens (Premarin) 2.5 mg po qd × 21 days
   - Medroxprogesterone acetate 10 mg po days 16–21
8. LH, FSH (see Normal Values, Section 2, page 20)
9. If no cause has been found, referral to an endocrinologist is appropriate.

Causes and Evaluation of Menorrhagia

Table 5-3   Possible Causes of Menorrhagia

Typically Presented As a Onetime Event
- Pregnancy
  Intrauterine
  Ectopic
  Gestational trophoblastic neoplasm (e.g., hydatidiform mole)
- Infections (usually related to PID, use of IUD, or following
  instrument-based intrauterine procedure)
  Endometritis
  Salpingitis

Typically Presented As an Ongoing, Cyclic Pattern
- IUD use
- Neoplasia
  Ovarian cysts
  Uterine fibroids (myoma)
  Adenomyosis (endometrial tissue located within the
  myometrium)
  Endometrial hyperplasia
  Polyps
  Carcinoma
- Coagulation disorders
  Inherited (e.g., von Willebrand's disease)
  Acquired (e.g., idiopathic thrombocytopenic purpura [ITP])
  Pharmacological (e.g., use of heparin, or even aspirin)
- Liver disorder (e.g., cirrhosis)
  Impaired metabolism of estrogen
  Decreased synthesis of fibrinogen and clotting factors
- Endocrine
  Hypothyroidism

Evaluation for menorrhagia in addition to history and physical exam:

1. Check hemoglobin, hematocrit, platelets
2. Pregnancy test if indicated
3. Screen for STDs and chronic cervicitis
4. Evaluate pelvis for masses, lesions
5. Consider endometrial biopsy if hyperplasia or cancer are suspected
6. Other possible labs include TSH, PT, PTT, LFTs
7. Sonogram to assess for fibroids, polyps, hyperplasia

Causes and Evaluation of Metrorrhagia

Table 5-4   Possible Causes of Metrorrhagia

- Pregnancy
  Intrauterine
  Ectopic
  Gestational trophoblastic neoplasm (e.g., hydatidiform mole)
- Infections (usually related to PID, use of IUD, or following instrument-based intrauterine procedure)
  Endometritis
  Salpingitis
- IUD use
- Post-tubal ligation (controversial)
- Ovulation
- Hormonal Causes
  Combined hormonal contraceptives, Depo-Provera, Norplant
  HRT
  Medications, herbs
  Thyroid disorder
- Neoplasia
  Ovarian cysts
  Uterine myomata (fibroids)

Adenomyosis (endometrial tissue located within the
myometrium)
Endometrial hyperplasia
Polyps
Carcinoma
- Coagulation disorders
Inherited (e.g., von Willebrand's disease)
Acquired (e.g., idiopathic thrombocytopenic purpura [ITP])
Pharmacological (e.g., use of heparin, or even aspirin)
- Organ disease   (e.g., liver or renal failure)

Evaluation for metrorrhagia, in addition to history and
physical exam:

1. Pregnancy test
2. Screen for STDs or other vaginal infections
3. Screen for genital trauma
4. Consider side effects of medications, herbal remedies,
   especially hormonal contraception or HRT
5. Endometrial biopsy as indicated, particularly with
   postmenopausal bleeding
6. Pelvic ultrasound
7. CBC, TSH, PT PTT, LFTs

Dysmenorrhea

Table 5-5   Pharmaceutical Regimens for Treatment
of Dysmenorrhea

Generic Drug	Sample Trade Drugs	Dosage*
Ibuprofen	Advil, Motrin, Nuprin	400 mg qid
Naproxen	Aleve, Anaprox, Naprosyn	275 mg qid
Fenamates	Ponstel	250 mg qid

Ketoprofen	Orudis	50 mg tid
Diclofenac	Cataflam	50 mg tid
Cyclooxygenase 2 inhibitors:[†]		
Celecoxib	Celebrex	200 mg bid
Rofecoxib	Vioxx	50 mg qd
Valdecoxib	Bextra	20 mg bid

*Medications should be initiated on the first day of symptoms and continued for 2 to 3 days.

[†]Cyclooxygenase 2 (COX-2) inhibitors are the most recent classification of drugs to receive FDA approval for the treatment of dysmenorrhea.

Painful menstruation arising in women with a history of pain-free cycles requires evaluation. Possible causes include:

- Endometriosis
- Polyps
- Uterine fibroids
- PID
- IUD
- Uterine cancer

Endometrial Biopsy

Indications are:

- Evaluate dysfunctional uterine bleeding.
- Evaluate thickened endometrium to rule out hyperplasia.
- Identification of uterine cancer or precancerous states
- Discover luteal defects or other pathology related to infertility.
- Evaluate AGUS or endometrial cells found on Pap.
- Assess the effect of HRT or Tamoxifen on the endometrium.

The most common reasons for most midwives to perform endometrial biopsy are the first two bullets. When planning an endometrial biopsy, the midwife should consider whether consultation or referral would better meet the woman's needs (for example, when endometrial cancer is a consideration, or when the woman is being evaluated for infertility).

See Chapter 82 of *Varney's Midwifery*, 4th edition, for information on the performance of this skill.

Polycystic Ovarian Syndrome (PCOS)

More correctly referred to as hyperandrogenism, PCOS affects as many as 5% of women, and is a leading cause of infertility. It has also been associated with Type II diabetes and cardiovascular disease. Not all women with PCOS present with symptoms, and some will have normal fertility.

Signs and symptoms include:

- Menstrual changes including oligomenorrhea and amenorrhea
- Obesity
- Hirsutism
- Acne
- Alopecia
- Insulin resistance
- Acanthosis nigrans
- Enlarged cystic ovaries on examination, or on ultrasound

Management can include weight loss, combined hormonal contraception for women not wishing to conceive, induction ovulation in the treatment of infertility. Metformin has been used in the long-term management of PCOS.

PMS

Essential evaluation includes:

- Timing of symptoms—PMS symptoms arise predictably in the last half of the menstrual cycle and resolve with the onset of menses. A prospective log is the only way to identify this.
- TSH to screen for hypothyroidism
- Depression screening
- Medical exam for enlarged thyroid, cardiac abnormalities, pelvic mass, other possible causes of symptoms

Management regimens:

- High-protein diet
- Regular exercise
- Decrease sugar, alcohol, caffeine during the luteal phase
- Pyridoxine (B6) supplementation 50 mg/day (can be increased up to 200 mg/day). However, some women will experience neuropathy with as little as 100 mg/day, so total B6 intake, such as from multivitamins, should be ascertained before the dose is increased above 50 mg.

Diagnosis and Management of PMDD

Unlike PMS, PMDD is a DSM IV defined psychiatric diagnosis, requiring 5 of 11 symptoms:

- At least 1 of:
  Sad, hopeless, or self-deprecating feelings
  Tension, anxiety, feeling on edge
  Labile mood with tearfulness

Irritability, anger, or increased interpersonal conflict

- And 1–4 of:
  Social withdrawal, decreased interest in usual activities
  Difficulty concentrating
  Fatigue, low energy
  Marked appetite changes, especially cravings or binge eating
  Sleep cycle disturbances
  Out of control feelings, overwhelmed
  Physical symptoms of PMS

Symptoms must be cyclical and occur in most cycles. Changes occur in the week prior to menses, resolve during menses, and are not present the week following menses.

Source: Adapted from American Psychiatric Association. (2000). *Diagnostic and statistical manual of mental disorders* (4th ed., Text Revision). Arlington, VA: American Psychiatric Publishing, Inc.

Assessment of Common Benign Breast Problems

Galactorrhea

Watery or milky breast discharge not associated with pregnancy and breastfeeding. Prolactin level usually shows elevation above the normal range (>20–25 ng/ml).

Causes include:

- Breast stimulation following pregnancy (as with lovemaking)
- Other stimulation of breast nerves (such as herpes zoster or trauma)
- Oral contraceptive use

- Medications, including tricyclic antidepressants, antihypertensives, and many others
- Stress
- Pituitary adenoma
- Hypothyroidism
- Renal disease

Ideally, if the galactorrhea is caused by stimulation or by medication use, stopping the stimulus will resolve the problem. When stopping a medication is not feasible, or when other causes are present, referral for physician management is indicated.

Benign Breast Disease

All persistent dominant breast masses require immediate evaluation and appropriate referral. A persistent dominant mass is one that can be identified as distinct from the surrounding tissue and lasts through the menstrual cycle.

Fibrocystic Breast Changes

Diagnosed by painful irregular breast contours found on examination, cyclic with the menses. May be single or multiple, up to several centimeters in diameter. Common among women 20–50 years old. Breast mammography/sonography is useful if the diagnosis is not completely clear. Any suggestion of a persistent mass requires follow-up.

Treatment:

- Supportive bra worn 24/7 while symptomatic
- Combined hormonal contraceptives
- Some experts suggest reducing methylxanthines (coffee, chocolate) and nicotine
- 3g/day of gamma-linoleic acid with evening primrose oil

- With physician consultation/referral diuretics, danazol (Danocrine, Cyclomen for severe cases)
- Aspiration of fluid
- Removal of cystic tissue

Fibroadenoma

Characteristics: firm, solid, freely moving, well-defined edge, rubbery texture, usually a single mass, usually painless. Most common among women in their teens and 20s. Diagnosis is with clinical examination and mammogram or ultrasound.

Management:

- Surgical removal—required for any rapidly growing lesion and for any new masses found in women over 35.
- Observation—for slow growing masses seen to be solid on sonogram, and with fine needle biopsy confirming diagnosis. Follow-up is at 6 month intervals, with breast specialist involved.

Fat Necrosis

Characteristics: firm, irregular in shape, tender, may have bruising around the area, skin retraction is possible, calcifications or tissue contraction seen on ultrasound. Usually caused by breast trauma.

Management:

- Refer for physician evaluation immediately. This mass cannot be distinguished from carcinoma of the breast without biopsy and excision.

Intraductal Papilloma

Characteristics: bloody, watery or serosanguinous nipple discharge, spontaneously appearing. Most masses are behind the areola, are small, soft, and difficult to palpate. Most common in perimenopausal women. Risk of breast cancer increases following this diagnosis.

Management:

- Refer for physician evaluation and excisional biopsy.

Assessment of Pelvic Problems

Table 5-6 Differential Diagnosis of Pelvic Pain

Acute	Chronic
Ovarian torsion	Endometriosis
Appendicitis	Vulvodynia (Chronic discomfort)
Ectopic pregnancy	Dyspareunia/vulvar pain
Pyelonephritis	PID/salpingitis
	Interstitial cystitis

Uterine Abnormalities

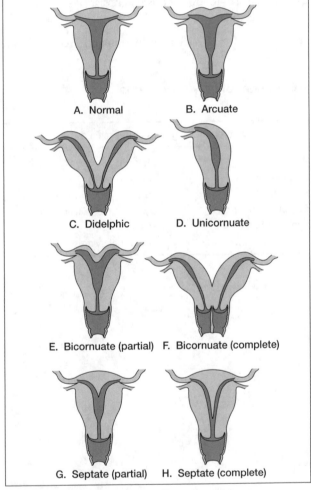

Figure 5-1   Developmental malformation of the uterus.

Classification of Fibroids

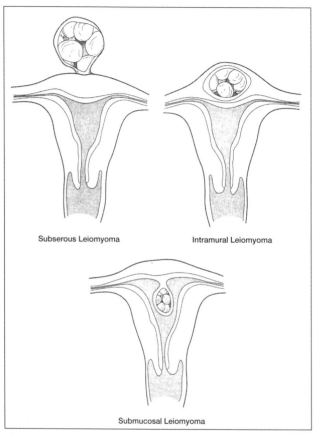

Figure 5-2   Classification of fibroids (leiomyomas) by location in relation to the uterus.

Assessment of Defects in the Vagina

Urethrocele

Descent of the urethra into the vagina as a result of thinning of the anterior fascia. Symptoms can include feeling of fullness, vaginal pressure, urgency, stress incontinence, incomplete bladder emptying. Seen as a bulging near the introitus when the posterior vaginal wall is depressed and the woman is told to bear down. Small urethroceles not interfering with voiding can be left alone. Pessaries, estrogen cream in older women, Kegel exercises can improve function. Definitive repair is surgical.

Cystocele

Descent of the bladder into the vagina as a result of weakened anterior fascia. Symptoms include vaginal fullness and pressure, urgency, stress incontinence, incomplete bladder emptying. Seen as a bulge into the anterior vagina on examination when the posterior vaginal wall is depressed, increasing in volume with straining. Kegel exercises and the use of pessaries, can offer relief. Definitive repair is surgical.

Rectocele

Thinning and loss of muscle support posteriorly, allowing protrusion of the rectum into the vagina. Patient complaints include vaginal fullness or heaviness, constipation, need to splint the posterior vaginal wall during the bowel movement. Seen as a bulging up from the rectum into the vagina with straining on exam, when the anterior wall is retracted upward. Kegel exercises, estrogen, and pessaries may be helpful in some cases. Definitive treatment is surgical.

Enterocele

Herniation of the pouch of Douglas into the upper vagina, containing small bowel. Occasionally identifiable separately from rectocele on examination. Treatment is surgical.

Uterine or cervical prolapse (Descensus)

Caused by trauma to endopelvic fascia or relaxation of the pelvic floor supports. Complaints include falling out sensation or fullness in the vagina, palpation of a mass at the introitus, pain, vaginal bleeding, difficulty with intercourse. Pessaries can be used in women with minimal descent. Surgery is required for more serious defects.

Table 5-7   Staging of Uterine/Cervical Prolapse

Stage 0	No prolapse
Stage 1	Most distal edge of prolapse is at least 1 cm above the hymen
Stage 2	Most distal edge of the prolapse is within 1 cm above or below the hymen
Stage 3	Most distal edge of the prolapse protrudes from the introitus no more than 2 cm less than the length of the vagina
Stage 4	Complete eversion of the lower genital tract

Source: International Continence Society Web site. Available at: http://www. continet.org/. Accessed on May 5, 2004.

Assessment of the Woman with DES Exposure

Diethylstilbestrol was used to prevent complications of pregnancy, including threatened abortion and recurrent miscarriage. It was withdrawn from the market in 1971. Risks associated with in utero exposure to DES include:

- Clear cell adenocarcinoma (CCA) of the vagina and cervix
- Reproductive tract structural differences
- Pregnancy complications
- Infertility

Although these women are past the identified period of greatest risk, the following assessment is recommended:

- Annual cervical and vaginal Pap smear
- Colposcopy for any abnormal or unexplained vaginal bleeding

Women who took DES during a pregnancy are at a slightly higher risk of breast cancer, and should be followed carefully with clinical breast examinations and regular mammography.

Assessment of Urinary Incontinence

Table 5-8 Risk Factors for Urinary Incontinence

Pregnancy/childbirth	Smoking
Obesity	Mental status changes
Medication use, including herbals	High-impact exercise or heavy lifting
Changes in fluid intake	Decreased pelvic muscle tone
Bladder or urethral abnormalities	History of fecal impaction
Urinary tract infections	Hypoestrogenicity
Diabetes	Immobility/stroke/decreased sensation
Renal disease	Pelvic surgery or trauma
Childhood nocturnal enuresis	Pelvic mass (e.g., fibroid, bladder cancer)

Stress Incontinence

Inability of the urethral sphincter to maintain function, demonstrated as involuntary loss of urine with effort, exertion, sneezing, or coughing.

Urge Incontinence

Involuntary leakage of urine immediately preceded by or accompanied by urgency.

Midwives who identify incontinence in women should screen for urinary tract infection, and for possible risk factors. Kegel exercises should be taught. Vaginal cones can also be used to reinforce strengthening of vaginal and pelvic floor muscles. Bladder training exercises can be used. Medical therapy for urge incontinence can be prescribed, such as Oxybutynin (Ditropan) and tolterodine (Detrol), antispasmodic medications that relax the smooth muscle of the bladder. Other medications that can be prescribed include:

- Anticholinergic agents (propantheline)
- Antispasmodic medications (oxybutynin, tolterodine, flavoxate)
- Tricyclic antidepressants (imipramine, doxepin)
- Calcium channel blockers (tolterodine)
- Beta agonist (terbutaline)

Consultation with or referral to the physician is warranted for severe cases.

Cancer Screening

Breast Cancer

Self-examination of the breast should be taught to every woman at the onset of sexual activity, but no later than age 20. The incidence of self-diagnosed breast cancer is low, however. Clinical breast examination should occur every year as part of routine health screening.

A woman's chance of being diagnosed with breast cancer is:

1 in 252	between ages 30 and 40
1 in 68	between ages 40 and 50
1 in 35	between ages 50 and 60
1 in 27	between ages 60 and 70
1 in 8	lifetime risk with current life expectancy

Source: American Cancer Society Web site. Available at: http://www. cancer. org. Accessed on May 5, 2004.

Table 5-9   Risk Factors Associated with Breast Cancer

- Older age (risk increases with each year of aging, especially after the age of 40)
- Early age at menarche (<12 years)
- History of never giving birth, or later age of giving first birth (≥30 years)
- No prior history of breastfeeding
- Caucasian American, African American
- Prior history of breast cancer
- Strong family history of breast cancer, especially in two or more first-degree relatives
- History of proliferative benign breast disease
- Prior history of having received thoracic radiation, especially prior to age 30
- History of nodular densities on postmenopausal mammograms
- Oophorectomy before age 35
- History of hormonal contraceptive or hormone replacement therapy use
- Alcohol use

Mammography Guidelines

The National Cancer Institute recommends:

- Women in their 40s should be screened every one to two years with mammography.
- Women aged 50 and older should be screened every year.
- Women who are at higher-than-average risk of breast cancer should seek expert medical advice about whether they should begin screening before age 40 and the frequency of screening.

Source: National Cancer Institute Web site. Available at: http://www. cancer.gov. Accessed on May 5, 2004.

The American Cancer Society continues to recommend yearly mammograms after age 40.

Cervical Cancer

It is essential when collecting a Pap smear to include both ectocervix and endocervix. The only exception is the woman whose cervix is absent after hysterectomy. Occasionally, stenosis at the cervix precludes an adequate specimen. This should be documented, as should any bleeding, irregularities in cervical appearance, or unusual discharge. Diagnosis of cervical cancer is made by colposcopy and biopsy, not by Pap smears.

Table 5-10 The 2001 Bethesda System (Abridged) (177)

Pap smear reports using the Bethesda Classification System will reflect the following language:

[Note that confusion remains a problem with interpreting results because the alternative terminology of the three category "CIN (cervical intraepithelial neoplasia)" reporting system or the descriptive "dysplasia" system still may be used by some laboratories, either as a substitute for the Bethesda terminology or as additional descriptors.]

Specimen Adequacy

Satisfactory for evaluation (presence/absence of endocervical/transformation zone component noted)

Unsatisfactory for evaluation (reason specified)

Specimen rejected/not processed (reason specified)

Specimen processed and examined, but unsatisfactory for evaluation of epithelial abnormality because of (reason specified)

General Categorization (optional)

Negative for intraepithelial lesion or malignancy

Epithelial cell abnormality

Other

Interpretation/Result

Negative for Intraepithelial Lesion or Malignancy

Organisms:

Trichomonas vaginalis

Fungal organisms morphologically consistent with *Candida* species

Shift in flora suggestive of bacterial vaginosis

Bacteria morphologically consistent with *Actinomyces* species

Cellular changes consistent with herpes simplex virus

Other non-neoplastic findings (optional to report)

Reactive cellular changes associated with:

Inflammation (includes typical repair)

Radiation

Intrauterine contraceptive device

Glandular cells status posthysterectomy

Atrophy

Epithelial Cell Abnormalities

Squamous cell

Atypical squamous cells (ASC)

of undetermined significance (ASC-US)

cannot exclude HSIL (ASC-H)

[All ASC is considered to be suggestive of SIL. Accordingly, the category of "ASCUS, favor reactive" has been eliminated. Also, when a report of "ASC" is given, it has been suggested by the American Society for Colposcopy and Cervical Pathology (ASCCP) that laboratory personnel conduct HPV DNA typing for high-risk viruses, if the clinician had requested "reflex to HPV hybrid capture" on the original laboratory request form. If "reflex" was not specifically requested by the clinician, some laboratories' staff will inquire on the written report if the clinician desires follow-up typing. However, it is important to note that reflex HPV DNA typing is only available if cervical cells were collected originally using liquid-based cytology.]

Low-grade squamous intraepithelial lesion (LSIL)

[encompassing old terminology of human papillomavirus/mild dysplasia/cervical intraepithelial neoplasia (CIN) 1]

High-grade squamous intraepithelial lesion (HSIL)

[encompassing old terminology of moderate and severe dysplasia, carcinoma in situ; CIN 2 and CIN 3]

Squamous cell carcinoma

Glandular cell

Atypical glandular cells (AGC) (endocervical or endometrial or not otherwise specified)—*formerly known as AGUS*

(atypical glandular cells of undetermined significance)

Atypical glandular cells, favor neoplastic (endocervical or not otherwise specified)

Endocervical adenocarcinoma in situ (AIS)

Adenocarcinoma

Other (list not comprehensive)

Endometrial cells in a woman ≥40 years of age

[Note that cervical cytology is primarily a screening test for squamous epithelial lesions and squamous cancer. It is unreliable for the detection of endometrial lesions and should not be used to evaluate suspected endometrial abnormalities.]

Automated Review and Ancillary Testing (included as appropriate)

For example, if a slide has been scanned by an automated computer system, the instrumentation used and the automated review result should be included in the cervical cytology report.

Educational Notes and Suggestions (optional)

Although not required, there has been evidence reported in the literature that laboratory staff suggestions included on a Pap report regarding further evaluation improves the likelihood that appropriate follow-up actually will occur.

Management Algorithm for Abnormal Pap Smears

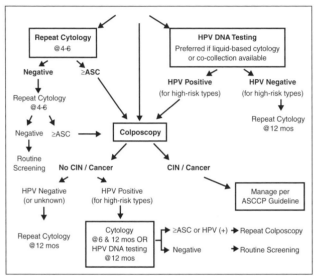

Figure 5-3   Management of women with atypical squamous cells of undetermined significance (ASC-US). © American Society for Colposcopy and Cervical Pathology.

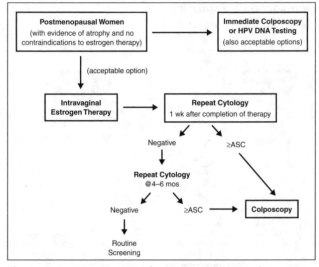

Figure 5-4 Management of women with atypical squamous cells of undetermined significance (ASC-US) in special circumstances. © American Society for Colposcopy and Cervical Pathology

Management of ASCUS Paps that favor high-grade lesions, and all LGSIL or HGSIL Pap results are referred for colposcopy. AGC-US results require colposcopy with endocervical sampling, and endometrial sampling for women over 35, except for atypical endometrial cells, which require only endometrial sampling at any age.

Endometrial Cancer

Table 5-11 Risk Factors Associated with Endometrial Cancer

- Age >50 years
- Early menarche or late menopause
- Polycystic ovary syndrome
- Obesity
- Nulliparity, infertility
- Family history
- Caucasian race
- European or North American country
- Use of unopposed exogenous estrogen (estrogen replacement therapy [ERT])
- Estrogen secreting tumors
- Diabetes
- Gallbladder disease
- Hypertension
- Prior history of pelvic radiotherapy
- History of breast cancer
- Use of tamoxifen for treatment of breast cancer

Endometrial cancer is the most common cancer of the lower female genital tract, affecting about 1 in 50 women in the United States.

Signs and symptoms include:

- Postmenopausal bleeding
- Abnormal perimenopausal bleeding

Endometrial biopsy can be performed by the midwife skilled in its use. If the biopsy sample is inadequate or if endometrial cancer is suspected based on symptoms or biopsy results, immediate referral to a gynecologist is

SECTION 5

required. Additional screening tests include vaginal ultrasound and fractional D&C.

Ovarian Cancer

Table 5-12   Risk Factors Associated with Ovarian Cancer

- Age ≥50 years
- Strong family history of ovarian cancer (first-degree relative [e.g., mother or sister] or multiple second-degree relatives)
- Evidence of mutations in the BRCA1 or BRCA2 genes
- More than 40 years of active ovulation (e.g., nulliparous never-user of oral contraceptives)
- Nulliparity
- Infertility
- Caucasian race
- Use of estrogen replacement therapy (ERT)
- Endometriosis
- High-fat, low-fiber diet deficient in multiple vitamins, including vitamins A, E, and beta-carotene
- Smoking
- Prolonged exposure to asbestos or talcum powder (the latter is controversial)

Note: Conflicting evidence regarding the above risk factors can be found in the literature, and strongly definitive risk factors for ovarian cancer have yet to be identified. Clinicians are encouraged to remain updated with the literature as more evidence becomes available.

Although less common than endometrial cancer, ovarian cancer is the leading cause of death among genital tract cancers. Most cases are not identified until the disease is advanced. The ovary is deep in the abdominal cavity and there are no early symptoms of disease. CA-125 is elevated in ovarian neoplasms, as well as several other malignancies; however, it is also elevated in a number of benign conditions, making it a poor tool for diagnosis. Vaginal ultrasound is also ineffective as a pure screening tool, but it is of assistance in making a diagnosis when an ovarian mass is suspected. The midwife should err on the side of caution by ordering vaginal ultrasound for any persistent adnexal mass, and obtaining consultation or arranging referral as indicated.

References

American Cancer Society Web site. Available at: http://www. cancer.org. Accessed on May 5, 2004.

American Society for Colposcopy and Cervical Pathology Web site. Available at: http://www.asccp.org. Accessed on May 5, 2004.

American Psychiatric Association (2000). *Diagnostic and statistical manual of mental disorders* (4th ed., Text Revision). Arlington, VA: American Psychiatric Publishing, Inc.

Bump, R. C., Mattiason, A., Bo, K., et al. (2003). The standardization of terminology of female pelvic organ prolapse and pelvic floor dysfunction. *American Journal of Obstetrics and Gynecology, 175*, 10-1.

Centers for Disease Control and Prevention Web site. Available at: http://www.cdc.gov. Accessed on May 4, 2004.

Hindle, W. (Ed.). (1999). *Breast care: A clinical guidebook for women's primary health care providers.* New York: Springer-Verlag.

International Continence Society Web site. Available at: http://www.continet.org. Accessed on May 5, 2004.

National Cancer Institute Web site. Available at: http://www. cancer.gov. Accessed on May 5, 2004.

Stenchever, M. A., Droegmueller, W., Herbst, A. L., & Mishell, D. R. (2001). *Comprehensive gynecology* (4th ed.). St. Louis, MO: Mosby.

Varney, H., Kriebs, J. M., & Gegor, C. L. (2003). *Varney's midwifery* (4th ed.). Sudbury, MA: Jones and Bartlett Publishers.

Infections of the Genital Tract

Common Vaginal Infections

Candidiasis (VVC)

Symptoms: thick white or cream colored discharge, occasionally separated in a watery liquid and adherent plaques. Acute vaginal itching. Occasionally external irritation or itching, or dysuria.

Diagnosis: Microscopy with KOH. Some clinicians can identify candida on saline wet mount, but this technique is not recommended.

VVC can be divided into uncomplicated and complicated infections, based on the following criteria:

Uncomplicated VVC

Sporadic or infrequent vulvovaginal candidiasis
Mild-to-moderate vulvovaginal candidiasis
Likely to be *C. albicans*
Non-immunocompromised women

Complicated VVC

Recurrent vulvovaginal candidiasis
Severe vulvovaginal candidiasis
Non-*albicans* candidiasis
Pregnant women
Women with uncontrolled diabetes, debilitation, or
    immunosuppression

145

Treatment:

Intravaginal Agents:

Butoconazole (Gynazole) 2% cream 5 g intravaginally for 3 days***

Butoconazole 2% cream 5 g (Butaconazole1-sustained release), single intravaginal application

Clotrimazole (Gynelotrimin) 1% cream 5 g intravaginally for 7-14 days***

Clotrimazole 100 mg vaginal tablet for 7 days

Clotrimazole 100 mg vaginal tablet, two tablets for 3 days

Clotrimazole 500 mg vaginal tablet, one tablet in a single application

Miconazole (Monistat) 2% cream 5 g intravaginally for 7 days***

Miconazole 100 mg vaginal suppository, one suppository for 7 days***

Miconazole 200 mg vaginal suppository, one suppository for 3 days***

Tioconazole (Gyno-Troysd) 6.5% ointment 5 g intravaginally in a single application***

Terconazole (Terazol) 0.4% cream 5 g intravaginally for 7 days

Terconazole 0.8% cream 5 g intravaginally for 3 days

Terconazole 80 mg vaginal suppository, one suppository for 3 days

Nystatin 100,000 unit vaginal tablet, one tablet for 14 days

Oral Agent:

Fluconazole (Diflucan) 150 mg oral tablet, one tablet in single dose

***Over-the-counter (OTC) preparations.

Note: Tioconazole is not available in the United States.

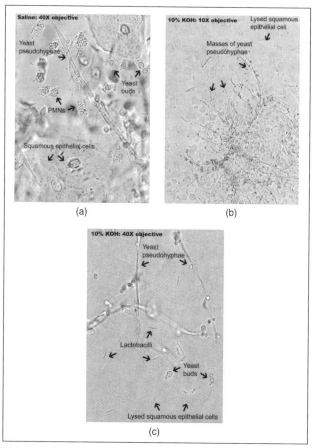

Figure 6-1 Candida pseudohyphae and budding spores under microscopic examination. (a) saline, 40×, (b) KOH, 10×, (c) KOH, 40×, PMNs = polymorphonuclear cells.

Source: Used with permission from Washington State Department of Health STD/TB Program, Seattle STD/HIV Prevention Training Center, and Cindy Fennell, MS, MT, ASCP.

Bacterial Vaginosis (BV)

Symptoms: malodorous thin, white discharge, burning. Associated with having multiple sexual partners, douching, and lack of vaginal lactobacilli.

Diagnosis: Amsel's criteria (3 of 4 required)

- Thin white discharge
- Vaginal pH >4.5
- Amine release with application of KOH to the specimen
- Clue cells seen on microscopy

Culture is relatively less useful, as many of the bacteria which cause BV also are part of the normal vaginal flora.

Treatment:

Metronidazole (Flagyl) 500 mg po bid for 7 days

Metronidazole gel (Metrogel) 0.75%, one full applicator (5 g) intravaginally, once a day for 5 days

Clindamycin (Cleocin) cream 2%, one full applicator (5 g) intravaginally at bedtime for 7 days. Not to be used in pregnancy.

Pregnancy regimens include:

Metronidazole 250 mg po tid for 7 days

Clindamycin 300 mg po bid for 7 days

Note: Metronidazole prescriptions should include a warning to avoid alcohol. Clindamycin cream causes latex rubber (condoms) to deteriorate.

Other regimens are available, but have lower cure rates for BV.

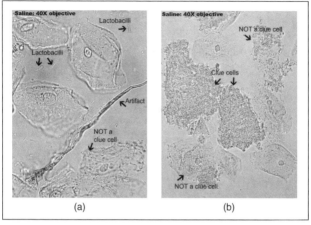

Figure 6-2 Microscopic diagnosis of bacterial vaginosis (BV). (a) no BV; note normal epithelial cells and presence of lactobacilli, (b) BV; note clue cells and lack of lactobacilli.

Source: Used with permission from Washington State Department of Health STD/TB Program, Seattle STD/HIV Prevention Training Center, and Cindy Fennell, MS, MT, ASCP.

Trichomonas Vaginalis

Symptoms: malodorous, frothy green to yellow discharge, copious in amount. Mild burning may be present. Occasionally no symptoms are offered.

Associated with having multiple sexual partners, douching, lack of lactobacilli.

Diagnosis: wet mount (less than 75% accurate due to difficulty in identifying dead protozoa), culture.

Treatment:

Metronidazole 2 g orally in a single dose
Metronidazole 500 mg po bid for 7 days

Single dose therapy is preferred.

Note: Metronidazole prescriptions should include a warning to avoid alcohol.

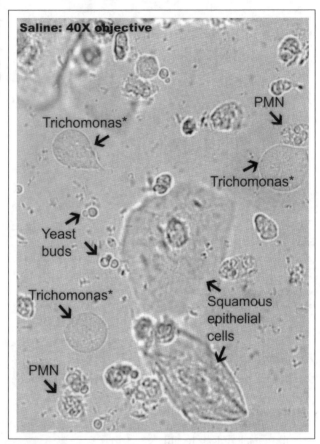

Figure 6-3 Trichomonads seen microscopically. Must be motile for identification.

Source: Used with permission from Washington State Department of Health STD/TB Program, Seattle STD/HIV Prevention Training Center, and Cindy Fennell, MS, MT, ASCP.

Risk Assessment for Sexually Transmitted Diseases

Table 6-1   STD Risk Assessment History

At what age did you start having sex?

How often do you have sex now?

Are you having sex with more than one partner?

How many partners have you had sex with in the last six
months?

Do you have sex with men, women, or both?

What sex is your current partner?

Does your partner have other partners? Are they the same sex
as your partner or the opposite sex?

Do you and your partner have sex while using alcohol or
recreational drugs?

Do either you or your partner use intravenous drugs? Do you or
your partner share needles?

Do you have anal intercourse?

What percentage of the number of times you have sex do you
use a condom or dental dam?

Do you have a history of a previous sexually transmitted
disease? What one(s)? When? Treatment? Cure?

Do you douche?

What is your occupation?

Source: Used with permission from Washington State Department of
Health STD/TB Program Training Center, and Cindy Fennell, MS, MT, ASCP.

Sexually Transmitted Infections

Gonorrhea

Symptoms: usually asymptomatic in women
Diagnosis: DNA PCR, culture. In some cases mucopurulent cervical discharge and pelvic tenderness suggests
the diagnosis. Partners of men complaining of penile

burning or discharge should be treated at the time of the visit.

Treatment:

> Ceftriaxone 125 mg IM in a single dose
> Ciprofloxacin 500 mg orally in a single dose*
> Ofloxacin 400 mg orally in a single dose*
> Levofloxacin 250 mg orally in a single dose*

> ***Plus, for any of the above, if chlamydia NOT ruled out:***

> Azithromycin 1 g orally in a single dose
> Doxycycline 100 mg po bid for 7 days*

*Not used in pregnancy.

Quinolones should not be used in communities with increased gonococcal resistance to quinolones, or if the infection is believed to have been transmitted in the Pacific region. Information about quinolone resistance can be gathered from the local health department or CDC. Spectinomycin 2 g in a single, IM dose is the treatment for resistant gonococcus.

Ceftriaxone is the preferred cephalosporin regimen. However, other single dose cephalosporins that are effective against uncomplicated gonorrhea include: cefixime 400 mg orally ceftizoxime 500 mg IM, cefoxitin 2 g, administered IM with probenecid 1 g orally, and cefotaxime 500 mg, administered IM.

Chlamydia

Symptoms: asymptomatic
Diagnosis: DNA-PCR, culture
Treatment (nonpregnant):

> Azithromycin 1 g orally in a single dose
> Doxycycline 100 mg po bid for 7 days

Women using these regimens do not need a test of cure except in pregnancy.

Alternative regimens include:

Erythromycin base 500 mg po qid for 7 days
Erythromycin ethylsuccinate 800 mg PO qid for
   7 days
Ofloxacin 300 mg po bid for 7 days
Levofloxacin 500 mg po for 7 days

Pregnancy

Azithromycin 1 g orally, single dose*
Erythromycin base 500 mg po qid for 7 days
Amoxicillin 500 mg po qid for 7 days

*The CDC lists Azithromycin as an alternative regimen. However, the benefit of directly observed or single dose treatment suggests priority use.

Alternative regimens in pregnancy include:

Erythromycin base 250 mg po qid for 14 days
Erythromycin ethylsuccinate 800 mg po qid for 7
   days
Erythromycin ethylsuccinate 400 mg po qid for 14
   days

Syphilis

Signs: Primary—firm, round chancre with moist, red
          appearance, non-tender. Appears 10-90 days
          after exposure and resolves in 3-6 weeks.
      Secondary—red-brown rash on trunk and extremi-
          ties, also on palms and soles of feet, patchy
          alopecia, condyloma lata, lymphadenopathy,
          malaise

Diagnosis: VDRL or RPR, followed by FTA-ABS
Treatment:

   Primary/secondary

Benzathine penicillin G 2.4 million units IM in a
single dose

Early latent syphilis (asymptomatic, less than 12
months since documented negative test)

Benzathine penicillin G 2.4 million units IM in a
single dose

Late latent syphilis or latent syphilis of unknown
duration

Benzathine penicillin G 7.2 million units total, administered as three doses of 2.4 million units IM each at 1-
week intervals

Pregnancy

Seropositive pregnant women are considered infected
unless an adequate treatment history is documented in the
medical records and sequential serologic antibody titers
have declined. Treatment during pregnancy is the same as
for nonpregnant women based on stage of syphilis determined at diagnosis. Women allergic to penicillin should be
desensitized and given the usual dose of penicillin. There
is not good evidence regarding the effectiveness of the
standard penicllin doses in preventing transmission. A
second dose of penicillin can be given one week after the
single dose regimen if desired.

Further information on syphilis in pregnancy can be
found in Section XX page XX on antepartal complications.

Herpes

Symptoms: clusters of multiple vesicular lesions. Some
primary and many secondary infections will produce few
or no visible lesions.
Diagnosis: culture, DNA-PCR
Treatment:

Primary

Acyclovir 400 mg orally three times a day for 7-10
days

Acyclovir 200 mg orally five times a day for 7-10 days

Famciclovir 250 mg orally three times a day for 7-10 days

Valacyclovir 1 g orally twice a day for 7-10 days

Recurrent

Acyclovir 400 mg orally three times a day for 5 days

Acyclovir 200 mg orally five times a day for 5 days

Acyclovir 800 mg orally twice a day for 5 days

Famciclovir 125 mg orally twice a day for 5 days

Valacyclovir 500 mg orally twice a day for 3-5 days

Valacyclovir 1.0 g orally once a day for 5 days

Supression (used in late pregnancy and for women with frequent recurrences)

Acyclovir 400 mg orally twice a day

Famciclovir 250 mg orally twice a day

Valacyclovir 500 mg orally once a day

Valacyclovir 1.0 gram orally once a day

Human Papillomavirus

Diagnosis: recognition of visible lesions on vulvar, perianal, perineal, vaginal surfaces. Biopsy. HPV testing on abnormal Pap test.

Treatment:

For external visible warts, any of:

Imiquimod 5% cream* applied at bedtime every other day for up to 16 weeks

Podofilox 0.5% solution or gel* twice a day for three days, then no treatment for four days, repeated for up to four weeks*

Podophyllin resin 10-25%* in a compound tincture of benzoin, applied weekly in the office. Air dry before patient leaves the exam table. Can be washed off after 4 hours.

Trichloroacetic acid (TCA) or bichloroacetic acid (BCA) 80-90%. Applied weekly, only to warts and allowed to dry, at which time a white "frosting" develops. Sodium bicarbonate, talc, or liquid soap can be used to reduce discomfort after treatment.

*Not approved for treatment during pregnancy.

Cryotherapy and surgical removal are options for large or persistent warts.

Internal warts are referred to the physician for treatment.

Chancroid

Symptoms: painful beefy open lesions, inguinal lymphadenopathy
Diagnosis: by exclusion, if herpes and syphilis tests are negative.

Treatment is with any of the following:

Azithromycin 1 g orally in a single dose
Ceftriaxone 250 mg intramuscularly (IM) in a single dose
Ciprofloxacin 500 mg orally twice a day for 3 days
Erythromycin base 500 mg orally three times a day for 7 days

Diagnosis of Pelvic Inflammatory Disease

- Nonspecific symptoms include vaginal bleeding, pain with intercourse, and vaginal discharge.
- Clinically most women have mucopurulent cervical discharge or WBCs on saline wet prep.
- Minimal diagnostic criteria for treatment are either uterine/adnexal tenderness or cervical motion tenderness.

- Additional diagnostic signs include oral temperature >101°F.
- Most women with PID have either mucopurulent cervical discharge or evidence of WBCs on a microscopic evaluation of a saline preparation of vaginal fluid. When neither of these signs are present, PID is unlikely.

Women who present with mild or nonspecific symptoms can be started on an oral regimen. If symptoms persist or worsen, physician consultation or referral for hospital admission are indicated within 72 hours of the initial dose.

Two oral regimens suggested by CDC are:

1) Ofloxacin 400 mg orally twice a day for 14 days, or

Levofloxacin 500 mg orally once daily for 14 days
with or without

Metronidazole 500 mg orally twice a day for 14 days

2) Ceftriaxone 250 mg IM in a single dose, or

Cefoxitin 2 g IM in a single dose and Probenecid, 1 g orally administered concurrently in a single dose, or,

Other parenteral third-generation cephalosporin (e.g., ceftizoxime or cefotaxime)
plus

Doxycycline 100 mg orally twice a day for 14 days
with or without

Metronidazole 500 mg orally twice a day for 14 days

Collection of Specimens for Microscopy

- Take a specimen of discharge from the posterior fornix or vaginal side wall.

- If checking this sample for vaginal pH, do so before placing the swab into saline
- Place sample in a droplet of saline on a microscope slide.

OR

- If placing the specimen in a test tube with a small amount of saline to transport, place a small droplet of the fluid on a microscope slide and cover.
- Always use a cover slip when examining wet specimens.
- View on both low and high power.
- KOH preparations can be made as described above.
- Check for "whiff" test as soon as the specimen is placed in the KOH solution.

Source: Centers for Disease Control and Prevention (2002). Sexually transmitted diseases guidelines 2002. *MMWR Recommendations and Reports*, *51*, RR-6.

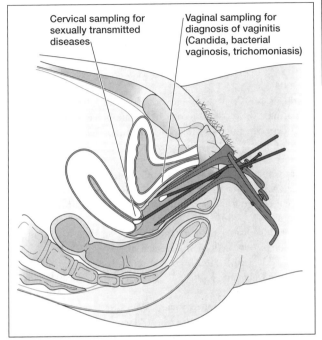

Cervical sampling for sexually transmitted diseases

Vaginal sampling for diagnosis of vaginitis (Candida, bacterial vaginosis, trichomoniasis)

Figure 6-4 Specimen collection.

Collection of Specimens for Culture/DNA testing

- Visualize the cervical os clearly.
- Place the sampling swab in the endocervix, rotate gently, and let it remain for 30 seconds, or as long as directed by the test's manufacturer.

See *Varney's Midwifery*, 4th edition, Chapters 58 and 59 for detailed explanations.

References

American Cancer Society Web site. Available at: http://www. cancer.org. Accessed on May 5, 2004.

American Society for Colposcopy and Cervical Pathology Web site. Available at: http://www.asccp.org. Accessed on May 5, 2004.

Bump, R. C., Mattiason, A., Bo, K., et al. (2003). The standardization of terminology of female pelvic organ prolapse and pelvic floor dysfunction. *American Journal of Obstetrics and Gynecology, 175,* 10–1.

Centers for Disease Control and Prevention. (2002). Sexually transmitted disease treatment guidelines 2002. *MMWR Recommendations and Reports, 51,* RR-6. Available at: http:// www.cdc.gov/STD/treatment/TOC2002TG.htm. Accessed on May 6, 2004.

Centers for Disease Control and Prevention Web site. Available at: http://www.cdc.gov. Accessed on May 5, 2004.

Hindle, W. (Ed.). (1999). *Breast care: A clinical guidebook for women's primary health care providers.* New York: Springer-Verlag.

International Continence Society Web site. Available at: http:// www.continet.org. Accessed on May 5, 2004.

National Cancer Institute Web site. Available at: http://www. cancer.gov. Accessed on May 5, 2004.

Stenchever, M. A., Droegmueller, W., Herbst, A. L., & Mishell, D. R. (2001). *Comprehensive gynecology* (4th ed.). St. Louis, MO: Mosby.

Varney, H., Kriebs, J. M., & Gegor, C. L. (2003). *Varney's midwifery* (4th ed.). Sudbury, MA: Jones and Bartlett Publishers. Chapters 14, 15, 58, 59, 82.

SECTION 7

Contraception

Family Planning Methods

Can be loosely grouped in the following categories:

- Natural family planning
- Barriers/spermicides
- Intrauterine devices
- Combined hormonal contraception
- Progesterone-only contraception
- Permanent sterilization

Criteria for choosing a method of contraception include:

- Acceptability
- Cost
- Safety
- Effectiveness
- Availability

When discussing choice of a method with women, all of the above should be considered. Documentation of counseling for choice of a contraceptive method includes the discussion of:

- Available methods
- Benefits (contraceptive and noncontraceptive)
- Risks
- Side effects
- Correct use

Emergency Contraception (EC)

- Is most effective within 72 hours of sex, can be used up to 120 hours after intercourse with 85% effectiveness
- Will *not* abort an existing pregnancy
- Has *no* medical contraindications other than an existing pregnancy, in which case EC will not work

Prescribing EC:

- Preven (0.05 mcg ethinyl estradiol, 0.25 mg levonorgestrel) 2 doses of 2 tabs each, 12 hours apart
- Plan B (0.75 mg levonorgestrel) 2 doses of one tab each, 12 hours apart
- 200 mcg ethinyl estradiol and 2 mg norgestrel OR 1 mg levonorgestrel in 2 doses, 12 hours apart

Examples (pills per dose):	
Ovral	2
Lo Ovral	4
Nordette	4
Alesse	5
Levlen	4
Levlite	5
TriPhasil	4 yellow

- Ovrette (norgestrel only) 2 doses of 20 pills each, 12 hours apart
- Mifepristone 600 mg single dose—*off label use*

Contraceptive Failure

The risk of accidental pregnancy when contraception is being used varies with the method's "perfect" effectiveness, or the pregnancy rate when the method is used correctly for every act of intercourse. Other effects on that perfect rate include user error, such as forgetting to insert a diaphragm or taking pills intermittently; the individual's physiology and metabolism, as when a hormonal method is less effective in obese women; and interactions with other medications.

Table 7-1   Comparison of Effectiveness: Number of Pregnancies per 100 Women During First Year of Use***

Method	Typical Use* (%)	Perfect Use** (%)	Risk Reduction for Sexually Transmitted Diseases
Continuous abstinence	0.00	0.00	complete
Outercourse	N/A****	N/A	good against HIV; reduces risk of others
Sterilization			
Men	0.15	0.1	none
Women	0.5	0.5	none
Norplant (implant)	0.05	0.05	none
IUD			
ParaGard (copper T 380A)	0.8	0.6	none
Mirena (copper T 380A)	0.1	0.1	none
Lunelle (injection)	N/A	0.05	none
Continuous breast-feeding	2.0	0.5	none

Method	Typical Use* (%)	Perfect Use** (%)	Risk Reduction for Sexually Transmitted Diseases
Depo-Provera (injection)	3.0	0.3	none
Combined oral contraceptive pills/Progestin only pills	8.0	0.3	none
NuvaRing (ring)	N/A	0.3	none
Ortho Evra (patch)	N/A	0.3	none
Male condom	15.0	2.0	good against HIV; reduces risk of others
Diaphragm	16.0	6.0	limited
Cervical cap			
Women who have not given birth	16.0	9.0	limited
Women who have given birth	32.0	26.0	limited
Fertility awareness-based methods			
Periodic abstinence	25.0		none
Postovulation method		1.0	none
Symptothermal method		2.0	none
Cervical mucus			
Ovulation method		3.0	none
Calendar method		9.0	none
Female condom	21.0	5.0	some
Withdrawal	27.0	4.0	none
Spermicide	29.0	15.0	none
No method	85.0	85.0	none

Emergency Contraception

- Emergency contraception pills: Treatment initiated within 72 hours after unprotected intercourse reduces the risk of pregnancy by 75–89%. (No protection against infection.) Can be initiated within 120 hours of unprotected intercourse.
- Emergency IUD insertion: Treatment initiated within 7 days after unprotected intercourse reduces the risk of pregnancy by more than 99%. (No protection against infection.)

Source: James Trussell, et al. Contraceptive effectiveness rates In: Hatcher, R. A., Trussell, J., Stewart, F., et al. (2000). *Contraceptive technology* (18th rev. ed.). New York: Ardent Media.

*"Typical use" refers to failure rates for women and men whose use is not consistent or always correct.

**"Perfect use" refers to failure rates for those whose use is consistent and always correct.

***Except for the breast-feeding (LAM) method for which rates are based on the number of pregnancies per 100 women during the first six months of use.

****N/A—Not available; no studies have yet been published.

Source: Planned Parenthood. Available at: http://www.plannedparenthood.org/bc/bcfacts2.html

Risk of Pregnancy with Newer Contraceptive Methods

- Oral contraceptives—Seasonale (4 cycles/year): 1.8% risk of pregnancy
- Female sterilization—Essure: 0.2% risk of pregnancy*

*Only 2 years of data available. Essure is not effective for the first 3 months after insertion, and requires HSG to confirm tubal occlusion.

Note: Perfect use of any method increases effectiveness. However, few couples use their contraceptive method perfectly, and typical use rates should be quoted. Typical and perfect use effectiveness are essentially the same for intrauterine devices and for sterilization techniques.

Source: Duramed prescribing information for Seasonale. Available at: http://www.seasonale.com. Conceptus prescribing information for Essure. Available at: http://www.essure.com.

Natural Family Planning (NFP)
Billings Method of NFP

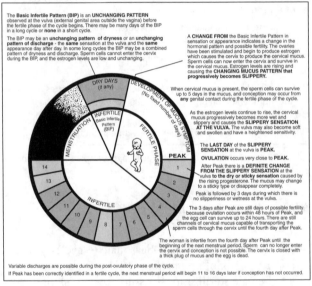

The Basic Infertile Pattern (BIP) is an **UNCHANGING PATTERN** observed at the vulva (external genital area outside the vagina) before the fertile phase of the cycle begins. There may be many days of the BIP in a long cycle or **none** in a short cycle.

The BIP may be an **unchanging pattern of dryness** or an **unchanging pattern of discharge** - the **same** sensation at the vulva and the **same** appearance day after day. In some long cycles the BIP may be a combined pattern of dryness and discharge. Sperm cells cannot enter the cervix during the BIP, and the estrogen levels are low and unchanging.

A **CHANGE FROM** the Basic Infertile Pattern in sensation or appearance indicates a change in the hormonal pattern and possible fertility. The ovaries have been stimulated and begin to produce estrogen which causes the cervix to produce the cervical mucus. Sperm cells can now enter the cervix and survive in the cervical mucus. Estrogen levels are rising and causing the **CHANGING MUCUS PATTERN that progressively becomes SLIPPERY.**

When cervical mucus is present, the sperm cells can survive up to 5 days in the mucus, and conception may occur from **any** genital contact during the fertile phase of the cycle.

As the estrogen levels continue to rise, the cervical mucus progressively becomes more wet and slippery and causes the **SLIPPERY SENSATION AT THE VULVA.** The vulva may also become soft and swollen and have a heightened sensitivity.

The **LAST DAY** of the **SLIPPERY SENSATION** at the vulva is **PEAK.**

OVULATION occurs very close to **PEAK.**

After Peak there is a **DEFINITE CHANGE FROM the SLIPPERY SENSATION** at the vulva **to the dry or sticky sensation** caused by the rising progesterone. The mucus may change to a sticky type or disappear completely.

Peak is followed by 3 days during which there is no slipperiness or wetness at the vulva.

The 3 days after Peak are still days of possible fertility because ovulation occurs within 48 hours of Peak, and the egg cell can survive up to 24 hours. There are still channels of cervical mucus capable of transporting the sperm cells through the cervix until the fourth day after Peak.

The woman is infertile from the fourth day after Peak until the beginning of the next menstrual period. Sperm can no longer enter the cervix and conception is not possible. The cervix is closed with a thick plug of mucus and the egg is dead.

Variable discharges are possible during the post-ovulatory phase of the cycle.

If Peak has been correctly identified in a fertile cycle, the next menstrual period will begin 11 to 16 days later if conception has not occurred.

Labels in figure: MENSTRUATION, DRY DAYS (if any), DEVELOPMENT OF MUCUS SYMPTOM (No fixed number of days), INFERTILE Basic Infertile Pattern (BIP), FERTILE PHASE, PEAK, INFERTILE, 1, 2, 3, 4, 5, 6, 7, 8, 9, 10, 11, 12, 13, 14

Figure 7-1   The Billings Ovulation Method of Natural Family Planning, 2000.

Source: Reproduced with permission of the Billings Family Life Centre. For further information visit: http://www.woomb.org.

Symptothermal Method of NFP

Combines basal body temperature tracking, cervical mucus examination, observation for signs of impending ovulation such as mittleschmerz, mood changes, increased libido that occur in some women.

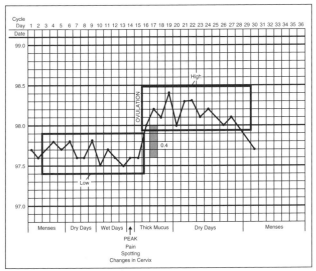

Figure 7-2 Symptothermal method.

Source: The Human Life and Natural Family Planning Foundation.

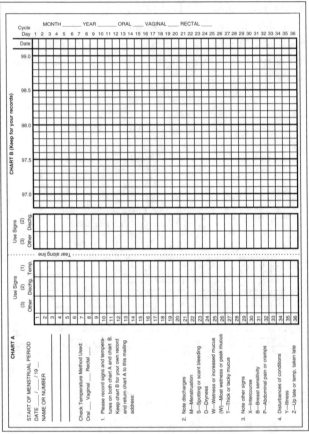

Figure 7-3 Chart for recording symptothermal method observations.

Source: The Human Life and Natural Family Planning Foundation.

Cervical Cap and Diaphragm—Woman-Controlled Barrier Methods

Correct use of the diaphragm or cervical cap requires that the woman be willing and able to master the insertion and removal procedures, and that she be confident of her ability to control the use of contraception in her relationship. Spermicide use is required for best effectiveness against unintended pregnancy.

Both the diaphragm and cap require office fitting, followed by practice at home before the method is depended upon for contraception.

Benefits include:

- No systemic effects
- Woman-controlled method
- May offer some protection against infections
- Convenient if sex is infrequent or intermittent

Contraindications include:

- Uterine prolapse
- Fistula
- Severe cystocele
- Severe anteflexion or retroflexion of the uterus

Risks include:

- Increased risk of UTI in some women
- Allergy to latex or spermicide
- Parous women will have decreased effectiveness with the cervical cap

Patient teaching includes:

- Checking for patency
- Care of diaphragm or cap
- Proper fit and insertion/removal techniques
- Use of spermicides to improve effectiveness

Intrauterine Devices (IUD)

Both the Cu T380A IUD (Paraguard) and the levonorgestrel-releasing intrauterine system (IUS) (Mirena) provide excellent long-term contraception for women who meet the criteria for use. Short-term use is not generally recommended because the cost of the device, insertion, and removal are relatively high if the woman does not plan to use the method for more than 1–2 years. However, there is no medical contraindication to short-term use. Neither IUD/IUS is an abortifacient. There is no long-term increase in infection rates for the IUD/IUS compared to other methods. Where the two differ is in contraindications, side effects, and noncontraceptive benefits.

Contraindications to IUD/IUS generally:

- Active, recent, or recurrent intrauterine infection
- Significant uterine abnormalities that distort the uterine cavity
- Pregnancy

Exercise caution with:

- High risk for STDs or PID
- Immune suppression
- Risk factors for HIV
- Undiagnosed abnormal vaginal bleeding
- Cervical or uterine cancer, including abnormal Pap smear with incomplete workup
- History of fainting or severe vasovagal response
- Poor access to health care for pelvic infections

Source: World Health Organization.

Contraindications to Copper T380A (absolute or relative):

- Copper allergy
- Heavy or irregular menstrual bleeding

Contraindications to levonorgestrel-releasing IUS:

- Progesterone contraindicated

Benefits, contraceptive or noncontraceptive:

- Long term, highly effective
- No conflict with breastfeeding
- No systemic side effects unless allergic to copper
- Levonorgestrel-releasing IUS decreases menstrual flow and dysmenorrhea

Prior to inserting an IUD/IUS, the clinician should verify that a pregnancy test is negative and there is no risk of preimplantation pregnancy. As a general rule, screening for gonorrhea, chlamydia, and vaginitis should be done within the last 30 days prior to the insertion visit. A normal Pap smear also should be verified.

IUDs are occasionally expelled, usually at the time of menses. If the woman desires to continue IUD use, another device can be inserted the same day.

Patient teaching includes:

- Warning signs include late or absent menses, pain on intercourse, abdominal pain, exposure to or symptoms of genital infections, fever and chills
- Check string and call if it is missing or suddenly longer
- Keep track of when the IUD should be removed
- Use condoms if not sure partner is monogamous

Combined Hormonal Contraception (CHC)—Pills, Patches, and Rings

Where we used to refer to combination OCs, now there are oral, transdermal, and vaginal methods for using combined estrogen and progesterone contraception.

SECTION 7

All of the combined products offer excellent contraception, ease of use, safety, and some degree of female control.

Noncontraceptive benefits of CHC:

- Reduction in risks of ovarian and endometrial cancer
- Decrease in fibrocystic breast changes
- Decrease in premenstrual symptoms
- Decrease in menstrual flow and dysmenorrhea
- Decreased risk of anemia if associated with heavy menses

Common side effects include:

- Decreased menstrual flow
- Nausea on initiation
- Decreased libido, depression
- Breast tenderness

Contraindications:

- Pregnancy; however, taking contraceptives in early pregnancy is not harmful to the pregnancy
- Thromboembolic disorders and thrombosis, present or by history
- Cerebrovascular accident, cerebrovascular disease, coronary artery disease
- Structural heart disease
- Breast cancer, estrogen-dependent tumors
- Long-term or progressive diabetes
- Liver damage, liver tumors, acute hepatitis
- Cholestatic jaundice during pregnancy or with prior pill use
- Migraine (can be ruled in for CHC by a neurologist)

- Hypertension
- Age 35 or older and smoking
- Prolonged immobility

Relative contraindications:

- Immediate postpartum use (2–3 weeks)
- Lactation
- Undiagnosed abnormal vaginal bleeding
- Medications that affect liver metabolism
- Gall bladder disease

Source: World Health Organization.

When teaching warning signs for CHC, be sure to review how these symptoms would differ from everyday experiences such as leg cramps after running in gym class.

Warning signs:

- Severe headache, especially one-sided or with numbness or dizziness
- Visual changes, inability to speak clearly
- Severe chest pain
- Severe abdominal pain
- Severe leg pain

Patient teaching includes:

- Correct use of the method
- Risks and benefits
- Minor side effects
- Major warnings
- What to do if the method is interrupted (e.g., forgotten pills)
- Smoking cessation
- Barrier use for prevention of infections including HIV, STDs

Table 7-2 Combined Hormonal Contraception Interactions with Selected Medications

Action of Medication	Recommendation
Reduced effectiveness of CHC	
Rifampin (Rifamycin, Rifadin)	Choose another contraceptive
Phenytoin (Dilantin) Primidone (Mysoline) Carbamazepine (Tegretol) Phenobarbitol (Donnatol)	If CHC is strongly indicated, a higher estrogen dose will be needed with seizure medications
Griseofulvin (Fulvicin) Tetracycline Penicillin	Use additional contraception such as condoms during course of therapy
Potentiation of CHC	
Vitamin C > 1 g/day	Increases EE by 50%, decrease vitamin dose to 1 g/day
Action potentiated by CHC	
Diazepam (Valium) Benzodiazepines (Librium, Ativan, Serax, Tranxene, Xanax)	Use with caution, greatest impairment during menstrual pause
Theophylline (Aerolate, Respibid, others)	Monitor theophylline levels
Tricyclic antidepressants (Elavil, others)	Monitor antidepressive effect
Corticosteroids, cortisone	Significance unknown
Beta-blockers (Inderal, Lopressor, others)	Monitor cardiovascular status
Effectiveness reduced by CHC	
Guanethidine (Ismelin, Esimel) Methyldopa (Aldomet, others) Oral anticoagulants	Use alternative contraceptive
Hypoglycemics (Diabinase, Orinase, others)	Monitor blood glucose
Acetaminophen	Monitor pain relief

Progestin-Only Contraception

Includes the minipill and medroxyprogesterone acetate (DepoProvera or "Depo")

Benefits:

- Can be used by lactating mothers, mildly hypertensive women, heavy smokers, and others who cannot use CHC due to estrogen effects
- Decrease in menstrual flow
- Decrease in pain from menstrual cycle, endometriosis
- Less risk of endometrial and ovarian cancer and PID
- Ease of use—minipills are always the same tablet, Depo requires little effort

Among common side effects or problems are:

- Irregular or absent menses
- Weight gain
- Breast tenderness
- Depression
- Decreased HDL
- Possibly decreased bone mass

Disadvantages of Depo, relative to the minipill, include increased risk of weight gain and slow return of fertility. Disadvantages of the minipill include the need for extreme accuracy in pill taking to prevent accidental pregnancy.

Contraindications*:

- Pregnancy
- Breast cancer
- Unexplained vaginal bleeding

Relative contraindications:

- Certain medications, especially those for epilepsy
- Liver tumors, cirrhosis, adenoma, acute hepatitis
- Cerebrovascular accident or disease

SECTION 7

- Uncontrolled hypertension
- Ischemic heart disease
- Progressive diabetes (neuropathy, nephropathy, retinopathy)

Source: World Health Organization.

*Many times, the contraindications for progestin-only methods reproduce the list of contraindications for estrogen-containing products. It is important to distinguish between estrogen-related risks and progestin-related risks when prescribing these products and counseling patients.

Warning signs:

- Severe lower abdominal pain
- Severe headaches
- Absent menses, when menses are usually present
- Heavy vaginal bleeding (with DepoProvera)

Patient teaching includes:

- Correct use of the method
- Risks and benefits
- Minor side effects
- Major warnings
- What to do if the method is interrupted (forgotten pills, late for injection)
- Use of barrier for protection against infections including HIV and STDs

In November 2004, the FDA issued a black box warning for DepoProvera. Loss of bone mass is associated with use of this contraceptive. Long-term use increases bone loss, which may be irreversible. Depo-Provera should be used for more than 2 years only if no adequate alternative is available. Calcium and vitamin D supplementation should be recommended to all women on DepoProvera.

Table 7-3 Relation of Side Effects to Hormone Content

	Reproductive System	Premenstrual Syndrome	General	Cardiovascular System
Estrogen Excess	Breast cystic changes	Bloating	Chloasma	Capillary fragility
	Cervical extrophy	Dizziness, syncope	Chronic nasal pharyngitis	Cerebrovascular accident
	Dysmenorrhea	Edema	Gastric influenza and varicella	Deep vein thrombosis
	Hypermenorrhea, menorrhagia, and clotting	Headache (cyclic)	Hay fever and allergic rhinitis	hemiparesis (unilateral weakness and numbness)
	Increase in breast size	Irritability	Urinary tract infection	Telangiectasias
	Mucorrhea	Leg cramps		Thromboembolic disease
	Uterine enlargement	Nausea, vomiting		
	Uterine fibroid growth	Visual changes (cyclic)		
		Weight gain (cyclic)		
Estrogen Deficiency	Absence of withdrawal bleeding	Nervousness		
	Bleeding and spotting during pill days 1 to 9	Vasomotor symptoms		
	Continuous bleeding and spotting			

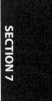

	Reproductive System	Premenstrual Syndrome	General	Cardiovascular System
Progestin Excess	Flow decrease, hypo-menorrhea Pelvic relaxation symptoms Vaginitis atrophic Cervicitis Flow length decrease Moniliasis		Appetite increase Depression Fatigue Hypoglycemia symptoms Libido decrease Neurodermatitis Weight gain (noncyclic)	Hypertension Leg vein dilation
Progestin Deficiency	Breakthrough bleeding and spotting during pill days 10 to 21			

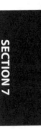

	Delayed withdrawal bleeding
	Dysmenorrhea (also estrogen excess)
	Heavy flow and clots (also estrogen excess), hypermenorrhea, menorrhagia
Androgen Excess	Acne
	Cholestatic jaundice
	Hirsutism
	Libido increase
	Oily skin and scalp
	Rash and pruritus
	Edema

Source: Adapted from Dickey, R. P. (2000). *Managing contraceptive pill patients* (10th ed.). Dallas, TX: Essential Medical Information Systems, Table 10, 102–103. Used with permission.

References

Billings Family Life Centre Web site. Available at: http://www. woomb.org.

Dickey, R. P. (2000). *Managing contraceptive pill patients* (10th ed.). Dallas, TX: Essential Medical Information Systems.

Hatcher R. A., Trussell, J., Stewart, F., et al. (2000). *Contraceptive technology*, (18th rev. ed.). New York: Ardent Media.

Varney, H., Kriebs, J. M., & Gegor, C. L. (2003). *Varney's midwifery* (4th ed.). Sudbury, MA: Jones and Bartlett Publishers.

World Health Organization Web site. Available at: http://www. who.int/en/.

SECTION 8

Caring for Older Women

Menopause is the permanent cessation of menses; the climacteric is the transition period of time during which reproductive function ceases. The term "perimenopause" is also used to refer to the years leading up to and following the menopause. The most common age range for menopause in the United States is 48–55, with a mean of 51 years. Premature ovarian failure is the term used for cessation of reproductive function and of menses prior to age 40. In addition to genetic predisposition, abdominal hysterectomy without oophorectomy increases this risk.

Anatomic and Physiologic Changes

Changes during the climacteric include:

- Decrease in number of maturing follicles and follicular resistance to FSH
- Continued ovarian production of androstenedione and testosterone
- Shift from estradiol to estrone as the primary circulating estrogen
- Increased variation in menstrual cycle and pattern of bleeding
- Hot flashes—recurrent periods of sweating, flushing, palpitations, anxiety
- Sleep disturbance—can be related to organic illness, hot flashes, emotional disturbance, breathing problems (e.g., sleep apnea)

- Vaginal/urinary tract tissue atrophy
- Increased facial hair, graying hair, occasionally hair loss
- Increased incidence of hypothyroidism

General Health Recommendations

- Increase exercise
- Decrease calorie and fat intake
- Stop smoking

Management of Hot Flashes

- Avoiding triggers in diet or environment
- Stress reduction techniques
- Maintaining cool temperature, dressing in layers so they can be removed as necessary
- Vitamin E 400 IU once or twice a day
- Ginseng tea
- Black Cohosh (Remifemin 20 mg) twice daily
- Possibly dietary sources of phytoestrogens, other herbal remedies—inadequate research available

Management of Atrophic Changes

- Hormone therapy—systemic or topical
- Vaginal lubricants/moisturizers
- Maintain sexual activity
- Vitamin E liquid or suppositories
- Increase fluids and household humidity
- Avoid petroleum-based oils (as opposed to vegetable-based)
- Avoid antihistamines and other dehydrating medications
- Avoid douches, sprays

Hormone Replacement Therapy (HRT)

*Current Recommendations for Use
of Hormone Therapy*

- Use only to control symptoms of perimenopause and in the smallest effective dose
- Use for the shortest reasonable period of time, realizing that this needs to be individualized
- Avoid prolonged use for health benefits, as the data increasingly suggest that these are outweighed by risks of increased thrombosis, stroke, and cancer
- Progestational agents are not used in women whose uterus has been removed

Counseling for HRT

- Long-term use of HRT is no longer recommended, as other medications can help prevent osteoporosis and there is no cardiac benefit
- The decision to use HRT should be based on the severity of symptoms as perceived by the woman, her preferences regarding medication use versus alternative therapies, her understanding of the risks and benefits, and her willingness to cooperate in lifestyle changes

Contraindications to HRT

- History of thromboembolus or thrombosis
- Estrogen-dependent tumor
- Impaired liver function
- Endometrial or breast cancer history mandates physician evaluation
- Hypertension and abnormal vaginal bleeding are two conditions that require evaluation and management prior to beginning HRT

Table 8-1 Estrogens

Conjugated Equine Estrogens (CEE)	Manufacturer	Route	Dose
Premarin	Wyeth-Ayerst	Oral caplets	0.3, 0.625, 0.9, 1.25, 2.5 mg
		Vaginal cream	0.625 mg/g (1 g 1–3 times a week)
PremPro (CEE plus MPA[a])		Oral caplets in blister pack	0.625 mg CEE plus 2.5 mg MPA; 0.625 mg CEE plus 5 mg MPA
Premphase (CEE plus MPA)		Oral caplets in blister pack	0.625 mg CEE for first 14 days of pill pack and 0.625 mg CEE plus 5 mg MPA next 14 days of pill pack

Estradiol (E)	Manufacturer	Route	Dose
Activella (E plus norethindrone)	Pharmacia and Upjohn	Oral tablets	1 mg E plus 0.5 mg norethindrone
Estrace	Bristol-Meyers, Squibb	Oral tablets	0.5, mg, 1.0 mg, 2.0 mg
		Vaginal cream	1 g 1–3 times a week
OrthoPrefest (E plus norgestimate	Ortho-McNeil	Oral tablets in blister pack (pulsed dosage)	3 days of 1 mg E (pink pills) followed by 3 days of combined 1 mg E plus 0.09 mg norgestimate; repeat

	Manufacturer	Route	Dose
Estring	Pharmacia and Upjohn	Insert vaginal ring for 90 days; reinsert new ring	2 mg
Estraderm	Novartis	Transdermal patch; change twice a week	0.05, 0.1 mg
Climara	Berlex	Transdermal patch; change once a week	0.025, 0.05, 0.075, 0.1 mg
Vivelle	Novartis	Transdermal patch; change twice a week	0.025, 0.0375, 0.005, 0.075, 0.1 mg
Esclim	WomenFirst	Transdermal patch; change twice a week	0.025, 0.0375, 0.05, 0.1 mg
Combipatch (E plus NETA[b])	Aventis	Transdermal patch; change twice a week	0.05 mg E plus 0.14 mg NETA; 0.05 mg E plus 0.25 mg NETA
Alora	Watson	Transdermal patch; change twice a week	0.05, 0.075, 0.1 mg

Esterified Estrogen

	Manufacturer	Route	Dose
Estratab	Solvay	Oral tablets	0.3, 0.625, 2.5 mg
Estratest (plus methyl-testosterone)	Solvay	Oral tablets	1.25 mg esterified estrogens plus 2.5 mg methyltestosterone

	Manufacturer	Route	Dose
Estratest HS (plus methyl-testosterone)	Solvay	Oral tablets	0.625 mg esterified estrogens plus 1.25 mg methyltestosterone
Estropipate	**Manufacturer**	**Route**	**Dose**
Ogen	Pharmacia and Upjohn	Oral tablets (also available in vaginal cream)	0.625, 1.25, 2.5 mg
Ortho-Est	WomenFirst	Oral tablets	0.625, 1.25 mg
Ethinyl Estradiol (EE)	**Manufacturer**	**Route**	**Dose**
FemHRT (EE plus NETA)	Pfizer	Oral tablets	5 mcg EE plus 1 mg NETA
Estinyl	Schering	Oral tablets	0.02, 0.05, 0.5 mg
Synthetic Conjugated Estrogen	**Manufacturer**	**Route**	**Dose**
Cenestin	Duramed/ Solvay	Oral tablets	0.625, 0.9, 1.25 mg

[a]Medroxyprogesterone acetate.

[b]Norethindrone acetate.

Table 8-2 Progestins

Medroxyprogesterone Acetate (MPA)

	Manufacturer	Route	Dose
Provera	Pharmacia and Upjohn	Oral tablets	2.5, 5, 10 mg
Cycrin	ESI Lederle Generics	Oral tablets	2.5, 5, 10 mg
Amen	Carnrick Laboratories	Oral tablets	10 mg
PremPro (CEE[a] plus MPA)	Wyeth-Ayerst	Oral tablets in blister pack	0.625 mg CEE plus 2.5 mg MPA; 0.625 mg CEE plus 5 mg MPA
Premphase (CEE plus MPA)	Wyeth-Ayerst	Oral tablets in blister pack	0.625 mg CEE for first 14 days of pill pack and 0.625 mg CEE plus 5 mg MPA next 14 days of pill pack

Micronized Progesterone

	Manufacturer	Route	Dose
Prometrium	Solvay	Oral tablets	100 mg BID for 12 consecutive days each cycle

Norethindrone

	Manufacturer	Route	Dose
Activella	Pharmacia and Upjohn	Oral tablets	1 mg E[b] plus 0.5 mg norethindrone

	Manufacturer	Route	Dose
Norethindrone Acetate (NETA)			
Combipatch	Aventis/Novartis	Transdermal patch	0.05 mg E plus 0.14 mg NETA; 0.05 mg EE[c] plus 0.25 NETA
FemHRT	Pfizer	Oral tablets	5 mcg EE plus 1 mg NETA
Norgestimate	**Manufacturer**	**Route**	**Dose**
OrthoPrefest	Ortho-McNeil	Oral tablets in blister pack (pulsed dosage)	3 days of 1 mg E (pink pills) followed by 3 days of combined 1 mg E plus 0.09 mg norgestimate

[a]Conjugated equine estrogens.

[b]Estradiol.

[c]Ethinyl estradiol.

Osteoporosis

Screening is by bone mineral density testing or dual-energy x-ray absorptiometry at age 65, or for younger postmenopausal women with an additional risk factor.

Risk Factors for Osteoporosis

- Advancing age
- Low body mass
- Smoking
- Sedentary life
- Genetic predisposition

Medications to Decrease Risks of Osteoporosis

- Bisphosphonates
  - Alendronate (Fosamax) 2.5 mg daily or 35 mg once a week for prevention, 5 mg daily or 70 mg once a week for treatment
  - Risendronate (Actonel) 5 mg daily for either prevention or treatment
- Selective estrogen receptor modulators
  - Raloxifene (Evista) 60 mg daily for prevention
- Calcitonin (Calcimar, Miacalcin) 200 IU daily intranasally

Other Preventive Measures for Osteoporosis

- Regular physical activity
- Calcium 1500 mg total intake/day
- Vitamin D supplementation 400–800 IU daily

The Examination of the Postreproductive-Age Woman

History

Instead of signs of reduced estrogen, some women present during the perimenopause with symptoms of estrogen excess, including uterine bleeding, bloating, growth of uterine fibroids, and endometriosis, any of which should be investigated. Assessment of the midlife woman should also focus on early detection of any of the major chronic diseases of midlife, including hypertension, heart disease, diabetes mellitus, and cancer.

As well as the usual history, the midwife needs to obtain historical information related to changes and specific risk factors associated with the following:

- Reproductive tract
- Urinary tract
- Breasts
- Vasomotor system (hot flashes, night sweats)
- Skeletal system
- Cardiovascular system
- Psychological changes

Additional screening includes:

- Impairments of vision
- Impairments of hearing
- Dental health
- Nutritional status
- Physical activities or limitations
- Injury prevention: seat belts, avoidance of drinking and driving
- Environmental risks
- Occupational, sexual, marital, relationship, and parental problems
- Use of cigarettes, alcohol, and other substances
- Contraceptive needs
- Immunization status

Physical Examination

In addition to the usual examination, attention should be paid to:

- Height measurement
- Skin assessment for lesions, loss of integrity
- Mouth, teeth, and gums
- Pelvic examination—consider using a smaller or Pederson speculum for comfort in the presence of vaginal atrophy or lack of sexual activity
- Rectum including assessment for stool guaiac

Laboratory and Other Tests

Tests for Routine Screening, Initial, or Annual Examinations

- Urinalysis/urine dipstick
- Pap smear with maturation index at least every 3 years—may be stopped after age 65–70 if all prior pap smears are normal
- Mammography: every 1 to 2 years between 40 and 49; annually from age 50
- Stool for occult blood
- Fasting plasma cholesterol, triglycerides, and lipid profile: every 3 to 5 years if normal.
- TSH at age 45 and then every other year

Other Tests Sometimes Ordered

- Pituitary gonadotropins to establish menopausal status
- Estrogen—used to evaluate menopausal status and the effects of hormone therapy on circulating levels of estradiol
- Fasting and two-hour postprandial glucose levels
- Liver function tests

- Endometrial biopsy
- Transvaginal ultrasonography
- Dual energy x-ray absorptiometry (DXA)

Frequency of Screenings

- Pap smears at least every 3 years until at least age 65
- Age 40–49: Annual examinations for breast and pelvic evaluation, scheduling screening mammograms. Complete physical every 5 years
- Age 50–59: Include annual testing for hypertension, weight assessment, lipid screening, colorectal screening. Consider thyroid and diabetes screening on an individual basis.
- Age 60–74: Visits every 1 to 2 years, adding influenza vaccine annually, and pneumococcal vaccine once

References

Varney, H., Kriebs, J. M., & Gegor, C. L. (2003). *Varney's Midwifery*, 4th ed. Sudbury, MA: Jones and Bartlett Publishers. Chapter 13.

Preconception Care

The preconception visit may be the single most important health care visit when viewed in the context of its effect on pregnancy.

— Caring for Our Future: The Content of Prenatal Care

Reasons and Opportunities for Preconception Care

Few women come for preconception care alone, but present for other health purposes; it is left to the midwife to be proactive in providing relevant information. The full range of possible topics for preconception care is far too wide to be included in every visit for every woman. However, integration of information to improve the health of the woman and her yet-to-be-conceived child can be achieved at most midwifery visits, including visits with a negative pregnancy test, STD screening, family planning, at annual exams, postpartum, substance abuse counseling, or smoking cessation.

Components of a Preconception Assessment

Health and Risk Assessment

In addition to the baseline history, physical and pelvic examination, laboratory tests, and adjunctive studies for a comprehensive health assessment, the following information pertinent to preconception needs can be assessed:

- Treatment of any medical illness
- Treatment of any mental illness
- Counseling/treatment for STDs
- HIV testing/counseling
- Discussion of treatment programs for substance abuse, tobacco, alcohol, prescription medications, and illicit drugs
- Self-evaluation of lifestyle, coping skills, and stress reduction
- Psychological, social, or economic support in the presence of
  - Depression or other mental health issues
  - Domestic abuse
  - Homelessness
  - Lack of resources for basic needs
- Nutritional counseling in the presence of
  - Underweight/malnutrition
  - Obesity
  - Inadequate dietary intake of any major food/nutritional source
  - Bulimia
  - Anorexia
  - Hypervitaminosis
  - Pica
- Vitamin/mineral supplements
- Fitness and exercise counseling/training
- Immunizations/vaccinations
- Genetic screening based on race, ethnicity, or family history
- A family planning method that is in accord with the woman's or the couple's childbearing plans

Additional Data to Be Obtained

- Exposure to household lead (lead poisoning) (Table 9-2)
- Occupational and environmental hazards (teratogens) (Tables 9-3, 9-4, 9-5)
- Involvement of the father-to-be, other family support
- Readiness for childbearing: psychological, financial, life goals (career, education)
- Need for dental care
- Need for mammography (for women over age 40 or who have a family history indicating need for early mammography)
- Need for special preparation in the presence of specific chronic illness
- Need for referral for further health assessment, social work assistance, mental health assessment/therapy

Folic Acid Supplementation

In 1992 the Centers for Disease Control and Prevention (CDC) recommended that all women of childbearing age take daily folic acid supplements to reduce the risk of having a baby with spina bifida or other neural tube defects. Most over-the-counter multivitamins have 0.4 mg of folic acid. Prescriptive prenatal vitamins are usually formulated with 1.0 g of folic acid and may be used during the preconception period. Ingesting a consistent quantity from food sources is difficult; supplementation is recommended. Dietary sources of folic acid are identified in Section 3. The CDC cautions against a total folate consumption of more than 1 mg per day due to risk of masking pernicious anemia.

Table 9-1   Folic Acid Prevention of Neural Tube Defects

To be taken at least one month prior to conception
and until 8 weeks gestation

All women of childbearing age	0.4 mg/day
During pregnancy	0.6 mg/day
History of a previous child with a neural tube defect	4.0 mg/day
Women with a seizure disorder	1.0 mg/day*

Source: From Centers for Disease Control and Prevention. Recommendations for the use of folic acid to reduce the number of cases of spina bifida and other neural tube defects. *MMWR Morb Mortal Week Rep.* 1992; 41(RR14):1-5.

*Source: Iqbal, M. M. Prevention of neural tube defects by periconceptual use of folic acid. *Pediatr Rev.* 2000;21:58-66.

See Section 4, Table 4-4 (page 65), for the FDA categories of drugs in pregnancy. See also Section 4, Table 4-5 (page 67), for medications that have moderate to high risk of teratogenicity.

Table 9-2   Assessing the Risk of High-Dose Exposure to Lead

Do you—

Live in or regularly visit a house with peeling or chipping paint built before 1960?

Live in or regularly visit a house built before 1960 with recent, ongoing, or planned renovation or remodeling?

Have a child being followed or treated for lead poisoning (that is, blood lead ≥ 15 µg/dL)?

Have a job or hobby that involves exposure to lead?

Live near an active lead smelter, battery recycling plant, or other industry likely to release lead?

Source: From Summers, L., and Price, R. A. Preconception care: An opportunity to maximize health in pregnancy. *J. Nurse-Midwifery* 38(4):196, 1993. Reprinted by permission.

Table 9-3 Chemical and Physical Agents That Are Reproductive Hazards for Women in the Workplace

Agent	Observed Effects	Potentially Exposed Workers
Cancer treatment drugs (e.g., methotrexate)	Infertility, miscarriage, birth defects, low birth weight	Health care workers, pharmacists
Certain ethylene glycol ethers such as 2-ethoxyethanol (2EE) and 2-methoxyethanol (2ME)	Miscarriages	Electronic and semiconductor workers
Carbon disulfide (CS2)	Menstrual cycle changes	Viscose rayon workers
Lead	Infertility, miscarriages, low birth weight, developmental disorders	Battery makers, solderers, welders, radiator repairers, bridge painters, firing range workers, home remodelers
Ionizing radiation (e.g., x-rays and gamma rays)	Infertility, miscarriages, birth defects, low birth weight, developmental disorders, childhood cancers	Health care workers, dental personnel, atomic workers
Strenuous physical labor (e.g., prolonged standing or heavy lifting)	Late pregnancy miscarriage, premature delivery	Many types of workers

Source: From Centers for Disease Control and Prevention/National Institute for Occupational Safety and Health. *The effects of workplace hazards on female reproductive health.* Pub. No. 90-104. February 1999.

Table 9-4 Disease-Causing Agents That Are Reproductive Hazards for Women in the Workplace

Agent	Observed Effects	Potentially Exposed Workers	Preventive Measures
Cytomegalovirus (CMV)	Birth defects, low birth weight, developmental disorders	Health care workers, workers in contact with infants and children	Good hygienic practices such as hand washing
Hepatitis B virus	Low birth weight	Health care workers	Vaccination
Human immuno-deficiency virus (HIV)	Low birth weight, child-hood cancers	Health care workers	Practice universal precautions
Human parvovirus (B19)	Miscarriage	Health care workers, workers in contact with infants, children	Good hygienic practices such as hand washing
Rubella (German measles)	Birth defects, low birth weight	Health care workers, workers in contact with infants, children	Vaccination before pregnancy if no prior immunity
Toxoplasmosis	Miscarriage, birth defects, developmental disorders	Animal care workers, veterinarians	Good hygienic practices such as hand washing
Varicella-zoster virus (chicken pox)	Birth defects, low birth weight	Health care workers, workers in contact with infants, children	Vaccination before pregnancy if no prior immunity

Source: From Centers for Disease Control and Prevention/National Institute for Occupational Safety and Health. *The effects of workplace hazards on female reproductive health.* Pub. No. 90-104. February 1999.

Table 9-5 Male Reproductive Hazards in the Workplace*

| | | Observed Effects | | |
Type of Exposure	Lowered Number of Sperm	Abnormal Sperm Shape	Altered Sperm Transfer	Altered Hormones/Sexual Performance
Lead	X	X	X	X
Dibromochloropropane	X			
Carbaryl (Sevin)		X		
Toluenediamine and dinitrotoluene	X			
Ethylene dibromide	X	X	X	
Plastic production (styrene and acetone)		X		
Ethylene glycol monoethyl ether	X			
Welding		X	X	
Perchloroethylene			X	
Mercury vapor				X

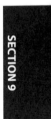

Type of Exposure	Observed Effects			
	Lowered Number of Sperm	Abnormal Sperm Shape	Altered Sperm Transfer	Altered Hormones/Sexual Performance
Heat	X		X	
Military radar	X			
Kepone†			X	
Bromine vapor†	X	X	X	
Radiation† (Chernobyl)	X	X	X	X
Carbon disulfide				X
2,4-Dichlorophenoxy acetic acid (2,4-D)		X	X	

*Studies to date show that some men experience the health effects listed here from workplace exposures. However, these effects may not occur in every worker. The amount of time a worker is exposed, the amount of hazard to which he is exposed, and other personal factors may all determine whether an individual is affected.

†Workers were exposed to high levels as a result of a workplace accident.

Source: From Centers for Disease Control and Prevention/National Institute for Occupational Safety and Health. *The effects of workplace hazards on male reproductive health.* Pub. No. 96-132. January 1997.

References

Varney, H., Kriebs, J. M., & Gegor, C. L. (2003). *Varney's midwifery* (4th ed.). Sudbury, MA: Jones and Bartlett Publishers. Ch. 5.

Centers for Disease Control and Prevention. (1992). Recommendations for the use of folic acid to reduce the number of cases of spina bifida and other neural tube defects. *MMWR Morb Mortal Week Rep, 41*, (RR14):1–5.

Centers for Disease Control and Prevention/National Institute for Occupational Safety and Health. (1999). The effects of workplace hazards on female reproductive health. February, Pub. No. 99–104.

Centers for Disease Control and Prevention/National Institute for Occupational Safety and Health. (1997). The effects of workplace hazards on male reproductive health. January, Pub. No. 96–132.

Iqbal, M.M. Prevention of neural tube defects by periconceptual use of folic acid. (2000). *Pediatr Rev, 21*, 58–66.

Public Health Service Expert Panel on the Content of Prenatal Care. (1989). *Caring for our future: The content of prenatal care.* Washington, DC: U.S. Public Health Service.

Reynolds, H.D. (1998). Preconception care: An integral part of primary care for women. *J Nurse Midwifery, 43*, 445–453.

Summers, L., Price, R.A. (1993). Preconception care: An opportunity to maximize health in pregnancy. *J Nurse Midwifery, 38*, 188–198.

SECTION 9

SECTION 10

Antepartum Care of the Pregnant Woman

Diagnosis of Pregnancy

Signs/Symptoms

Although many of these signs and symptoms are non-specific, their appearance in reproductive age women with no evidence of illness suggests the need for pregnancy testing, particularly when several are present.

Table 10-1   Signs of Pregnancy—By History or Examination

Presumptive	Probable	Positive
Abrupt cessation of menses	Positive pregnancy test	Fetal heart tones
Persistent BBT elevation without infection	Abdominal enlargement	Identification of IUP on sonogram
Persistent intermittent nausea and vomiting	Palpation of fetus	
Increased salivation	Ballottement	
Enlargement, tingling, tenderness of breasts and nipples	Fetal movement	
	Uterine enlargement, change in shape	
	Piskacek's sign	
	Hegar's sign	

Presumptive	Probable	Positive
Darkening of nipples and areolae	Goodell's sign	
Appearance of Montgomery's tubercles	Palpation of Braxton-Hicks uterine contractions	
Breast nodularity		
Presence of colostrum		
Frequent urination		
Fatigue		
Changes in skin pigmentation (linea negra, chloasma), formation of striae, vascular spiders		
Chadwick's sign		
Quickening		

Related Terms

Chadwick's sign	Bluish or purplish discoloration of the vulva and vaginal mucosa, including the vaginal portion of the cervix
Goodell's sign	Softening of the cervix
Hegar's sign	Softening and compressibility of the uterine isthmus.
Piskacek's sign	Asymmetrical enlargement of the uterus due to implantation close to one cornual area. Occurs at eight to ten weeks.

Pregnancy Tests

Hormonal pregnancy tests are based on the production of human chorionic gonadotropin (hCG), which is present in the maternal plasma after implantation occurs, 6 to 12 days after ovulation.

Urine Tests

Once implantation occurs and hCG is present in maternal plasma, it is excreted in the urine. A positive test is possible when there is a concentration of hCG in the urine of at least 25mIUs. This usually occurs by the time of the missed menses or 12 to 14 days after conception.

The same tests used in offices are available over the counter or from medical supply distributors. Women should be encouraged to read and closely follow the manufacturer's instructions.

A positive urine pregnancy test has a 99.5% predictive value for pregnancy. False negatives can occur due to a low concentration of hCG that may be caused by dilute urine, inaccurate dates, ectopic pregnancy, or spontaneous abortion.

Serum beta-hCG

The presence of beta-hCG in the blood can be detected at 5mIU, 7 to 12 days after conception (within one day of implantation). After implantation, the hCG level increases exponentially, doubling approximately every 2 days until it peaks at 8 1/2 to 10 weeks' gestation from the LMP. The hCG levels then decline rapidly between 12 and 16 weeks.

Serial testing requires two values, approximately 48 hours apart.

- Causes of low or falling beta-hCG:
  - Spontaneous abortion
  - Viable pregnancy after 12 weeks
- Causes of slow rising or leveling beta-hCG:
  - Ectopic pregnancy
  - Missed abortion

- Causes of very rapid increase in beta-hCG:
  - Multiple gestation
  - Hydatidiform mole
  - Choriocarcinoma

False-negative immunologic pregnancy tests occur in about 2% of all tests, usually resulting from performing the test too early in pregnancy or, occasionally, too late in the pregnancy (after the middle of the pregnancy).

False-positive results (rare) may be caused by massive proteinuria or during the onset of menopause when pituitary gonadotropins rise.

Initial Antepartum History

Components of the General Antepartum History

- Identifying information
- Past medical and primary care history
- Family history
- Menstrual history, including LMP
- Genetic history
- Obstetric history
- Gynecologic history
- Sexual history
- Contraceptive history

Present Pregnancy History

- Headaches
- Dizziness/syncope
- Visual disturbances
- Fever
- Fatigue
- Nausea/vomiting
- Heartburn

- Breast changes/colostrum
- Shortness of breath
- Abdominal pain
- Back pain
- Vaginal discharge/bleeding
- Dysuria
- Urinary frequency
- Constipation
- Hemorrhoids
- Leg cramps
- Varicosities
- Edema (ankle, pretibial, face, hands)
- Infections (flu, other viruses)
- Medications
- Exposure to x-ray
- Accidents
- Relationship status: support from significant other for pregnancy, presence or history of emotional, physical, or sexual abuse
- Sexual satisfaction: sexual changes and the feelings of both partners about those changes
- Feelings about the pregnancy: effect on her life and her body image; feelings about the baby
- Quickening (date of)
- Any complaints, discomforts, or other concerns other than those already discussed

Investigation of Positive Responses

- When during the pregnancy this occurred; duration; recurrences
- Specific location (if applicable)
- Severity (if applicable)
- Associated symptoms
- Factors aggravating or relieving the symptoms

- Medical help sought (date and name of provider); diagnosis and treatment (if applicable)
- Treatment or relief measures (medically or self-prescribed) and their effectiveness

Determination of Gravidity/Parity

When using a 2-digit system of Gravida/Para:

Gravida   Number of times a woman has been pregnant. If she is currently pregnant, include this pregnancy.

Para   Number of pregnancies that terminated in birth of a fetus that reached viability. If a woman has a multiple pregnancy, it is still counted as one pregnancy. If the fetus is stillborn, but past the age of viability, it is included in the parity.

When using a 4-digit system, the classic notation of parity includes the following:

First digit   Number of term pregnancies a woman has delivered (>37 weeks); if there is a multiple birth, this is still counted as one pregnancy.

Second digit   Number of preterm births (viable pregnancies <37 weeks gestation)

Third digit   Number of pregnancies ending in spontaneous or induced abortion prior to the time when a fetus is developed enough to survive (usually considered to be less than 20 weeks or 500 grams [*Williams Obstetrics*, p. 856])

Fourth digit   Number of children currently alive

Related Terms

Nullipara	A woman who has not completed a pregnancy beyond the point of viability
Primipara	A woman who has given birth to one pregnancy (regardless of number of fetuses) with a duration beyond the point of viability
Multipara	A woman who has given birth to two or more pregnancies (regardless of number of fetuses) with a duration beyond the point of viability
Nulligravida	A woman who has never been pregnant
Primigravida	A woman in the course of her first pregnancy
Multigravida	A woman who is now pregnant with her second or greater pregnancy

Initial Antepartal Physical and Pelvic Exam

A screening physical assessment at the initial visit should include at least the following exam components:

- Blood pressure, pulse
- Height and weight (current and pre-pregnancy)
- Head and neck
- Thyroid
- Breasts
- Heart and lungs
- Liver and spleen
- Presence of abdominal masses
- CVAT
- Lower extremities

Table 10-2 Obstetric Abdominal Exam

- Observations of any scars or bruises and inquiry to obtain explanation of them
- Observation of linea nigra
- Observation of abdominal striae
- Determination of the lie, presentation, position, and variety of the fetus
- Measurement of the fundal height
- Auscultation of the fetal heart tones
- Estimation of fetal weight
- Observation or palpation of fetal movement

A complete pelvic examination is performed, including speculum and bimanual as well as evaluation of the bony pelvis by clinical pelvimetry. Rectovaginal exam may be done if required to further evaluate findings.

Any positive findings or relevant maternal history may indicate the need for a physical exam in greater detail.

Dating of Pregnancy

To date the pregnancy with accuracy, the EDD should agree using two of these three methods:

1. "Sure" dates—the woman knows the date of the first day of her last normal menstrual period and has regular cycles—by Naegele's rule
2. Uterine sizing
3. Ultrasound

Calculating from "Sure" Dates by Naegele's Rule

- Add 7 days to the first day of the LMP
- Subtract 3 months from that date
- Be certain to use actual number of days in the month when crossing over to another month

Example:

5/28	(LMP of May 28)
+ 7	days
6/4	(June 4—May has 31 days)
− 3	months
=3/4	(March 4 of the next year, as 9 months have been added)

Uterine Sizing

A pregnancy between 6 and 16 weeks can be accurately dated within 1–2 weeks when the pelvic exam is not limited by maternal body habitus, pelvic masses, or a severely retroflexed uterus. (See Figure 10-1.) If there is a significant difference between the expected uterine size according to menstrual dating, an ultrasound examination is indicated.

Table 10-3 Uterine Sizing by Bimanual Exam in the Singleton Pregnancy

Gestational Age	Uterine Shape	Uterine Size Equivalent
6 weeks	Slight globular shape, softening of the isthmus	Handball or tangerine
8 weeks	Overall globular shape with some uterine irregularity, particularly around one cornua (Piskacek's sign)	Baseball or small orange
10 weeks	Globular shape, Piskacek's sign may be present	Softball or large orange
12 weeks	Uterus at pelvic brim	Medium grapefruit

SECTION 10

Table 10-4   Accuracy of Dating by Ultrasound

Gestational Age (weeks)	Ultrasound Measurements	Range of Accuracy
<8	Sac size	±10 days
8–12	Crown rump length	±7 days
12–15	Crown rump length BPD	±14 days
15–20	BPD, HC, FL, AC	±10 days
20–28	BPD, HC, FL, AC	±2 weeks
>28	BPD, HC, FL, AC	±3 weeks

BPD = biparietal diameter

HC = head circumference

FL = femur length

AC = abdominal circumference

The Perinatal Collaborative Project and the National Institutes for Health (NIH) have recommended using a range of accuracy of ±11 days prior to 20 weeks and ±2 weeks of gestational ages greater than 20 weeks to take into consideration the variability in the accuracy of ultrasounds at different institutions.

Source: Used by permission of Eva Pressman, MD, Johns Hopkins University School of Medicine.

Table 10-5   Criteria and Range of Accuracy for Dating Pregnancy

Criteria	Range of Accuracy
Basal body temperature chart with coital record, ovulation, and temperature elevation, combined with previous menstrual record	±2–5 days [3]
First trimester ultrasound	±3–5 days [4]

Serum beta hCG <10,000, 2 values, 1 week apart, rising appropriately	±3–5 days [5]
LMP that is certain, normal, regular, and consistent with a first trimester examination	±1–2 weeks [6]
Second trimester ultrasound	±1–2 weeks [7]
Third trimester ultrasound	±2–3 weeks [7]
Physical examination after 20 weeks	±2–3 weeks [8]

Return Antepartum Visits

After the initial OB visit when a complete data base is collected, the revisits are opportunities to continue to collect data necessary to manage the duration of the pregnancy and to plan for the birth and care of the newborn.

Chart Review

- Name
- Age
- Parity
- Weeks gestation by best known dates
- Any significant finding from:
  - Obstetrical history
  - Past medical and primary care history
  - Family history
  - Present pregnancy history
  - Initial physical examination
  - Initial pelvic examination
- Previously identified problems, treatment, and evaluation of effectiveness of the treatment
- Problem list update
- Any concerns and desires of the woman and her family
- Specific current medications, treatments, and dietary requirements

- Laboratory reports from previous visits:
  - Normality of results
  - Need to repeat or follow up any tests
  - Need for further investigation and testing

Interval History

- Any concerns or questions voiced by the woman or her significant others
- Headaches
- Dizziness
- Visual disturbances
- Fever/chills
- Nausea/vomiting
- Fetal movement
- Abdominal pain/contractions
- Back pain
- Dysuria
- Vaginal discharge/leaking fluid
- Vaginal bleeding
- Constipation/hemorrhoids/diarrhea
- Varicosities/leg ache
- Leg cramps
- Edema (ankle, pretibial, hands, face)
- Exposure to infectious disease
- Appropriate use of prescribed medications and vitamins
- Relationship changes, evidence of substance abuse
- Any medical care since last visit (emergency room, dentist, other care providers) for what diagnosis, treatment, continuing care

In addition, review information with women related to specific timing in pregnancy, e.g., triple screening, quickening, arranging for classes to prepare for childbirth, parenting, and breastfeeding.

Physical Examination

At each antepartal revisit:

- Blood pressure (compare with initial visit baseline blood pressure and readings through pregnancy)
- Weight (compare with prepregnancy weight, interval, and the overall weight gain and the pattern of weight gain)
- Obstetric abdominal exam (See Table 10-1)
- CVA tenderness
- Exam of hands for edema
- Exam of lower extremities for:
  - Ankle and pretibial edema
  - Varicosities
  - Quadriceps (knee-jerk) DTRs and Homan's sign when indicated
- Breast exam if the woman plans to breastfeed by 36 weeks to ascertain the need for measures to help bring out flat or inverted nipples

Table 10-6   Approximate Expected Fundal Height at Various Weeks of Gestation

Weeks of Gestation	Approximate Expected Fundal Height
12	Level of the symphysis pubis
16	Halfway between symphysis pubis and umbilicus
20	1–2 fingerbreadths below umbilicus
24	1–2 fingerbreadths above umbilicus
28–30	One-third of the way between umbilicus and xyphoid process (three fingerbreadths above umbilicus)
32	Two-thirds of the way between umbilicus and xyphoid process (three to four fingerbreadths below xyphoid process)
36–38	One fingerbreadth below xyphoid process
40	Two to three fingerbreadths below xyphoid process if lightening occurs

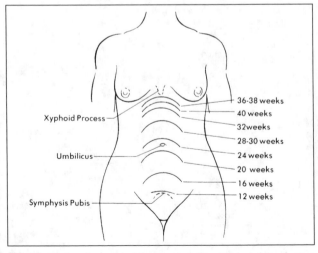

Figure 10-1   Approximate normal fundal heights during pregnancy.

Leopold Maneuvers

Leopold maneuvers (Figure 10-2) and the combined Pawlik's grip (Figure 10-3) is conducted for the following purposes:

- Evaluation of uterine irritability, tone, tenderness, consistency, and contractility
- Evaluation of abdominal muscle tone
- Detection of fetal movement
- Estimation of fetal weight
- Determination of fetal lie, presentation, position, and variety
- Determination of whether the head is engaged

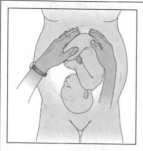

Figure 10-2 Leopold maneuvers: Palpation of fetus in left occiput anterior position.

A. First maneuver. Curve fingers of both hands around top of fundus. What is in the fundus?

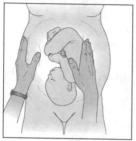

B. Second maneuver. Place both hands on sides of uterus. Where are the baby's small parts?

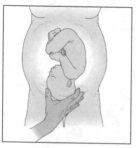

C. Third maneuver. With thumb and middle finger of one hand press gently but deeply into the mother's abdomen immediately above the symphysis pubis and grasp the presenting part. What is the presenting part?

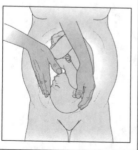

D. Fourth maneuver. Place both hands on sides of lower uterus, press deeply and move fingertips towards pelvic inlet. Where is the cephalic prominence? Is the presenting part engaged?

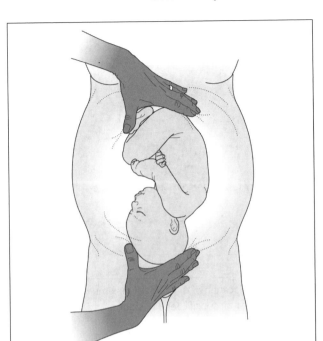

Figure 10-3   Combined Pawlik's grip. Combine Leopold's third maneuver with one hand, and palpation of the fundus using the other hand. Compare the two poles for final determination of lie and presentation.

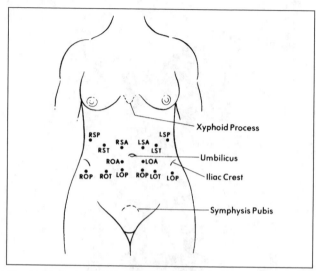

Figure 10-4   Location of the point of maximum intensity of the fetal heart tones for specific fetal positions.

Table 10-7   Causes of Apparent Size/Dates Discrepancies

Trimester	Size Less Than Dates	Size Greater Than Dates
First	Inaccurate dates	Inaccurate dates
	Missed abortion	Inaccurate measurement
	Ectopic pregnancy	Full bladder or bowel
	Maternal build	Multiple pregnancy
		Uterine fibroids
		Ovarian cysts
		Maternal build
Second	Inaccurate dates	Inaccurate dates
	Inaccurate measurement	Inaccurate

Fetal anomaly (GU, renal agenesis)	measurement
	Multiple pregnancy
Chromosomal abnormality	Fetal anomaly (CNS, GI [tracheo-esophageal fistula])
Placental pathology	
Oligohydramnios	
Fetal death	
Severe, early onset IUGR related to chronic maternal illness (i.e., diabetes, lupus, sickle cell anemia)	Chromosomal abnormality
	Polyhydramnios
	Early macrosomia
Fetal infection (parvovirus, CMV, rubella, toxoplasmosis)	
Elevated MSAFP/hCG	
Third	IUGR	Macrosomia
	SGA—genetically small infant, normally grown	LGA—genetically large infant, normally grown
	Placental pathology (previa, abruption, infarction, circumvallate)	Gestational diabetes
		Breech presentation
	Fetal death	Placenta previa
	Oligohydramnios	Polyhydramnios
	Transverse or obligue lie	Excessive maternal weight gain
	Poor maternal weight gain	

Pelvic Examination

After the initial examination, the midwife performs some or all of the following components of a pelvic examination, as indicated:

- A speculum examination if the woman complains of vaginal discharge:
  - Look for visual signs of vaginal infection, and obtain material for a diagnostic wet smear slide

- ○ Obtain specimen for GC and chlamydia diagnostic testing
- ○ Evaluate treatment for vaginal infection (test of cure)
- Repeat Pap smear, if needed
- GC and chlamydia diagnostic testing in the third trimester if indicated by history or by local regulations
- Rule out premature rupture of membranes
- Clinical pelvimetry late in the third trimester if the pelvis needs to be reevaluated
- Preterm labor (see Section 11)
- May perform a 36-week evaluation, including a repeat of clinical pelvimetry; obtaining specimens for diagnostic testing of GC, chlamydia, and GBS; and evaluation of cervical status.
- May do a vaginal exam at the fortieth week to determine cervical "ripeness" (readiness) for labor.

Antepartum Laboratory Tests and Adjunct Studies

Initial Visit

- Pap smear
- Gonorrhea culture
- Chlamydia culture
- Blood type (ABO)
- Antibody screen/antibody titer
- Sickle cell prep or hemoglobin electrophoresis (if indicated)
- VDRL, RPR, or STS
- Hepatitis B surface antigen
- Rubella titer
- Varicella antibody screen (if a woman denies previous varicella infection)

- Hemoglobin and hematocrit (some settings add CBC with differential, SMA 4, or SMA 12)
- Urinalysis for protein, glucose, and microscopic exam. Many settings also perform a urine culture.

All women should be offered the following:

- HIV testing (and counseling)
- Maternal serum alpha-fetoprotein (MSAFP) or multiple marker testing (to be done between 15 and 18 weeks' gestation) OR first trimester bio-chemical markers
- Screening ultrasound for gestational age and anatomy review at 18 to 20 weeks

Revisit Laboratory Tests and Adjunctive Studies

- Urine dipstick test for protein and glucose
- Urine dipstick test for ketones if indicated
- Diabetes screening at 26 to 28 weeks
- Screening for vaginal and rectal group B strepto-coccus (GBS) colonization at 35 to 37 weeks' gestation
- Repeat hemoglobin and hematocrit at 28 weeks
- Practice and institutional policies vary regarding repeating laboratory tests or repeating them only if indicated by history, physical, and laboratory findings. This includes hemoglobin and hemato-crit, VDRL, gonorrhea, chlamydia, and antibody titers for Rh-negative women prior to receiving prophylactic Rh immune globulin at 28 weeks (Section 11).

Assessment for Structural and Genetic Abnormality

Maternal Serum alpha-Fetoprotein (MSAFP) and Triple Screen

Triple screen (MSAFP, hCG, estradiol) or quad screening (including inhibin A) offer improved identification of chromosomal anomalies over MSAFP alone. MSAFP is elevated when the fetus has an open neural tube defect and is decreased with Down's syndrome or other chromosomal anomaly. Offer MSAFP or the multiple marker screen to all women at 15 to 18 weeks menstrual age. If first trimester chemical markers are drawn, perform only the MSAFP in the second trimester.

Normal values are based on:

- Gestational age
- Maternal age
- Weight
- Race
- Diabetes, if present
- Multiple gestation

Table 10-8   Major Reasons for MSAFP Elevations

Underestimation of gestational age

Multiple gestations

Neural tube defects

Ventral wall defects (omphalocele, gastroschisis)

Renal anomalies (renal agenesis, urethral obstruction)

Severe oligohydramnios

Ectopic (including abdominal) pregnancy

Fetal-maternal hemorrhage (may occur spontaneously or
   following CVS or amniocentesis)
Underweight mother
Black race
Increased placental size

Source: Thomas, R. L., Blakemore, K. J. (1990). Evaluation of elevations in
maternal serum alpha-fetoprotein: A review. *Obstet Gynecol Surv*, *45*,
269–283. Reprinted with permission.

Table 10-9   Risk of Down Syndrome by Maternal Age

Maternal Age	Risk for Down Syndrome	Risk for any Chromosomal Abnormality
21	1/1667	1/526
23	1/1429	1/500
25	1/1250	1/476
27	1/1111	1/455
29	1/1000	1/417
31	1/909	1/385
33	1/625	1/317
35	1/385	1/204
37	1/227	1/130
39	1/137	1/82
41	1/82	1/51
43	1/50	1/32
45	1/30	1/20
47	1/18	1/12
49	1/11	1/7

Source: Gabbe, S. G., Niebyl, J. R., Simpson, J.L. (2001). *Obstetrics: Normal
and problem pregnancies,* (4th ed.). New York: Elsevier.

Table 10-10 Indications for Prenatal Diagnosis and Counseling

Couples at increased risk
- Maternal age >35 years
- Either parent with chromosomal translocation or inversion
- Either parent with aneuploidy
- Previous child with chromosome abnormality
- Women with dizygotic twins at age 31 or older

Family history of birth defects and/or mental retardation
- Congenital heart disease
- Neural tube defect
- Cleft lip and/or palate
- Multiple congenital anomalies
- Mental retardation

Family history of known or suspected Mendelian genetic disorder
- Cystic fibrosis
- Hemophilia A
- Hemophilia B
- Duchenne muscular dystrophy
- Becker muscular dystrophy
- Fragile X

Ethnicity
- African population:
  - Sickle cell disease
  - Sickle Trait
- Mediterranean/Indian:
  - beta-thalassemia
  - Other hemoglobinopathies
- Ashkenazi Jewish:
  - Tay-Sachs disease

Exposure to possible teratogens
- Alcohol
- Cocaine
- Radiation
- Lead

Use of potentially teratogenic medications

• Anticonvulsants	DES
• Retinoids	Tetracycline
• ACE inhibitors	Thalidomide
• Coumarin	Methotrexate

• Androgens (anabolic steroids, danocrine)

Infectious agents

- Toxoplasmosis
- Rubella
- Cytomegalovirus
- Parvovirus B19
- Syphilis

Medical illnesses

- Insulin-dependent or uncontrolled diabetes mellitus
- Epileptic disorder: antiseizure medications

Abnormally low or high MSAFP

Fetal abnormalities diagnosed by sonogram

Consanguinity

Multiple pregnancy losses, stillbirth, infertility

Assisted reproductive technologies

Anxiety

Source: Bauman, P., McFarlin, B. (1994). Prenatal diagnosis. *J Nurse-Midwifery, 39,* (2 suppl), 37S.

Table 10-11 Age-Related Detection Rates and False-Positive Rates for Women Ages 16 to 44 with Risk Cutoff of 1:300

Age (y)	Detection Rate of AFP, hCG, and Unconjugated Estriol	False-Positive Rate
16	44.3%	3.1%
18	44.3%	3.1%
20	44.7%	3.2%
22	45.2%	3.2%
24	46.5%	3.6%

Age (y)	Detection Rate of AFP, hCG, and Unconjugated Estriol	False-Positive Rate
26	48.5%	4.1%
28	51.6%	4.7%
30	56.0%	6.1%
32	62.0%	8.7%
34	69.5%	12.5%
36	78.0%	19.0%
38	85.5%	28.6%
40	91.6%	40.9%
42	95.7%	55.3%
44	98.1%	70.0%

Source: Reynolds, T. M., Nix, A. B., Dunstan, F. D. & Dawson, A. J. (1993). Age-specific detection and false-positive rates: An aid to counseling in Down's syndrome risk screening. *Obstet Gynecol, 81,* 449.

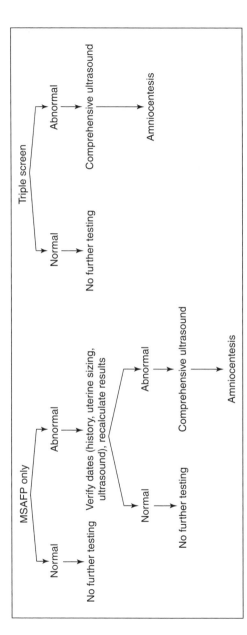

Figure 10-5 Management of abnormal MSAFP/triple screen test results. Most abnormal results are caused by inaccurate assessment of gestational age.

Additional Screening Tests for Structural and Chromosomal Anomalies

- Maternal serum pregnancy associated plasma protein (PAPP-A) and hCG:
  - Performed in the first trimester
  - Increased PAPP-A with decreased hCG present in Down's syndrome
- Nuchal Translucency Screening:
  - Ultrasound exam of fetal neck
  - 10–14 weeks gestation
- Enlarged sonolucent area at back of fetal neck is associated with chromosomal anomalies
- Risk can be calculated using triple screen markers or first trimester markers to increase accuracy

Diagnostic Genetic Testing

Table 10-12 Invasive Diagnostic Genetic Testing

Test	Timing	Advantages	Disadvantages/Comments
Chorionic villus sampling (CVS) Sampling of chorionic villi for chromosomal analysis	10-15 weeks menstrual age	Early diagnosis Rapid results (48 hours initially, then final results in 10-14 days)	Slight increase in pregnancy loss (0.8%) compared to amniocentesis Limb reduction defects reported when performed at 8–9 weeks, not a risk at 10 weeks or later MSAFP testing still needed for neural tube defect screening MSAFP can be falsely elevated by CVS Requires extensive operator experience
Early amniocentesis Sampling of sloughed fetal cells for chromosomal analysis and biochemical markers (acetylcholinesterase) for open neural tube defects	Prior to 15 weeks as an alternative to CVS	Early results This is not a widely used technique	Increased risk of pregnancy loss compared to both CVS and amniocentesis after 15 weeks Risk of amnionitis, rare reports of fetal injury

Test	Timing	Advantages	Disadvantages/Comments
Amniocentesis Sampling of sloughed fetal cells for chromosomal analysis and biochemical markers (acetylcholinesterase) for open neural tube defects	15 weeks gestation or later Generally performed between 15–20 weeks, but can be done at anytime until term	High degree of accuracy Results in 2–3 weeks, but FISH technology can be used for rapid results	Low risk of fetal loss (0.5–1.0%)
Cordocentesis/ Percutaneous Umbilical Blood Sampling (PUBS) Directly samples fetal blood cells for chromosomal analysis	Third trimester	Rapid karyotyping of fetus by DNA	Used only for small number of very high-risk pregnancies Risks include spontaneous abortion, rupture of membranes, preterm labor, infection, bleeding, fetal trauma, and isoimmunization

Rh(D) negative women should receive Rh immune globulin to prevent iso-immunization

Table 10-13   Indications for Obstetrical Ultrasound

Estimated gestational age for patients with uncertain clinical dates
Evaluation of fetal growth
Vaginal bleeding of undetermined etiology in pregnancy
Determination of fetal presentation
Suspected multiple gestation
Adjunct to amniocentesis
Significant uterine size/clinical dates discrepancy
Pelvic mass
Suspected hydatidiform mole
Suspected ectopic pregnancy
Adjunct to special procedures, e.g., fetoscopy, cordocentesis, chorionic villus sampling, in vitro fertilization, cervical cerclage placement
Suspected fetal death
Suspected uterine abnormality
Localization of intrauterine contraceptive device
Surveillance of ovarian follicle development
Biophysical evaluation for fetal well-being
Observation of intrapartum events, e.g., version/extraction of second twin
Manual removal of placenta
Suspected polyhydramnios or oligohydramnios
Suspected abruptio placentae
Adjunct to external cephalic version
Estimation of fetal weight
Abnormal serum alpha-fetoprotein value
Follow-up observation of identified fetal anomaly
Follow-up evaluation of placental location for identified placenta previa
History of previous congenital anomaly
Serial evaluation of fetal growth in multiple gestation
Evaluation of fetal condition in late registrants for prenatal care

Source: National Institutes of Health. (1984). *Diagnostic ultrasound imaging in pregnancy: Report of a consensus development conference sponsored by the National Institute of Child Health and Human Development.* Washington, DC: NIH, 3–13. DHHS publication NIH 86-667.

Table 10-14   Components of a Basic Obstetrical Ultrasound Examination

First Trimester Sonography

Scanning may be performed abdominally or vaginally, dependent on gestational age and information required. The following assessments should be made:

Gestational sac location (intra- or extra-uterine)
Identification of embryo
Crown-rump length
Presence or absence of fetal cardiac activity (identify rate when possible)
Fetal number
Evaluation of the uterus and adnexal structures for size, shape, and location

Second and Third Trimester Sonography

Unless technically impossible, the following aspects should be assessed during a basic ultrasound examination:

Fetal number
Fetal presentation
Documentation of fetal cardiac activity
Placental localization
Amniotic fluid volume assessment (single pocket measurement or amniotic fluid index)
Gestational age dating, using at least two fetal parameters (biparietal diameter, abdominal circumference, femur length)
Detection and evaluation of maternal pelvic masses
Survey of fetal anatomy for gross malformations (cerebral midline, 4-chamber heart, stomach, kidneys, bladder, and identification of all fetal limbs)

Source: American College of Nurse-Midwives (1996). *Limited obstetrical ultrasound in the third Trimester.* Clinical bulletin. Washington, DC: ACNM. Reprinted by permission.

Table 10-15   Indications for Limited Scans

A limited ultrasound examination may be appropriate and
desirable in certain circumstances—for example, when
specific information is required or the clinical situation is
urgent. A limited examination may be useful for the following
tasks:

Assessment of amniotic fluid volume
Conducting fetal biophysical profile
Conducting ultrasound-guided amniocentesis
Guidance of external cephalic version
Confirmation of fetal life or death
Localization of placenta
Confirmation of fetal presentation

Source: American College of Nurse-Midwives (1996). *Limited obstetrical
ultrasound in the third Trimester.* Clinical bulletin No. 1. Washington, DC:
ACNM. Reprinted by permission.

Table 10-16   Minimum Components of Limited Obstetrical
Ultrasound, Second and Third Trimester

Fetal number
Fetal cardiac activity
Fetal lie
Placental location
Biophysical profile parameters
Amniotic fluid volume

Source: American College of Nurse-Midwives (1996). *Limited obstetrical
ultrasound in the third Trimester.* Clinical bulletin No. 1. Washington, DC:
ACNM. Reprinted by permission.

SECTION 10

Nutrition in Pregnancy

Weight Gain

The Institute of Medicine's Subcommittee on Nutritional Status and Weight Gain During Pregnancy proposed that gestational weight gain be based on a woman's prepregnancy body mass index (BMI) (Section 3) as shown in Table 10-17.

Table 10-17   Recommended Total Weight Gain Ranges for Pregnant Women,[a] by Prepregnancy Body Mass Index (BMI)[b]

	Recommended Total Gain	
Weight-for-Height Category	kg	lb
Low (BMI < 19.8)	12.5–18	28–40
Normal (BMI of 19.8 to 26.0)	11.5–16	25–35
High[c] (BMI > 26.0 to 29.0)	7.0–11.5	15–25

[a]Young adolescents and black women should strive for gains at the upper end of the recommended range. Short women (< 157 cm, or 62 in.) should strive for gains at the lower end of the range.

[b]BMI is calculated using metric units.

[c]The recommended target weight gain for obese women (BMI > 29.0) is at least 6.0 kg (15 lb).

Source: National Academy of Sciences. (1990). *Nutrition during pregnancy.* Washington, DC: National Academy Press.

Higgins Intervention Methodology

Determine normal weight requirements on Table 10-18. The ideal weight and activity level are then located on the 1948 Canadian Dietary Standard (Table 10-19), and the woman's nonpregnant calorie and protein requirements are ascertained.

Table 10-18 Metropolitan Life Insurance Company Desirable Weights for Women

Height (includes 2-inch heels)	Small Frame (range in pounds and average)	Medium Frame (range in pounds and average)	Large Frame (range in pounds and average)
4'10"	92–98 (95)	96–107 (101.5)	104–119 (111.5)
4'11"	94–101 (97.5)	98–110 (104)	106–122 (114)
5'0"	96–104 (100)	101–113 (107)	109–125 (117)
5'1"	99–107 (103)	104–116 (110)	112–128 (120)
5'2"	102–110 (106)	107–119 (113)	115–131 (123)
5'3"	105–113 (109)	110–122 (116)	118–134 (126)
5'4"	108–116 (112)	113–126 (119.5)	121–138 (129.5)
5'5"	111–119 (115)	116–130 (123)	125–142 (133.5)
5'6"	114–123 (118.5)	120–135 (127.5)	129–146 (137.5)
5'7"	118–127 (122.5)	124–139 (131.5)	133–150 (141.5)
5'8"	122–131 (126.5)	128–143 (135.5)	137–154 (145.5)
5'9"	126–135 (130.5)	132–147 (139.5)	141–158 (149.5)
5'10"	130–140 (135)	136–151 (143.5)	145–163 (154)
5'11"	134–144 (139)	140–155 (147.5)	149–168 (158.5)
6'0"	138–148 (143)	144–159 (155.5)	153–173 (163)

Source: 1959 Actuarial Tables. Courtesy of the Metropolitan Life Insurance Company.

SECTION 10

Table 10-19 Canadian Dietary Standard for Female Adults[a]

Ideal Body Weight (lb)	Sedentary Activities		Moderate Activities		Heavy Activities	
	Calories	Protein	Calories	Protein	Calories	Protein
80	1600	40	1900	40	2400	40
85	1650	43	1950	43	2450	43
90	1700	45	2000	45	2500	45
95	1750	48	2050	48	2550	48
100	1800	50	2100	50	2600	50
105	1875	51	2175	51	2675	51
110	1950	53	2250	53	2750	53
115	2025	54	2325	54	2825	54
120	2100	55	2400	55	2900	55
125	2150	57	2450	57	2950	57
130	2200	58	2500	58	3000	58
135	2250	59	2550	59	3050	59
140	2300	60	2600	60	3100	60
145	2350	63	2650	63	3150	63
150	2400	65	2700	65	3200	65
155	2450	68	2750	68	3250	68
160	2500	70	2800	70	3300	70

[a]1948.

After 20 weeks' gestation, add 500 calories and 25 gms of protein to the daily nonpregnant calorie and protein requirements.

If the pregnancy is a multiple gestation, add 500 calories and 25 grams of protein for each fetus. For a mother 19 years of age or less, refer to the U.S. Recommended Daily Allowance (RDA) calorie and protein requirements (Table 10-20).

Table 10-20 Calorie and Protein Requirements for Women under 19, U.S.

Age	Calories	Protein
13–15	2600	80 g
16–19	2400	75 g

Source: Food and Nutrition Board, National Academy of Sciences—National Research Council (1958).

Table 10-21 Additional Corrective Allowances for Implementation of Higgins Methodology

Nutritional Status	Definition	Corrective Allowances
Undernutrition	A deficit in protein between the normal pregnancy requirements and actual dietary intake	Protein—the number of gm of protein deficit is added to the daily normal pregnancy requirements Calories—for each gm of protein deficit, 10 cal are added to the daily normal pregnancy requirements
Underweight	Pre-pregnant weight 5% or more under the ideal weight from Table 10-18	Protein—20 gm per day Calories—500 cal per day Both protein and calories are added to daily pregnancy requirements This allowance will permit a weight gain of 1 lb/week.
Nutritional stress	The existence of one or more of: —Pernicious vomiting —Pregnancy spacing < 1 year —Poor obstetric history —< 10 lb gain by 20 wks gestation —Serious emotional upset	Add 1200 cal and 20 gm protein for each stress condition (up to 400 cal and 40 gm protein maximum added to normal pregnancy requirements

Table 10-22 Average Nonpregnant Adolescent
Female Weight Gain

Age	Average Weight Gain per Year
11–13	11 lb
13–15	8 lb
15–17	3 lb
17–19	1 lb

Table 10-23 Summary Format for Calculating Calorie
and Protein Requirements During Pregnancy

	Calories	Protein (g)
Nonpregnant requirements	_____	_____
Addition for pregnancy (after 20th week)	500	25
Undernutrition corrective allowance	_____	_____
Underweight corrective allowance	_____	_____
Nutritional stress corrective allowance	_____	_____
TOTAL	_____	_____

Immunizations in Pregnancy

Table 10-24 Immunizations During Pregnancy

Vaccine	Consider Use If Indication Exists	Contra-indicated	Comments
Hepatitis A			Safety in pregnancy not determined; theoretic risk is low
			Risk should be weighed against risk for hepatitis A in women at high risk for exposure
Hepatitis B	X		Recommended for pregnant and breastfeeding women at risk for hepatitis B virus infection
Influenza (Inact.)	X		Women who will be pregnant during the influenza season should be vaccinated in any trimester
Influenza (LAIV)		X	Use inactivated influenza vaccine in pregnancy
Measles		X	See Rubella comment
Mumps		X	See Rubella comment
Pneumococcal			Safety during the first trimester has not been evaluated, but no adverse events have been reported in newborns whose mothers were vaccinated during pregnancy

Polio (IPV)		Vaccination of pregnant women should be avoided on theoretical grounds. If at risk for infection, IPV can be given.
Rubella	X	Measles-mumps-rubella (MMR) vaccine should not be administered to pregnant women. Because risk to the fetus cannot be excluded for theoretical reasons, women should be counseled to avoid pregnancy for 28 days after vaccination. If a pregnant woman is vaccinated or if she becomes pregnant within 4 weeks after MMR vaccination, counsel regarding the theoretical basis of concern for the fetus; however, MMR vaccination during pregnancy should not be a reason to terminate pregnancy
Tetanus/Diphtheria	X	Td toxoid is indicated routinely for pregnant women. Previously vaccinated pregnant women who have not received a Td vaccination within the last 10 years should receive a booster dose
Varicella	X	Effects on the fetus are unknown; therefore, pregnant women should not be vaccinated. Nonpregnant women should avoid pregnancy for 1 month. A pregnant household member is not a contraindication to vaccination. If a pregnant woman is vaccinated or she becomes pregnant within 4 weeks, counsel

Vaccine	Consider Use If Indication Exists	Contra-indicated	Comments
Anthrax			regarding the theoretical concern for the fetus. Varicella vaccination during pregnancy should not ordinarily be a reason to terminate pregnancy. VZIG [Varicella Zoster Immune Globulin] should be strongly considered for susceptible, pregnant women who have been exposed.
			No studies are published regarding use of anthrax vaccine in pregnancy. Vaccinate against anthrax if the benefits outweigh the potential risks to the fetus.
BCG		X	Although no harmful effects to the fetus have been associated with BCG vaccine, its use is not recommended during pregnancy
Japanese Encephalitis			No specific data is available on the safety of JE vaccine in pregnancy. Vaccination poses a theoretical risk to the fetus, so should not be routinely administered during pregnancy. Pregnant women traveling where risk of JE is high should be vaccinated when theoretical risks are outweighed by risk of infection to mother and fetus.
Meningococcal	X		The vaccine has been shown to be both safe and efficacious when given to pregnant women

Rabies	X	Consequences of inadequately treated rabies exposure are grave. No fetal abnormalities are associated with rabies vaccination, therefore, postexposure prophylaxis is indicated in pregnancy. If risk of exposure to rabies is substantial, preexposure prophylaxis may be indicated during pregnancy.
Typhoid (Parenteral & Ty21a)	X	No data have been reported on the use of any of the three typhoid vaccines among pregnant women
Vaccinia (Smallpox)	X	Vaccinia vaccine should not be administered to pregnant women for routine indications. Not known to cause congenital malformations, but has been reported to cause fetal infection on rare occasions, almost always after primary vaccination of the mother. Pregnant women with a definite exposure to smallpox virus (e.g. face-to-face, household, or close-proximity contact with a smallpox patient) should be vaccinated. Smallpox infection among pregnant women can result in more severe infection than in nonpregnant women. Risks to mother and fetus from clinical smallpox substantially outweigh potential risks of vaccination.

Vaccine	Consider Use If Indication Exists	Contra-indicated	Comments
Yellow Fever			The safety of yellow fever vaccination during pregnancy has not been established. Administer only if travel to an endemic area is unavoidable and if an increased risk for exposure exists. For specific indications and need for serologic testing, call the Division of Vector-Borne Infectious Diseases (970-221-6400) or the Division of Global Migration and Quarantine (404-639-1600) at CDC

Source: Guidelines for Vaccinating Pregnant Women from Recommendations of the Advisory Committee on Immunization Practices (ACIP). (October 1998, updated June 2004). Centers for Disease Control and Prevention (CDC) Department of Health and Human Services (DHHS). Available online at: http://www.cdc.gov/nip/publications/preg_guide.htm.

Exercise in Pregnancy

Exercise History (Prenatal)

Name: _____ Date: _____ Due Date: _____

For the year prior to your pregnancy, which of the following things did you do regularly?

Aerobic exercise

No. of sessions/week _____ Approx. length of each session _____

What was your target heart rate range? _____ bpm

What was your RPE (rate of perceived exertion) range? (Circle lowest and highest intensity)

Very light   Light   Fairly light   Somewhat hard   Hard   Very hard   Very, very hard

List your activities (running, aerobic dancing, etc.): _____

Strength activities (weight lifting, calisthenics, etc.)

No. of sessions/week _____ Hip and knee flexors/extensors and ab/abductors

_____ Chest and back; shoulders and arms

_____ Abdominals; spine (core strength)

_____ Pelvic floor

Flexibility activities (yoga, stretching, dance, etc.)

No. of sessions/week _____

Combination activities (advanced dance, martial arts, basketball, etc.)

No. of sessions/week _____   List your activities: _____

Relaxation (progressive relaxation, autogenic training, hypnosis, etc.)

No. of sessions/week _____

Centering (mediation, dance, t'ai chi, etc.)

No. of sessions/week _____

Do you have one or more children in the 1- to 5-year-old range who are very active? (circle one) Yes   No

If so, how much time do you spend with her/him/them? _____

Do you have a physically demanding job? (circle one)   Yes   No   Is it stressful?   Yes   No

Are you on your feet a lot? (circle one)   Yes   No   Describe your work activities: _____

Describe your exercise and/or physical activities since the start of this pregnancy: _____

Figure 10-6 Exercise history (prenatal).

Source: © 1996 Anne Cowlin.

Medical Screening Form for Prenatal Exercise Participants

Name: _____   Date: _____

TO THE CARE PROVIDER: Review these conditions and indicate if any now exist or existed previously. Add any notes you think may be helpful to the fitness instructor.

Contraindications for Exercise

_____ Placenta previa

_____ Premature rupture of membranes (PROM)

_____ Incompetent cervix

_____ Chronic heart disease

_____ Premature labor

_____ Preeclampsia, eclampsia, or PIH

_____ Tearing or separation of placenta (abruptio)

_____ Fever (or presence of infection)

_____ Acute and/or chronic life-threatening condition

Conditions That May Benefit from Exercise

_____ Diabetes

_____ Gestational diabetes

_____ Hyperinsulinemia

_____ Overweight

_____ Discomforts

_____ Depression

_____ Weakness

_____ Lack of stamina

_____ Elevated blood pressure

Conditions for Assessment

_____ Marginal or low-lying placenta

_____ History of IUGR

_____ Diabetes or hyperinsulinemia

_____ Irregular heartbeat or mitral valve prolapse

_____ Anemia

_____ Multiple gestations

_____ Thyroid disease

_____ Three or more spontaneous abortions

_____ Excessive over- or underweight

_____ Extremely sedentary lifestyle

_____ Asthma

Warning Signs or Symptoms

_____ Edema of face and hands

_____ Severe headaches

_____ Hypertension

_____ Dizziness or disorientation

_____ Palpitations or chest pain

_____ Difficulty walking

_____ Nausea

_____ Bleeding or fluid discharge

_____ Regular strong contractions

_____ Cramps

_____ Fever

Figure 10-7 Medical screening form for prenatal exercise participants.

Source: © 1985, 1995, 2002 Anne Cowlin.

Third Trimester Fetal Assessment
Fetal Movement Counting

All women benefit from understanding that the fetus will develop its own behavior pattern. If a woman notices a decrease or cessation in fetal movement, she should report this finding to the midwife. There are no specific "normal" numbers of fetal movements. A number of different time and number guidelines for fetal movement counting exist. Each clinician should choose and consistently use a single method.

Table 10-25   Count-to-Ten Movement Counting Method

1. Schedule one count session daily.
2. Schedule session for the same time each day—e.g., at 8:00 a.m., or select a time when you have the time to count and when the fetus is usually active.
3. Chart how long it takes to reach 10 movements.
4. There must be at least 10 movements identified in 10 hr.
5. If there are fewer than 10 movements in 10 hr, if it takes an increasing time to reach 10 movements, or if no movements are felt within 10 hr, call your midwife.

A Simple Method of FMC

1. Put 10 pennies in a cup.
2. Turn the pennies out onto the table.
3. Put a penny back in the cup every time the baby moves.
4. If the pennies are not all back in the cup within 2 hours, call the midwife.

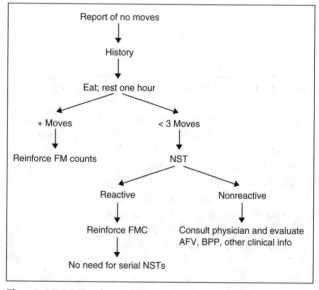

Figure 10-8   Fetal movement assessment paradigm for response to a woman's report of decreased fetal movement.

Source: Gegor, C. L., Paine, L. L., & Johnson, T. R. B. (1991) Antepartum fetal assessment: A nurse-midwifery perspective. *J Nurse-Midwifery.* 36, 157.

Indications for Antepartum Testing

Table 10-26   Obstetric Indications for Antepartum Testing

Suspected intrauterine growth restriction (IUGR) in this
pregnancy
History of IUGR in previous pregnancy
Pregestational diabetes
Gestational diabetes
Chronic hypertension
Pregnancy-induced hypertension
Preeclampsia
Multiple gestation
Oligohydramnios
Post dates
Rh isoimmunization
Preterm rupture of membranes (PROM)
Decreased fetal movement
Previous stillbirth

Table 10-27   Maternal Indications for Antepartum Testing

Antiphospholipid syndrome
Hyperthyroidism (poorly controlled)
Hemoglobinopathies (hemoglobin SS, SC, or S-thalassemia)
Cyanotic heart disease
Systemic lupus erythematosus
Chronic renal disease
Type I diabetes mellitus
Hypertensive disorders

SECTION 10

Nonstress Test (NST)

Table 10-28   Performance of the NST

---

1. Place woman in a side-lying position (left or right side).
2. Initiate external electronic fetal monitoring (both FHR and contraction monitoring).
3. Identify the baseline FHR (minimum of 3 min).
4. Continue monitoring for a minimum of 20 min.

Note: A fetal event marker is not required for performance of the NST. FHR accelerations are associated with fetal movement, and maternal perception of this movement is not required.

Table 10-29   Interpretation Criteria for the NST

Interpretation	Criteria
Reactive	At least two accelerations of the FHR within a 20-min period that are off the baseline for at least 15 sec and that have a minimum amplitude of 15 bpm
Nonreactive	FHR tracing that fails to demonstrate adequate number or amplitude of FHR accelerations within any 20-min period
Inconclusive	A tracing of FHR that is uninterpretable because of difficulty obtaining the EFM tracing, or a tracing that does not demonstrate an FHR baseline (common with very vigorous fetuses)

Table 10-30   Common Causes of Nonreactivity of the NST

Fetal Causes	**Maternal Causes**
Gestational age (28–32 weeks)	Disease (e.g., diabetes, hypertension)
Deep sleep state	Medications (e.g., beta-blockers, CNS depressants, tocolytics, steroids)
Hypoxia	Illicit drug use
Oligohydramnios	Smoking
CNS or cardiac anomalies	Chorioamnionitis
Circadian rhythms	Dehydration

Table 10-31   Management of Results of the NST

- If the NST is reactive, the frequency of subsequent testing depends on the indication for testing.
- If the NST is non-reactive, further testing is indicated with a biophysical profile (BPP) or a contraction stress test (CST).
- If the NST is inconclusive, prolonging the NST for a total of 45 minutes may clarify the tracing, or one can test further with a BPP.

Contraction Stress Test

Table 10-32   Contraction Stress Test Indications/ Contraindications

Indications
As follow-up to non-reassuring NST
High risk for IUGR
Post dates
Insulin-dependent diabetes
Ultrasound not available to perform a BPP

Relative contraindications

Gestational age less than 37 weeks

Multiple gestation

Risk-benefit consideration is necessary to weigh possible
consequences of unintended labor from contractions with
the need for information regarding fetal status.

Absolute contraindications

Clinical situations when labor would be dangerous

Previous classical cesarean section

History of myomectomy entering the uterine cavity

Placenta previa

Current risk for preterm labor

Table 10-33   Procedures for Inducing Contractions for the CST

Breast Stimulation

Stimulation of one nipple, through the clothing

2 min stimulation

5 min resting

Do not stimulate through a contraction

If not successful within 45 min, perform OCT

Oxytocin Challenge Test (OCT)

Intravenous infusion, D5/0.2NS keep-vein-open rate

Oxytocin solution: 10 units pitocin in 500 cc D%/0.2NS per
infusion pump

Titrate oxytocin from 1 mIU/min

Increase 1 mIU/min every 15 min

Continue until adequate contraction pattern or abnormal FHR
patterns

Table 10-34 CST Interpretation Criteria

Procedure

Establish FHR baseline prior to initiation of CST.

Prior to interpretation of FHR patterns, the EFM strip must demonstrate 3 contractions within 10 min.

Minimum contraction duration is 40 sec off the baseline (unnecessary for the woman to perceive the contractions).

Interpretation

Negative (reassuring): FHR baseline stable, without evidence of late decelerations

Positive (nonreassuring): Repetitive late decelerations

Equivocal:

Unable to obtain satisfactory tracing

Hyperstimulation

Nonrepetitive late decelerations

Table 10-35 Management of CST Results

- If the CST is negative (reassuring), another CST is not necessary for 7 days.
- If the CST is positive (non-reassuring), the results should be interpreted within the context of the overall clinical picture, because this test has a 30% false-positive rate. This assessment determines whether to follow up with a BPP, to repeat the CST within 24 hours, or to take immediate steps to deliver the baby.
- If the CST is equivocal, with the results confounded by hyperstimulation or non-repetitive decelerations, the CST should be repeated within 24 hours or a BPP should be done immediately. If the BPP results are reassuring, the CST need not be repeated.

SECTION 10

Biophysical Profile

Table 10-36 Indication for BPP and Suggested Frequency of Testing

Diagnosis	Frequency of BPP/NST	Begin at Gestational Age (weeks)
IUGR or suspected uteroplacental insufficiency	Weekly/twice weekly	28
Diabetes, insulin dependent	Weekly/twice weekly	28
Diabetes, gestational, diet only	Weekly	36
Hypertension, chronic	Weekly	34–36
Hypertension, uncontrolled, PIH	Weekly/twice weekly	28
Twins, normal growth	Weekly	34–36
Twins, discordant growth	Weekly/twice weekly	28
PROM	Twice weekly or daily	Onset of PROM
Previous loss	Weekly	34 (or 2 wks earlier than previous loss occurred)
Postdates ≥41 weeks	Twice weekly	40–41

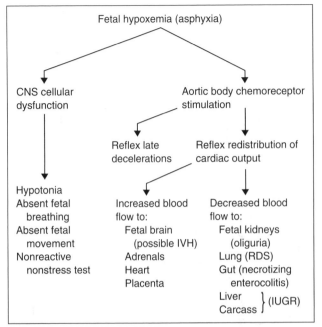

Figure 10-9   Biophysical effects of hypoxia on the fetus.

CNS: central nervous system; IUGR: intrauterine growth retardation; IVH: intraventricular hemorrhage; RDS: respiratory distress syndrome

Source: Druzin, M. L. (1992). *Antepartum fetal assessment.* Boston: Blackwell Scientific. Reprinted by permission.

Table 10-37 Manning Criteria for Biophysical Profile (BPP) Scoring

Biophysical Variable	Normal (Score = 2)	Abnormal (Score = 0)
Fetal tone	At least one episode of active extension with return to flexion of fetal limb(s) or trunk; opening and closing of hand considered normal tone	Either slow extension with return to partial flexion or movement of limb in full extension or absent fetal movement, or partially open fetal hand.
Gross body movement	Two or more discrete body/limb movements in 30 min (episodes of active continuous movement considered a single movement)	Less than two episodes of body/limb movements in 30 min
Fetal breathing movements	At least one episode of ≥ 20 sec duration in 30 min observation	No episode of ≥ 20 sec duration in 30 min
Reactive fetal heart rate	At least two episodes of acceleration of ≥ 15 bpm and >15 sec duration in 20 min	One or no accelerations or acceleration <15 bpm in 20 min
Amniotic fluid volume	At least one pocket of amniotic fluid measuring ≥ 2 cm in vertical axis	Either no amniotic fluid pockets or a pocket < 2 cm in vertical axis

Source: Manning, F. A. (1999). Fetal biophysical profile. *Obstet Gynecol Clin North Am., 26,* 560. Reprinted by permission.

Table 10-38 Obstetrical Management Based on BPP Results

BPP Score	Interpretation	Percent Risk of Asphyxia (umbilical venous blood pH 7.25)	Risk of Fetal Death (per 1000/week)	Recommended Management
10/10	Nonasphyxiated	0	0.565	Conservative management
8/10 (normal AFV)	Nonasphyxiated	0	0.565	Conservative management
8/8 (NST not done)	Nonasphyxiated	0	0.565	Conservative management
8/10 (decreased AFV)	Chronic compensated asphyxia	5–10	20–30	If mature (> 37 wks), deliver; serial testing (twice weekly) in the immature fetus
6/10 (normal AFV)	Possible acute asphyxia	0	50	If mature (> 37 wks), deliver; repeat test in 24 hr in immature fetus; if < 6/10, deliver
6/10 (decreased AFV)	Chronic asphyxia w/ possible acute asphyxia	>10	>50	Factor in gestational age; if > 32 wks, deliver; if < 32 wks, test daily

BPP Score	Interpretation	Percent Risk of Asphyxia (umbilical venous blood pH 7.25)	Risk of Fetal Death (per 1000/week)	Recommended Management
4/10 (normal AFV)	Acute asphyxia likely	36	115	Factor in gestational age; if > 32 wks, deliver; if < 32 wks, test daily
4/10 (decreased AFV)	Chronic asphyxia w/ acute asphyxia likely	>36	>115	If > 26 wks, deliver
2/10 (normal AFV)	Acute asphyxia nearly certain	73	220	If > 26 wks, deliver
0/10	Gross severe asphyxia	100	550	If > 26 wks, deliver

Source: Manning, F. A. (1999). Fetal biophysical profile. *Obstet Gynecol Clin North Am., 26,* 565. Reprinted by permission.

Modified Biophysical Profile (NST and AFI)

The reactive NST = 2 points

Reactivity proves the fetus is moving (2 pts), and has tone (2 pts)

Therefore, the reactive NST is equivalent to a BPP score of 6

Amniotic fluid index (AFI) of >5.0 cms = 2 pts

A reactive NST plus an AFI > 5.0 has the same predictive value as a BPP score of 8/10.

If the NST is nonreactive or the AFI is < 5.0, a full BPP must be done.

Amniotic Fluid Volume

Table 10-39   Procedure for Performing an Amniotic Fluid Index

---

1. Place woman in supine position with slight left tilt.
2. Identify four quadrants of maternal abdomen.
3. Scan with the transducer placed perpendicular to the floor, aligned longitudinally with the maternal spine.
4. Measure vertical depth of largest clear pocket of amniotic fluid in each quadrant.

Note: The AFI is equal to the sum of the four quadrants.

Normal Values for AFI at term

Rule of Thumb at term

< 5.0 cm = oligohydramnios
>23.0 cm = polyhydramnios

References

Varney, H., Kriebs, J. M., & Gegor, C. L. (2003). *Varney's Midwifery* (4th ed.). Sudbury, MA: Jones and Bartlett Publishers. Ch. 5, 6, 9, 21, 22, 23, 24, 53.

American College of Nurse-Midwives. (1996). *Limited obstetrical ultrasound in the third trimester.* Clinical bulletin. Washington, DC: ACNM.

American College of Nurse-Midwives. (1997). *Early-onset group B strep infection in newborns: Prevention and prophylaxis.* Clinical bulletin No. 2. Washington, DC: ACNM.

Bauman, P., McFarlin, B. (1994). Prenatal diagnosis. *J Nurse-Midwifery, 39,* suppl, 37.

Centers for Disease Control and Prevention. (2004). *Guidelines for vaccinating pregnant women: From recommendations of the advisory committee on immunization practices.* Accessed online at: http://www.cdc.gov/nip/publications/preg_guide.htm.

Centers for Disease Control and Prevention, National Center for Infectious Diseases. (2004). *Travelers' health: Pregnancy, breast feeding, and travel.* Accessed online at: http://www/cdc.gov/travel/pregnant.htm#table_6_3.

Centers for Disease Control and Prevention. (2002). Prevention of perinatal group B streptococcal disease. *MMWR Morb Mortal Wkly Rep, 51,* (RR-11), 4.

Cunningham, F. G., Gant, N. F., Leveno, K. J., et al. (2001). *Williams obstetrics* (21st ed.). New York: McGraw-Hill.

Druzin, M. L. (1992). *Antepartum fetal assessment.* Boston: Blackwell Scientific.

Gabbe, S. G., Niebyl, J. R., & Simpson, J. L. (2001). *Obstetrics: Normal and problem pregnancies* (4th ed.). New York: Elsevier.

Gegor, C. L., Paine, L. L., & Johnson, T. R. B. (1991). Antepartum fetal assessment: A nurse-midwifery perspective. *J Nurse-Midwifery, 36,* 157.

Higgins, A. C. (1973). Montreal Diet Dispensary study. In Nutritional supplementation and the outcome of pregnancy. Proceedings of a workshop conducted on November 3–5, 1971. Washington, DC: National Academy of Sciences.

Institute of Medicine, Committee on Nutritional Status During Pregnancy and Lactation. (1990). *Nutrition during pregnancy.* Washington, DC: National Academy Press.

Manning, F. A. (1999). Fetal biophysical profile. *Obstet Gynecol Clin North Am, 26,* 560, 565.

Moore, T. R., Cayle, J. E. (1990). The amniotic fluid index in normal human pregnancy. *Am J Obstet Gynecol 162,* 1168–1173.

National Academy of Sciences. (1990). *Nutrition during pregnancy.* Washington, DC: National Academy Press.

National Institutes of Health. (1984). Diagnostic ultrasound imaging in pregnancy: Report of a consensus development conference sponsored by the national institute of child health and human development. Washington, DC: NIH. DHHS publication NIH 86–667.

National Research Council, Food and Nutrition Board, Commission on Life Sciences. (1989). *Recommended Daily Dietary Allowances* (10th ed.). Report of the Subcommittee on the Tenth Edition of the RDAs. Washington, DC: National Academy Press.

Reynolds, T. M., Nix, A. B., Dunstan, F. D., & Dawson, A. J. (1993). Age-specific detection and false-positive rates: An aid to counseling in Down's syndrome risk screening. *Obstet Gynecol, 81,* 449.

Thomas, R.L., & Blakemore, K.J. (1990). Evaluation of elevations in maternal serum alpha-fetoprotein: A review. *Obstet Gynecol Surv, 45,* 269–283.

US Public Health Service Expert Panel on the Content of Prenatal Care. (1989). *Caring for our future: The content of prenatal care.* Washington, DC: U.S. Public Health Service, Dept of Health and Human Services.

SECTION 11

Antepartum Complications

Spontaneous Abortion (SAB)

Natural termination of pregnancy by expulsion of the products of conception prior to 20 weeks gestation or 500 grams in weight. 10–15% of all clinically diagnosed pregnancies are lost.

Causes

- Genetic abnormality (75-90%)
- Abnormal progesterone levels
- Thyroid abnormalities
- Uncontrolled diabetes
- Uterine anomalies
- Infection
- Autoimmune diseases

Related Terms

Threatened abortion	Vaginal bleeding during the first half of pregnancy
Inevitable abortion	Pregnancy loss is almost certain to occur and cannot be stopped
Incomplete abortion	All products of conception are not expelled with the fetus at the time of the abortion
Missed abortion	Pregnancy is retained for a prolonged period of time following fetal death

Habitual abortion   Spontaneous loss of three or
                           more consecutive pregnancies

Database for First Trimester Vaginal Bleeding
History

- LMP and regularity of menses
- Dates confirmed by exam or sonogram
- Pregnancy test results: urine or blood, date positive
- Previous pregnancy history:
  - Incidence of SAB or ectopic pregnancy
- Contraceptive history
- History of bleeding:
  - Onset
  - Whether continuous or intermittent
  - Amount of bleeding
  - Whether dark or bright red
  - Presence of tissue, clots, or fluid
- Pain or cramping:
  - Onset
  - Location (lower front, right or left side, back, rectal, shoulder, painful breathing)
  - Nature of pain (mild, intense, sharp, dull)
  - Improved or worsened by change in activity?
- Fever or urinary tract symptoms
- Recent UTI or STD
- Change in pregnancy symptoms (worsening nausea, suddenly improved nausea, improved breast tenderness)
- Most recent intercourse:
  - Timing
  - Any impact on pain or bleeding

If the woman is known to the practice and reports that bleeding is slight without abdominal or back pain, she may be seen the next day. Offer instructions for minor first trimester bleeding (see Table 11-1). If she reports moderate or heavy bleeding, lower abdominal, back, or generalized pelvic pain, is febrile or has symptoms of hypotension, recommend immediate evaluation in the office or the emergency room.

Table 11-1   Patient Instructions for Minor First Trimester Bleeding

---

- Rest: There is no requirement to change your activity level but be very aware of symptoms as they occur. If bleeding and/or cramping escalate, try to be in an environment where you can rest, be watchful of any bleeding, and have supportive persons with you. Bed rest has been shown to have no effect on the outcome of the pregnancy.
- Pelvic rest: Do not have sexual intercourse; do not douche or insert tampons or anything else into your vagina (except for progesterone suppositories if you have been using them prior to the bleeding).
- Do not engage in any sexual activity that leads to orgasm; orgasm causes contraction of the uterus.
- Notify the midwife immediately of the following:
  - An increase in vaginal bleeding
  - Lower abdominal cramps or back pain
  - Pelvic pain other than cramping
  - A gush of fluid from the vagina
  - A fever of more than 100.4°F

Physical Exam

Vital signs (BP, pulse, temp)
  Abdominal exam including:

- Palpation for tenderness/pain
- Fundal height or other masses
- Assessment for rebound tenderness
- Bowel sounds (diminished in appendicitis)
- CVA tenderness (pyelonephritis can present with referred pelvic pain)
- Auscultation for FHT if greater than 10 weeks gestation

Speculum examination

- Screen for vaginitis and cervicitis with cultures and a wet prep if indicated.
- Observe the cervical os for dilation, presence of fluid, blood, clots, pus, fetal parts or membranes.

Bimanual examination for

- Uterine size
- Cervical effacement, dilatation
- Adnexal masses or pain
- Cervical motion pain

Laboratory/Imaging Studies as Indicated

- Hemoglobin and hematocrit
- Blood type and Rh factor
- Pregnancy test
- Sonogram
- Serial serum quantitative B-hCG or progesterone
- Vaginal or urine cultures

Serum B-hCG Values

- First positive after implantation of the embryo
- Viable IUPs increase twofold in 48-hours
- Decreasing values are consistent with a nonviable pregnancy
- Values increasing at a slow rate may indicate ectopic pregnancy
- Transvaginal ultrasound should visualize a gestational sac by 1500 mIUs/ml
- Transabdominal ultrasound should visualize a gestational sac by 6000 mIUs/ml

Serum Progesterone Values

- If ≥ 25 ng/ml:
  - Ectopic pregnancy can be ruled out
  - Nearly 100% indicative of a viable IUP
  - If ≤ 5 ng/ml, pregnancy is nonviable; does not rule out ectopic pregnancy
  - If 5–25 ng/ml, further evaluation indicated

First Trimester Ultrasound

- Identifies:
  - Intrauterine vs. extrauterine pregnancy
  - Gestational age (accurate within 5 days)
  - Number of fetuses
  - Cardiac activity (by 6 weeks' menstrual age—once identified, rate of SAB drops to 3%)
  - Adnexal masses (ectopic pregnancy, ovarian cyst, dermoid cyst)
  - Uterine fibroids
  - Presence of fluid in the cul-de sac
  - Subchorionic bleeding—a cause of bleeding without pregnancy loss

- ○ Incomplete abortion with retained products of conception
- ○ Molar pregnancy

Management of SAB

Table 11-2 Management Options for Inevitable Spontaneous Abortion

---

Options if the woman:
- Is in the first trimester
- Does not have excessive bleeding or pain
- Has normal vital signs
- Is not severely emotionally distressed
- Has a hematocrit of at least 30%
- Has no medical contraindications

Option One: Await SAB without medical intervention	**Option Two:** Operative (D&C) termination of pregnancy
Requires presence of another adult	If any assessment data are outside the limits above
Monitor temperature every 4 hours	**or**
Call midwife if:	If the woman prefers medical/surgical termination, arrange for the consulting physician to evaluate the woman and consider completion of the SAB by D&C.
• Temp > 100.4° or chills	
• Soaking through a sanitary pad in ≤ 1 hour	
• Passing clots larger than a 50-cent piece	
Call when abortion is complete	

Incomplete Abortion

Consult MD to complete evacuation of the uterus and to avoid or treat infection.

Missed Abortion

When confirmed, refer for medical management

Habitual Abortion

Refer for:

- Genetic counseling
- Endocrinologic workup
- Exam for anomalies of the genital tract (e.g., bicornuate uterus, vaginal septum)

Follow-up Care:

- Repeat B-hCG in 2 weeks or until levels return to zero
- Support through the grieving process
- Counsel for contraception and future pregnancy planning

Regardless of the category of spontaneous abortion, all postabortal Rh-negative mothers with negative antibody titers should receive Rh immune globulin (e.g., RhoGAM) within 72 hours of the abortion.

Ectopic Pregnancy

Occurs whenever the blastocyst implants anywhere outside the uterine endometrium. 95% of ecotopic pregnancies are tubal. Signs and symptoms vary widely.

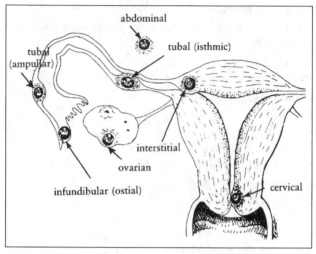

Figure 11-1 Possible sites of an ectopic pregnancy.

Source: The Boston Women's Health Collective (1998). *Our bodies, ourselves.* New York: Touchstone/Simon & Schuster.

Risk Factors

- Pelvic infections
- Intrauterine contraceptive devices
- Previous ectopic pregnancy
- Prior tubal surgery

Early Symptoms

- Vaginal bleeding or spotting
- Mild lower abdominal pain
- Fewer presumptive signs of pregnancy (due to lower levels of B-hCG)

Emergent Symptoms

- Vaginal bleeding or spotting
- Lower abdominal pain ranging from mild to sudden, sharp, stabbing, tearing

- Hypotension and other signs of shock
- Pain in the neck or shoulder due to diaphragmatic irritation from blood in the peritoneal cavity
- Diarrhea and rectal pressure due to irritation from blood in the abdomen

Data collection is the same as first trimester bleeding. Specific signs and symptoms that may allow diagnosis before catastrophic rupture of the ectopic. None of these are diagnostic, nor are they always present.

- Painful pelvic examination; cervical motion
- Palpation of a soft, pliable pelvic mass posterior or lateral to the uterus
- Uterine deviation to the side
- Expulsion of the decidual lining of the uterus (decidual cast)

Laboratory Findings

- Urine pregnancy tests may be negative due to very low B-hCG levels.
- Serum B-hCG levels may be lower than anticipated for gestational age, or serial B-hCG levels will rise slowly.
- White blood cell (WBC) count may be normal or elevated.
- Transvaginal ultrasound examination should identify an intrauterine gestational sac by the time the B-hCG is 1500 mIUs. If no IUP is identified, and/or if there is an extrauterine mass, ectopic pregnancy should be considered.

Management of Ectopic Pregnancy

- Refer for medical management when the midwife confirms or suspects an ecotpic pregnancy.

- Medical management of ectopic pregnancy with methotrexate has diminished the need for surgical intervention and improved preservation of tubal function.
- Surgical intervention can be performed laparoscopically or as an open abdominal procedure depending on the symptoms.

Hydatidiform Mole

This is a genetically abnormal pregnancy with developmental anomaly of the placenta. Placental villi become a mass of clear, cystlike vesicles hanging in clusters from thin pedicles, resembling a bunch of grapes. Usually a benign neoplasm, but has the potential to become choriocarcinoma.

- Complete hydatidiform mole (CHM)—Entirely paternal genetically, usually diploid 46, XX; all vesicles with no fetal tissue apparent
- Partial hydatidiform mole(PHM)—Usually triploid (e.g., 69, XXY), with both villus changes and fetal tissues

Risk Factors

- Age > 45 years
- Asian ethnicity
- Previous molar pregnancy

Symptoms

Rapid growth of abnormal placental tissue causes very elevated B-hCG which may stimulate some symptoms:

- Persistent, often severe, nausea and vomiting
- Vaginal bleeding: spotting or profuse bleeding

- Large-for-dates uterus
- Shortness of breath
- Enlarged, tender ovaries (theca lutein cysts)
- No fetal heart tones
- Fetal parts not evident with palpation
- Preeclampsia or eclampsia before 24 weeks gestation

Management

- Ultrasound is diagnostic for molar pregnancy.
- Once suspected or confirmed, referral to medical management is required.
- Surgical evacuation of the uterus is necessary.
- Follow-up includes serial hCG levels for 6 months to 1 year to assure return to normal and to monitor for possible choriocarcinoma.
- Pregnancy is contraindicated for 1 year following molar pregnancy.

Hyperemesis Gravidarum

Excessive nausea and vomiting during pregnancy of greater intensity and duration than common first trimester nausea and vomiting. Associated with ketonemia, weight loss, dehydration and blood chemistry abnormalities. May occur in any trimester, usually begins in the first and persists in varying degrees throughout gestation.

Signs, Symptoms, and Effects

- Vomiting not controlled by treatment measures for morning sickness
- Pernicious vomiting
- Poor appetite
- Poor nutritional intake

- Weight loss
- Dehydration
- Electrolyte imbalance
- Acidosis due to starvation
- Alkalosis resulting from loss of hydrochloric acid in the vomitus
- Hypokalemia

History

- Frequency of vomiting episodes
- Relationship of vomiting to food intake (amount and type)
- Dietary history (food and fluid choices, amounts, timing, reaction)
- Medication history (medication reactions)
- Elimination (frequency, amount, constipation, diarrhea)
- Blood in vomitus (peptic ulcer or esophagitis produced by repeated vomiting)
- Fever or chills
- Exposure to viral infection
- Exposure to contaminated food
- Abdominal pain
- History of eating disorders
- History of diabetes
- Previous abdominal surgery
- Amount of rest
- Family support
- Anxieties regarding the pregnancy

Physical Examination

- Weight (and relationship to previous weights)
- Temperature, pulse, respirations
- Skin turgor

- Moistness of mucous membranes
- Condition of tongue (swollen, dry, cracked)
- Abdominal palpation for: organomegaly, tenderness, distention
- Bowel sounds
- Sweet odor to breath
- Assessment of fetal growth

Laboratory

- Urine dipstick for ketones
- Urinalysis
- BUN and electrolytes
- Liver function tests (rule out hepatitis, pancreatitis, and cholestasis)
- TSH and T4 (rule out thyroid disease)

Assessment

Poor tissue turgor, dry tongue and mucus membranes, increased pulse and respirations, decreased urinary output, and increased urine specific gravity are all symptoms indicating that the woman is dehydrated. If the urine dip is positive for ketones, the breath has a sweet odor, or she has lost weight, the woman has had too few calories and is acidotic. If there are no symptoms of dehydration or acidosis, the woman may not have hyperemesis.

Management

- IV fluids with 5% dextrose solution at 200 ml/hour for the first liter, then 125-150 ml/hr
- NPO or minimal sips of clear fluid and ice chips
- Initiate oral fluids gradually. If nausea or vomiting resume, revert to NPO. If the fluids are tolerated, increase gradually.

- Dip all urine samples for ketones.
- Once the ketones have cleared, assess maternal status for maintenance.
- Many women will be able to tolerate oral fluids and food after initial IV therapy. Maintenance with oral antiemetics may be recommended.
- If unable to tolerate oral fluids or food after an initial course of treatment, consult the MD.

Table 11-3 Antiemetics for Management of Nausea and Vomiting in Pregnancy

Medication	Pregnancy Category	Route	Dosage	Comments
Pyridoxine (Vitamin B6) Alone or with:	A	Oral	10–25 mg tid to qid	These may be used alone or in combination for treatment of mild nausea and vomiting in pregnancy; available OTC*
Doxylamine (Unisom)	A	Oral	12.5 mg bid to tid and 25 mg qhs	
Diphenhydramine (Benadryl)	A	Oral	25 mg q 4 h prn	Available OTC
Promethazine (Phenergan)	C	IV	25 mg q 4 h	
		Rectal suppository	25 mg q 4 h	
		Oral	12.5–25 mg q 4–6 h	
Prochlorperazine (Compazine)	Not Rated	IM	10 mg q 3–4 h	Use only for severe nausea and vomiting when benefit outweighs risk. Refer to full prescribing literature.
		Rectal suppository	2.5–10 mg q 3–4 h	
		Oral	5–10 mg tid to qid	

Medication	Pregnancy Category	Route	Dosage	Comments
Metoclopramide (Reglan)	B	Oral	10 mg qid	Do not combine with phenothiazines due to possible extrapyramidal effects
Ondasetron (Zofran)	B	IV	5–10 mg q 8 h	For severe nausea and vomiting
		IM	4 mg single dose	
		IV	4–8 mg q 8–12 h, infuse over 15 minutes	
		Oral	4–8 mg q 8 h	
Methyl-prednisolone	C	Oral	16 mg tid for 3 days, then tapered over 2 weeks	For recalcitrant hyperemesis

*OTC = Over the counter

Incompetent Cervical Os (Incompetent Cervix)

Cervical effacement and dilation without pain in the second or early third trimester leading to pregnancy loss.

Risk Factors

- History of fetal loss at 14 weeks gestation or more
- History of cervical laceration
- Overdistension of the cervix with prolonged second stage in a previous pregnancy
- DES exposure
- Previous cervical conization with a large amount of tissue removed

History

- Signs and symptoms surrounding previous loss (e.g., bleeding, abdominal cramping/contractions, suprapubic pain, low back pain, vaginal or lower abdominal pressure, vaginal discharge without signs or symptoms of vaginal infection, ruptured membranes) and when they occurred in relation to delivery
- Gestational age at time of each consecutive loss
- Congenital abnormalities of previously aborted fetuses
- Family history of early fetal loss
- History of cervical trauma with previous delivery
- History of any other cervical trauma or surgery on the cervix

Pelvic Examination

- Speculum examination for:
  - Cervical discharge

- ○ Cervical length
- ○ Evidence of previous cervical laceration
- ○ Observation of any cervical dilation, bulging or rupture of membranes or fetal parts at or through the os
- Bimanual examination for:
  - ○ Consistency and length of the cervix
  - ○ Dilatation of the internal and external cervical os
  - ○ Palpable membranes
  - ○ Position and station of the presenting part

Management

- If there is concern for an incompetent cervix based on history and/or current symptoms, physician consultation is required.
- Based on clinical scenario, medical management may include:
  - ○ Weekly or biweekly vaginal ultrasound to measure cervical length
  - ○ Cervical cerclage

Tuberculosis

Screening

- Screen pregnant women as noted in Table 11-4.
- Screening tests, classification of reactions, and classification of tuberculosis are found in Section 4.

Diagnosis

- All pregnant women with a positive skin reaction should have a chest x-ray with her abdomen shielded.
- Positive radiologic findings should be followed by a series of three sputum cultures for AFB.

- Positive x-ray findings and or positive AFB cultures require medical consultation for treatment.

Management

- Pregnant women must be given adequate therapy as soon as TB is suspected.
- Preferred initial treatment regimen is isoniazid, rifampin, and ethambutol (ethambutol may be excluded if primary isoniazid resistance is unlikely).
- Streptomycin should not be used because of potential harmful effects on the fetus.
- Pyrazinamide should not be used routinely because its effect on the fetus is unknown.
- To prevent peripheral neuropathy, give pyridoxine (vitamin B 6) with isoniazid.
- Breastfeeding during TB therapy is not contraindicated. Women are encouraged to breastfeed their infants. Medication transferred to the infant via breast milk cannot be construed as treatment of the newborn.
- Families of women with a positive PPD should be screened.
- Tuberculosis is a reportable disease.

Table 11-4   High Risk Groups That Should Be Screened for Tuberculosis Infection

Persons at Higher Risk for TB Exposure or Infection

- Close contacts of persons known or suspected to have TB (e.g., those sharing the same household)
- Foreign-born persons, including children, from areas that have a high TB incidence or prevalence (e.g., Asia, Africa, Latin America, Eastern Europe, Russia)
- Residents and employees of long-term residential facilities (e.g., correctional institutions, nursing homes, mental institutions, and shelters for the homeless)
- Health care workers who serve high-risk clients
- High-risk racial or ethnic minority populations, defined locally as having an increased prevalence of TB (e.g., Asians and Pacific Islanders, Hispanics, African Americans, Native Americans, migrant farm workers, or homeless persons)
- Children exposed to adults in high-risk categories
- Persons who inject illicit drugs; any other locally identified high-risk substance users (e.g., crack cocaine users)

Persons at Higher Risk for TB Disease Once Infected

- Persons with HIV infection
- Persons infected with *M. tuberculosis* within the past 2 years
- Persons with medical conditions that increase risk for disease if infection occurs—e.g., diabetes
- Persons who inject illicit drugs; other groups of high-risk substance users (e.g., crack cocaine users)
- Persons with a history of inadequately treated TB

Source: National Center for HIV, STD, and TB Prevention. (2001). *Core curriculum on tuberculosis: What the clinician should know.* Available online at: http://www.cdc.gov/nchstp/tb/ pubs/corecurr.

Hepatitis

Hepatitis can present as an active infection or be identified as a chronic infection through lab studies during routine prenatal care. Refer to Section 4 for identification, treatment, and prevention of hepatitis.

Rubella

The rubella virus is particularly virulent during pregnancy. Infection after 20 weeks rarely causes defects. Effects of rubella in the first trimester include:

- Spontaneous abortion
- Stillbirth
- IUGR
- 52% incidence of fetal transmission and congenital rubella syndrome (CRS):
  - Cataracts
  - Cardiac defects
  - Deafness
  - Glaucoma
  - Microcephaly
  - Other defects of the eyes, ears, heart, brain, and CNS

Screening in Pregnancy

A rubella antibody titer for immunity should be routine at the new OB visit:

- Titer 1:10 or above = immunity
- Titer below 1:10 = non-immune—offer rubella immunization postpartally
- Titer 1:64 or above = suggestive of current infection

Prevention

- Most US cases are in young Hispanic adults born outside the United States.
- Most infants with CRS are born to foreign-born mothers.
- Ensure immunity in women of childbearing age, especially those at highest risk for exposure.
- Determine rubella-immune status of all women of childbearing age.
- Offer rubella vaccination to all nonimmune persons (nonpregnant).

Vaccination Postpartum

Rubella vaccination is not recommended during pregnancy as the attenuated live virus has a theoretical risk of malformations. Offer rubella vaccine to nonimmune women immediately postpartum. Breastfeeding is not a contraindication to vaccination. See Table 10-24.

Cytomegalovirus

Table 11-5   CDC Recommendations for CMV During Pregnancy

1. Practice good personal hygiene, especially hand washing with soap and water, after contact with diapers or oral secretions (particularly with a child who is in day care).
2. Pregnant women working with infants and children should be informed of the risk of acquiring CMV infection and the possible effects on the unborn child.
3. Women who develop a mononucleosis-like illness during pregnancy should be evaluated for CMV infection.

4. Routine laboratory screening is not recommended; however, laboratory testing for antibody to CMV can be performed to determine if a woman has already had CMV infection.
5. Recovery of CMV from the cervix or urine of women at or before delivery does not warrant a cesarean section.
6. The demonstrated benefits of breastfeeding outweigh the minimal risk of acquiring CMV.
7. There is no need to screen for CMV or exclude CMV-excreting children from schools or institutions because the virus is frequently found in healthy children and adults.

Source: Centers for Disease Control and Prevention. (2002). National Center for Infectious Diseases. Cytomegalovirus (CMV) infection. Available online at: http://www.cdc.gov/ncidod/diseases/cmv.htm.

Toxoplasmosis

Table 11-6 CDC Recommendations for Prevention of Toxoplasmosis

1. To prevent toxoplasmosis and other foodborne illnesses, food should be cooked to safe temperatures. A food thermometer should be used to measure the internal temperature of cooked meat to ensure that meat is cooked all the way through. Beef, lamb, veal roasts, and steaks should be cooked to at least 145°F, and pork, ground meat, and wild game should be cooked to 160°F before eating. Whole poultry should be cooked to 180°F in the thigh to ensure doneness.

2. Fruits and vegetables should be peeled or thoroughly washed before eating.

3. Cutting boards, dishes, counters, utensils, and hands should always be washed with hot soapy water after they have contacted raw meat, poultry, seafood, or unwashed fruits or vegetables.

4. Pregnant women should wear gloves when gardening and during any contact with soil or sand because cat waste might be in soil or sand. After gardening or contact with soil or sand, they should wash their hands thoroughly.

5. Pregnant women should avoid changing cat litter if possible. If no one else is available to change the cat litter, use gloves, then wash hands thoroughly. Change the litter box daily because *Toxoplasma* oocysts require several days to become infectious. Pregnant women should be encouraged to keep their cats inside and not adopt or handle stray cats. Cats should be fed canned or dried commercial food or well-cooked table food, not raw or undercooked meats.

6. Health education for women of childbearing age should include information about meat-related and soilborne toxoplasmosis prevention. Health care providers should educate pregnant women at their first prenatal visit about food hygiene and prevention of exposure to cat feces.

Source: Centers for Disease Control and Prevention. (2000). Preventing congenital toxoplasmosis. *MMWR, 49,* (RR02), 55–57.

Varicella

Table 11-7 Management of Care for the Woman with Varicella Based on Patient Exposure or Route of Infection

Exposure/Infection Route	Management of Care
Household member exposed to varicella (e.g., child in day care)	1. Determine history of varicella in exposed household member. 2. Conduct serologic test for immunity in woman. 3. Have woman avoid contact with exposed household member until incubation period ends without evidence of infection.
Direct exposure to varicella (child with varicella infection)	1. Conduct serologic test for immunity. 2. Administer VZIG within 96 hr of exposure if woman's immunity is negative or unknown.
Varicella infection in mother in first 20 weeks of pregnancy	1. Provide symptomatic relief with mild analgesics and antipyretics. 2. If woman is experiencing fulminant disease with high fever, extensive rash, and/or pulmonary symptoms, refer to physician for intravenous acyclovir. 3. Consult MD for ultrasound and possible fetal blood sampling (identify fetal infection).
Varicella infection in mother after 20 weeks but no later than 10 days before delivery	1. Provide symptomatic relief with mild analgesics and antipyretics. 2. If woman is experiencing fulminant disease with high fever, extensive rash, and/or pulmonary symptoms, refer to physician for intravenous acyclovir. 3. Infants will receive passive immunity from mother.

Exposure/Infection Route	Management of Care
Varicella in mother beginning in the period 6 days before delivery	1. Give VZIG to mother. 2. Prepare for the possibility of tocolysis. 3. Give VZIG to infant at birth. 4. May need to isolate infant from mother, even if no maternal rash. 5. Possibly pump breast milk for infant, to minimize infant's contact with any maternal lesions.
Varicella in mother beginning within first 72 hr postpartum	1. Treat infant with VZIG. 2. Treat mother with VZIG if rash has not appeared (may reduce risk of serious infection). 3. Isolate mother and baby together. 4. Pump breast milk for infant, to minimize infant's contact with any maternal lesions.
Exposure of mother/baby to varicella after 72 hr postpartum	1. Determine serologic status of mother (immune mother passes antibodies to fetus/newborn). 2. Treat infant of nonimmune mother with VZIG or notify infant health care provider. 3. Avoid mother/baby contact with infected individual.

Source: Centers for Disease Control and Prevention. (2002). National Immunization Program. Varicella. In *Epidemiology and prevention of vaccine—Preventable diseases* (7th ed.). Atlanta, GA: CDC.

Parvovirus B19 (Fifth Disease, *Erythema Infectiosum*)

Table 11-8   Management of Care of the Woman with Parvovirus B19 During Pregnancy

Symptoms:
- Prior to rash: mild fever, malaise, myalgias, and headache
- Then, flushed red face, with "slapped cheek" pattern
- Symmetric, maculopapular, lacelike, pruritic rash may then appear on the trunk and move peripherally to the arms, buttocks, and thighs.
- Adult women may experience arthralgia and arthritis.
- May rarely cause transient red-cell hypoplasia or aplastic crisis.

Transmission:
- Primarily respiratory secretions
- Exposure to blood or blood products
- Vertical transmission from mother to fetus

Period of greatest contagion:
- Transmission risk highest prior to the onset of symptoms
- Transmission rare after onset of rash
- Once symptoms are present, there is no need for isolation of children or of pregnant women.

Incubation period:
- 4 to 21 days from exposure to onset of symptoms
- Rash and joint symptoms may not appear for 14 to 21 days after exposure.

Risk factors:
- Common in elementary and middle school children
- Spreads easily among family members
- Teachers and other school workers

Diagnosis and management:
- Parvovirus B19-specific IgM and IgG
- IgM antibody indicates infection within the past 2 to 4 months

- IgG antibody indicates previous infection and immunity; no further testing required
- Negative IgG—nonimmune; repeat in 3 to 4 weeks
- Seroconversion—monitor fetus weekly by ultrasound for fetal hydrops, placentomegaly, and IUGR
- Physician consultation

Pregnancy-related course:
- 20–30% percent placental transfer rate
- Affected fetuses may experience aplastic anemia, nonimmune hydrops, and rarely death
- Fetal hydrops is present in 18%; fetal death rate is 3–9%
- Most severe when the infection occurs in the first half of pregnancy
- Congenital anomalies are not associated with parvovirus.

Urinary Tract Infections (UTI)

Identification and treatment of UTIs during pregnancy is critical, as they are associated with preterm labor, low birth weight, hypertension, preeclampsia, and maternal anemia. Minor bladder infections left untreated have a high incidence of developing into pyelonephritis.

- Asymptomatic bacteriuria is a lower urinary tract infection without symptoms that occurs in up to 11% of pregnancies. Urine culture at the first OB visit will identify many of these infections. Screen women with an increased risk of UTIs, e.g., sickle cell trait, sickle cell anemia, or diabetes, with monthly urine cultures. Treatment is the same as for cystitis.
- Cystitis is inflammation of the bladder, usually due to a bacterial infection.

History

Risk factors for lower urinary tract infections:

- History of UTIs
- Sickle cell trait
- Sickle cell anemia
- Diabetes

Symptoms

- Urinary urgency
- Urinary frequency
- Dysuria
- Nocturia
- Lower abdominal (suprapubic) pain
- Hematuria (possible)

Laboratory

- Dipstick urine—for WBCs, nitrates, or protein greater than trace
- Urinalysis—for WBCs, RBCs, bacteria

If either or both of the above are positive, send a clean catch urine for culture and sensitivity.

- Bacteriuria—>100,000 bacteria/ml of the same species

Management of Cystitis
and Asymptomatic Bacteriuria

- Antibiotic therapy can decrease the risk of pyelonephritis, preterm labor, and low birth weight infants.
- If culture results are available, select an antibiotic to which the organism is sensitive.

- If the woman is symptomatic and has a positive dipstick or U/A, begin empiric therapy and make changes if necessary when culture and sensitivities are available (see Table 11-9).
- Repeat urine culture 1 to 2 weeks after completion of antibiotic therapy.
- Group B streptococcus bacteriuria should be treated antepartally and in labor.

Suppressive therapy:

- Maintenance dose of antibiotic for duration of pregnancy (see Table 11-9)
- Use when two courses of treatment have not cured asymptomatic bacteriuria or cystitis
- Monitor with monthly urine cultures

Table 11-9 Antibiotic Treatment of Lower Urinary Tract Infections

Medication	Pregnancy Category	Dosage	Duration	Comments
Amoxicillin	B	500 mg po tid	7–10 days	
Ampicillin	B	250 mg po qid	7–10 days	
Cephalexin (Keflex)	B	250 mg po qid or 500 mg po bid	7–14 days	
Cefuroxime (Ceftin)	B	250 mg po bid	7–10 days	
Nitrofurantoin (Macrodantin)	B	100 mg po qid	7–10 days	Take with food, contraindicated after 36 weeks, and with G6PD
Trimethoprim/ sulfamethoxazole (TMP/SMX) (Bactrim DS)	C	160mg / 800 mg po bid	7–10 days	Contraindicated after 36 weeks, and with G6PD
Sustained release nitrofurantoin (Macrobid)	B	100 mg po bid	7 days	Contraindicated after 36 weeks, and with G6PD
Suppression				
Sustained release nitrofurantoin (Macrobid)	B	100 mg qhs	Ongoing	Contraindicated after 36 weeks, and with G6PD
Cephalexin (Keflex)	B	250–500 mg po qhs	Ongoing	

Acute Pyelonephritis

Pyelonephritis is a bacterial infection of one or both kidneys. It is the primary nonobstetric indication for hospitalization of pregnant women. The complications of pyelonephritis—preterm labor and delivery, adult respiratory distress syndrome, hemolysis resulting in anemia, and septic shock—can be life-threatening for mother and fetus.

Physiologic Risk Factors

- Compression of the ureters at the pelvic brim by the uterus
- Dilatation and decreased tone of the ureters due to hormonal effects (probably progesterone)
- Urinary stasis caused by ureteral compression and relaxation
- Dilatation of the renal pelves and calyces
- Decreased bladder tone and urine stasis in the immediate puerperium

Medical Risk Factors

- Asymptomatic bacteriuria or cystitis
- Sickle cell disease or sickle cell trait
- Gestational or pregestational diabetes

Symptoms

- Fever—temperature usually 100.4°F or above
- Shaking chills
- Hematuria
- Myalgia
- Nausea, vomiting, and loss of appetite
- Urinary urgency, frequency, dysuria due to associated cystitis

- Low back (lumbar) pain
- CVA tenderness
- Generalized abdominal pain
- Suprapubic pain

Laboratory

- Urinalysis
- Clean catch or catheterized urine culture and sensitivity
- CBC with differential

Positive findings include:

- Bacteriuria
- Pyuria-WBCs $\geq$ 10/hpf
- Hematuria
- Proteinuria
- Increased serum WBC and a left shift in the differential

Management

- Consult with the physician for management
- Hospitalization:
  - Intravenous therapy for dehydration and electrolyte imbalance
  - Intravenous antibiotic therapy
- Consider suppression therapy with antibiotics or nitrofurantoin until delivery
- Repeat urine culture at 6 to 8 weeks postpartum

Anemias and Hemoglobinopathies

- Anemia is either a decrease in the number of red blood cells (RBCs) or decrease in concentration of hemoglobin in the circulating blood.

- The usual definition of anemia is a hemoglobin level < 12.0 gm/dl in nonpregnant women and < 10.0gms/dl in pregnant women.
- Physiological changes in pregnancy affect normal blood counts:
  - Increase in maternal blood volume
    - Primarily an increase in plasma volume
    - Small increase in number of red blood cells
  - Disproportion of erythrocytes to plasma causes a lowered hemoglobin level
    - Greatest during the second trimester
  - Plasma volume decreases toward term while increase in RBCs continues

History

- Iron deficiency anemia
- Sickle cell disease
- Self or family history of thalassemia
- Idiopathic thrombocytopenic purpura (ITP)
- Bleeding disorders
- Medications used
- Previous pregnancy with increased bleeding (from episiotomy, cesarean incision, previous blood therapy, or bruising from IV sites)
- Any previous infant with bleeding problems, e.g., after circumcision
- History of HELLP syndrome
- HIV infection (associated with anemia and an ITP-like syndrome)
- Dietary history (e.g., foods with high iron content, pica)

Symptoms

- Often asymptomatic
- Fatigue, drowsiness, malaise
- Dizziness, weakness
- Headaches
- Sore tongue
- Skin pallor, pale fingernail beds
- Pale mucous membranes, e.g., conjunctivae
- Loss of appetite, nausea, and vomiting

Laboratory

- Anemia is a sign of underlying illness rather than a disease entity itself.
- Initial laboratory evaluation determines the red cell size: microcytic, normocytic, or macrocytic.
- Further laboratory evaluation may be necessary to determine the specific anemia within a category (e.g., folate deficiency or B_{12} deficiency in macrocytic anemia).

Table 11-10 Anemias by Red Blood Cell Size Category

Microcytic Anemias (Decreased Red Cell Size)

Iron deficiency anemia

Thalassemias

Hemoglobin E disorders

Lead toxicity

Chronic disease (infection, neoplasm)

Normocytic Anemias (Normal Red Cell Size)

Increased red blood cell loss or destruction

- Acute blood loss

Hemolytic disorders
- Hemoglobin SS disease (sickle cell disease)
- Hemoglobin C disorders
- Spherocytosis
- Glucose-6-phosphate dehydrogenase (G6PD) deficiency
- Acquired hemolytic anemias (medication side effect)
- Autoimmune hemolytic anemias

Decreased red blood cell production
- Aplastic anemia (life-threatening bone marrow failure)
- Chronic disease (liver disease, renal failure, infection, neoplasm)

Overexpansion of plasma volume (pregnancy, overhydration)

Macrocytic Anemias (Increased Red Cell Size)

Vitamin B12 deficiency

Folic acid deficiency

Hypothyroidism

Alcoholism

Chronic liver or renal disease

Medication side effect

Iron Deficiency Anemia

- Accounts for 95% of anemias related to pregnancy
- Microcytic

Risk Factors

- Poor dietary intake
- Chronic blood loss

Management

- Dietary counseling:
  - Iron is more readily absorbed from foodstuffs than from oral iron medication (see Table 11-11).

- Heme iron contained in meat, fish, and poultry is more completely absorbed than iron in plant and dairy foods
- See food sources with high iron content in Section 3.
- Supplement with iron, folic acid (≥400 mcg), and vitamins
  - See Table 11-12 for amounts of elemental iron in frequently prescribed iron preparations.
  - If hemoglobin levels do not increase, ascertain if the woman is taking her iron supplement.
  - Offer dietary or medication changes that may help the woman tolerate iron use.
- Laboratory evaluation—when the hemoglobin falls below 10 g/dl, initiate the following laboratory tests:
  - Complete blood count (CBC) with differential
  - Reticulocyte count
  - Serum iron
  - Serum ferritin
  - Total iron-binding capacity (TIBC)
  - Platelet count
  - Hemoglobin electrophoresis
- If iron deficiency anemia, continue iron replacement and monitor for improvement.
- If another anemia than iron deficiency is suspected, evaluate lab results according to Table 11-13.
- Physician consultation is recommended when iron deficiency anemia is recalcitrant, or if another etiology is identified or suspected.

Table 11-11   Tips to Increase Absorption of Iron

1. Take iron supplements between meals or 30 minutes before meals.
2. Avoid calcium ingestion with iron (milk, antacid, prenatal supplements).
3. Take with vitamin C (orange juice, vitamin C supplement).
4. Cook foods in a minimal amount of water, for the shortest possible time.
5. Eat meat, poultry, and fish—foods in which iron is absorbed and utilized more readily than the iron in other foods.
6. Eat a wide variety of foods.

Table 11-12   Oral Iron Preparations

Preparation	Typical Dose	Elemental Iron/Dose
Ferrous sulfate	325 mg tid	65 mg
Ferrous sulfate, exsiccated (Feosol)	200 mg tid	65 mg
Ferrous gluconate	325 mg tid	36 mg
Ferrous fumarate (Hemocyte)	325 mg bid	106 mg

Table 11-13 Laboratory Diagnosis, Evaluation, and Management of Anemia in Pregnancy

			Management	
Laboratory Test	Result	Interpretation	Additional Data Needed	Treatment
Hemoglobin	<10.0 g/dL	True anemia (hypochromic)	Management based on other indices	
Reticulocyte count	Elevated above 2.5%	Increased marrow activity due to blood loss or hemolysis	Review history for blood loss, hemolysis	
			Order stool for ova and parasites	
	Absent to low (<0.5%)	Marrow failure due to iron or folate deficiency or effect of medications	Review medications for risk of marrow depression side effect	Change medication
				Supplement with iron and folic acid
Mean corpuscular hemoglobin (MCH)	Decreased	Iron deficiency (hypochromic)		Supplement with iron
Mean corpuscular volume (MCV)	Low value MCV <80 ft	Iron deficiency (microcytic)		Supplement with iron

Management

Laboratory Test	Result	Interpretation	Additional Data Needed	Treatment
	High value MCV >95 ft	Confirms iron deficiency if serum ferritin is also low		
		Folate or vitamin B_{12} deficiency (macrocytic)	Order serum folate	If serum folate is low, supplement with folic acid
				If serum folate is high or normal, consider vitamin B_{12} deficiency
				Consult with physician for further evaluation
Serum iron	Elevated slightly	Mobilization of iron stores		Supplement with iron
	Low	Depleted iron stores		Supplement with iron

Test	Result	Interpretation	Action
Serum ferritin	Elevated	Iron overload, inflammatory diseases, alcoholism, inflammatory liver diseases	Consult physician for further evaluation
	Normal or elevated	Chronic disease, thalassemia	Consult MD for further evaluation
	Low	Iron stores depleted	Supplement with iron
Total iron-binding capacity (TIBC)	Elevated	Response to fall in serum iron	Supplement with iron
Platelets	Mild decrease (100,000–149,000/mm³)	Thrombocytopenia Gestational most likely	No treatment needed; Consult physician for further evaluation; Antiplatelet antibody screen, peripheral smear; Recheck platelet counts each trimester, 36 weeks, and in labor
	Moderate decrease (50,000–99,000/mm³)	Thrombocytopenia Gestational most likely	As above; No treatment needed; Consult physician for further evaluation and collaborative management

Management

Laboratory Test	Result	Interpretation	Additional Data Needed	Treatment
	Profound decrease ($<$50,000/mm^3)	Thrombocytopenia Gestational, ITP, HELLP	As above Preeclampsia labs	Medical management
Hemoglobin electrophoresis	AA	Normal		Inform woman
	AS	Sickle cell trait Carrier		Inform woman Genetic counseling Monitor for urinary tract infections
	SS	Sickle cell disease		Inform woman Consult physician for further evaluation and collaborative management

Sickle Cell Trait, Sickle Cell Disease (Hemoglobin S Disease), and Sickle C Disease (Hemoglobin C Disease)

All African American women should be screened for sickle cell trait at the initial prenatal visit with a Sickledex or hemoglobin electrophoresis

Sickle Cell Trait (Hemoglobin AS)

- Recommend sickle cell screening of father of the baby
- If mother *and* father are sickle cell trait positive, or if the father's status is unknown, recommend genetic counseling to rule out sickle cell disease in the fetus.
- Increased risk of urinary tract infections during pregnancy—screen monthly with a urine culture.

Sickle Cell Disease (SS and SC Hemoglobin)

- Pregnancy increases the frequency and intensity of sickle cell crises
- Collaboration with and possible referral to the consulting physician is required

Glucose-6-Phosphate Dehydrogenase (G6PD) Deficiency

- X-linked genetic disease affecting an enzyme (G6PD) associated with red blood cells
- Common in persons of Mediterranean and African descent
- Hemolysis occurs when the individual receives oxidant drugs, e.g., sulfa and sulfa derivatives, nitrofurantoin (Macrodantin), toluidine blue, and methylene blue.

Management

- Avoid drugs (and fava beans) that may cause hemolysis in high risk populations.
- Prompt diagnosis and treatment of infections minimizes the risk of hemolysis.
- Surgery can precipitate an episode of hemolysis.
- Offer genetic counseling and prenatal testing to women with G6PD deficiency.
- Notify the consulting physician if operative delivery is needed or if the woman requests postpartum surgical sterilization.

Thalassemia in Pregnancy

Accurate diagnosis of type of anemia is critical. Take care not to decide that all anemia is related to iron deficiency. With the thalassemias, folic acid supplementation may be useful, but iron supplementation is not indicated and may cause hemosiderosis, an over-accumulation of iron. In addition, genetic counseling is indicated as this is a genetically inherited condition. (See Section 4.)

Gestational Idiopathic Thrombocytopenic Purpura

Thrombocytopenia is a decrease in the platelet count below 150,000/ml. Gestational thrombocytopenia is the most common cause of decreased platelets in pregnancy.

- Increased plasma volume during pregnancy has a slight dilutional effect, but platelets should not drop below 150,000/ml.
- Usually mild (platelets 100,000 to 150,000/ml) with no serious complications for mother or fetus

Immune thrombocytopenic purpura (ITP), thrombotic thrombocytopenic purpura (TTP), and hemolytic uremic syndrome (HUS) are uncommon but must be ruled out when platelets are abnormally low.

Diagnosis

If the platelet count is low, or if there is a history of bleeding problems during previous pregnancies, request:

- Antiplatelet antibody screening
- A peripheral smear
- Coagulation studies

Management

- Consultation with a physician is required.
- Treatment is not usually necessary.
- Rarely, fetal platelets may be depressed:
  - Internal scalp electrodes are not to be used unless the benefit outweighs the risk.
  - Avoid both fetal scalp blood sampling and operative vaginal birth if at all possible.
  - Vacuum-assisted vaginal birth is contra-indicated.

Cardiac Disease

Normal Physiologic Changes of Pregnancy

Antepartum

- Cardiac output increases up to 40%:
  - Increase begins early in pregnancy and peaks by 24 weeks.
- Mean arterial pressure falls in the first trimester, is lowest in second trimester, increases to non-pregnant levels by term.

Intrapartum

- Cardiac output increases almost 50% during contractions.
- Pain and anxiety cause tachycardia and catecholamine response.
- Heart rate, blood pressure, and cardiac output all increase with contractions, with the magnitude increasing as labor progresses.

Postpartum

- Cardiac output is highest immediately postpartum.
- Blood from the uterus is returned to central circulation and can be protective against effects of hemorrhage.
- During the first 2 weeks postpartum, extravascular fluid is mobilized and diuresis ensues.
- Decompensation during postpartum fluid mobilization is common in women with mitral stenosis and cardiomyopathy.
- Unsuspected cardiac disease may be diagnosed postpartum when the woman reports increasing symptoms of pulmonary edema.

When women are vulnerable to cardiac disorders, the stresses of normal physiologic changes may precipitate cardiac decompensation. The midwife must be aware of the signs and symptoms of cardiac disease in order to refer the woman for appropriate diagnosis and management. (See Section 4 for the New York Heart Association (NYHA) Classification of Cardiac Disease.)

Screening for Cardiac Disease in Pregnancy

History

- Known cardiac disease
- Symptoms more pronounced than in normal pregnancy
- Pathologic murmur

Signs and symptoms of cardiac disease in pregnancy

- Palpitations
- Racing heart rate
- Shortness of breath with exertion
- Dyspnea
- Chest pain

Physical Examination Findings

- Systolic flow murmur present in 80% of pregnant women due to increased flow volume in the aorta and pulmonary artery:
  - Grade I or II, midsystolic, heard best at the cardiac base, is not associated with any other abnormal physical exam findings.
  - Normal physiologic split-second heart sound is heard in patients with a flow murmur.
- Any diastolic or systolic flow murmur that is loud ($\geq$Grade 3/6) or radiates to the carotids is abnormal.

Diagnostic Studies

If cardiac disease is suspected:

- Echocardiogram
- Chest x-ray if CHF suspected

Mitral Valve Prolapse

- Most common cardiac disorder in pregnancy
- Incidence up to 12%
- Etiology—genetic, rheumatic heart disease, connective tissue disorders
- Normal course of pregnancy unless complicated by mitral regurgitation, Marfan's or Ehler-Danlos syndrome
- Consider antibiotic prophylaxis (Figure 11-2)
- Systolic "click" murmur
- May develop tachyarrhythmia

Diagnosis

- Echocardiogram to confirm MVP and to rule out mitral regurgitation

Management

Antibiotic prophylaxis is not required for cesarean section or vaginal birth with MVP without mitral regurgitation or thickened leaflets. With additional cardiac complications, or chorioamnionitis or postpartum infection, treat with an antibiotic for eradication of enterococci. If antibiotic prophylaxis is required due to mitral valve regurgitation with mitral valve prolapse or another risk category, refer to Table 11-14 for the drug of choice.

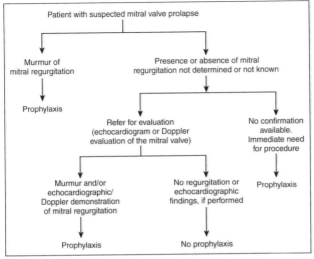

Figure 11-2 Clinical approach to determination of the need for prophylaxis with suspected mitral valve prolapse.

Source: Dajani, A.S., Taubert, K.A., Wilson, W., et al. (1997). Prevention of bacterial endocarditis: Recommendations by the American Heart Association. *JAMA, 227,* (22), 1794-1801. Reprinted by permission of the American Medical Association.

Table 11-14 Recommended Prophylaxis for OB/Gyn Procedures

Risk Status	Medication/Dosage
High	Initial dose within 30 min of starting procedure: Ampicillin 2 gm IM or IV; and Gentamicin 1.5 mg/kg (not to exceed 120 mg) IM or IV
	6 hr later: Ampicillin (only) 1 gm IM or IV
Moderate	2 hr before the procedure:
	Amoxicillin 2 gm orally
	or

Within 30 min of procedure:
Ampicillin 2 gm IM or IV

If Penicillin Allergic

High   To be completed 30 min before procedure:
Vancomycin 1 gm IV over 1–2 hr and
Gentamicin 1.5 mg/kg (not to exceed
120 mg) IM or IV

Moderate   To be completed 30 min before procedure:
Vancomycin 1 gm IV over 1–2 hr

Source: Dajani, A.S., Taubert, K.A., Wilson, W., et al. (1997). Prevention of bacterial endocarditis: Recommendations by the American Heart Association. *JAMA, 227,* (22), 1798. Reprinted by permission of the American Medical Association.

Peripartum Cardiomyopathy

An uncommon cardiac complication that presents in the last weeks of pregnancy through the first month postpartum; can occur in women without risk factors. CNM role is awareness of possible symptoms and early referral for medical examination.

- Incidence—uncommon, but mortality 25-50%
- Etiology—unknown
- Clinical features/signs and symptoms—pulmonary edema, dyspnea, cough, orthopnea, tachycardia, hemoptysis

Diagnostic Criteria

- Heart failure during the last month of pregnancy through 5 months postpartum
- Absence of prior heart disease
- No identifiable alternative cause
- Echocardiographic indication of left ventricular failure

Thyroid Disorders

Table 11-15   Effects of Abnormal Thyroid Levels in Pregnancy

Hyperthyroid

Maternal	*Fetal*
Miscarriage	Neonatal hyperthyroidism
Preterm labor/delivery	IUGR
Congestive heart failure	SGA
Thyroid storm	Prematurity
PIH	Stillbirth
Abruptio placentae	
Infection	

Hypothyroid

Maternal	*Fetal*
Hyperemesis-like syndrome	Congenital malformation
PIH	Low birth weight
Abruptio placentae	Fetal anemia (<26%)
Postpartum hemorrhage	Stillbirth
Postpartum depression-like syndrome	

Diagnosis

Table 11-16   Indications for Thyroid Testing in Pregnancy

Family History
Autoimmune thyroid disease (Hashimoto's disease)

Current Medical Diagnosis
Hypothyroidism with thyroid supplementation
Hyperthyroidism with thyroid suppression
Presence of goiter
Presence of thyroid nodule
Type I diabetes mellitus

Previous History
High-dose neck radiation
Graves' disease (hyperthyroid)
Thyroid cancer
Postpartum thyroid dysfunction
Infant with thyroid disease

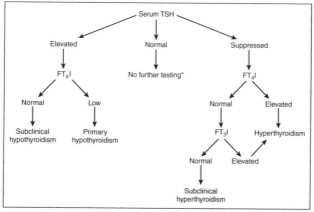

Figure 11-3 Algorithm for the diagnosis of thyroid disease.

Source: From Mestman, J.H. Endocrine diseases in pregnancy. In Gabbe, S.G., Niebyl, J.R., & Simpson, J.L. (2002). *Obstetrics: Normal and problem pregnancies* (4th ed.). New York: Churchill Livingstone. Reprinted by permission.

Management

Consultation is required for abnormal testing results and need for medication. (See Section 4.)

Asthma

Associated with

- Increased perinatal mortality
- Hyperemesis gravidarum
- Preterm delivery
- Chronic hypertension
- Preeclampsia
- Low birth weight infants
- Vaginal hemorrhage

The incidence and severity of these adverse effects may be mitigated by good control. The clinical course of asthma is unpredictable in pregnancy.

- Rule of 1/3s: 1/3 improve, 1/3 worsen, 1/3 are unaffected

Management
Antepartum

Commonly used medications considered to be safe in pregnancy:

Inhaled bronchodilators

- Albuterol (Proventil)
- Metaproterenol (Alupent)
- Terbutaline sulfate aerosol (Brethaire)

Oral bronchodilators

- Theophylline (Theo-Dur, Slo-Bid)
- Terbutaline sulfate (Breathine)

Anti-inflammatory agents

- Beclomethasone (Vanceril, Beclovent)
- Flunisolide (Aerobid)
- Prednisone

Influenza vaccination is recommended.

Upper respiratory infections

- May trigger asthma attacks
- Must be treated aggressively
- Use antibiotics if bacterial infection is suspected

Intrapartum/Immediate Postpartum

- Continue use of regular medications
- To help prevent bronchospasm:
  ○ Adequate hydration
  ○ Adequate pain management

- Avoid morphine and meperidine (Demerol) which can produce bronchospasm
- Management of hemorrhage (see Section 13 for dosages):
  ○ Prostaglandin E2 (PGE2), (dinoprostone)
  ○ Misoprostol (Cytotec)
  ○ Avoid 15-methyl prostaglandin F 2 alpha (PG F2 a (Hemabate, Carboprost, Prostin/ 15M), that may trigger bronchospasm

See Section 4 for more information regarding asthma.

Multifetal Pregnancy

The diagnosis of a multifetal pregnancy must be made as early in pregnancy as possible. This enables the woman to adjust to the situation as well as to optimize the potential for a good outcome.

Incidence, Etiology, and Physiology

2% of all spontaneous pregnancies and an increased number from assisted reproductive technologies are multifetal.

Monozygotic Twins

- From a single, cleaved ovum
- 1/3 of all multiple pregnancies
- 4/1000 births
- Unrelated to age, race, or parity
- May be mono-amnionic or diamnionic
- Perinatal Mortality Rate (PMR) of diamnionic, monochorionic twins = 25%
- PMR of monoamnionic, monochorionic twins = 50–60%

Dizygotic Twins

- Result from 2 fertilized ovum
- Are dichorionic and diamniotic
- PMR is 8.9%
- May be familial connection
- Increased incidence in African Americans
- Decreased incidence in Asian populations
- Increased incidence with age, parity, weight, and height

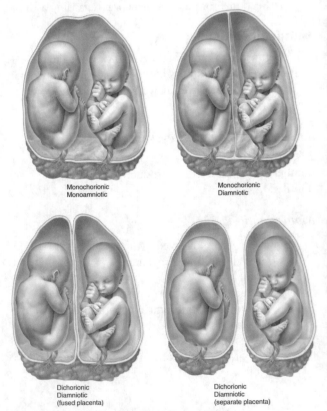

Monochorionic
Monoamniotic

Monochorionic
Diamniotic

Dichorionic
Diamniotic
(fused placenta)

Dichorionic
Diamniotic
(separate placenta)

Figure 11-4 Placentation in twin pregnancies.

Twin gestations are at increased risk for:

Fetal anomalies   Preterm labor and birth
Early pregnancy loss   Gestational diabetes
Stillbirth   Preeclampsia
IUGR   Malpresentation
Placenta previa   Dysfunctional labor

Diagnosis
History

- Familial history of twins
- Use of assisted reproductive technologies
- Severe nausea and vomiting (associated with rapidly increasing hCG levels)
- Episode(s) of vaginal bleeding in this pregnancy

Physical Examination

- Large-for-dates uterine size, fundal height, and abdominal girth
- Rapid uterine growth during the second trimester
- Abdominal palpation of three or more large parts and/or multiple small parts
- Auscultation of more than one clearly distinct fetal heart tone (differing by more than 10 bpm and separate from the maternal pulse)

Laboratory Studies

- MSAFP may be elevated to several times the norm for singleton pregnancies
- Ultrasound is utilized to:
  - Accurately date the pregnancy
  - Determine fetal number
  - Carefully assess fetal anatomy

○ Determine amnionicity and chorionicity of placentation

Management

- Develop a management plan with the consultant physician at the time of diagnosis and at agreed upon times during the pregnancy.
- Anticipate birth in the hospital with the physician present.
- Higher order multiples (triplets and greater) require medical management.

In Addition to Routine Prenatal Care

- Individualize schedule of visits related to course of pregnancy and risk factors identified
- Counsel for maternal nutrition factors critical to the development of the fetuses:
  ○ Add protein and calories for each fetus
  ○ Monitor weight gain, anticipating an average total weight gain of 35 to 45 pounds for the normal weight woman
  ○ Increase iron and vitamin supplementation as needed
- Schedule ultrasound at least monthly beginning at 20 to 24 weeks:
  ○ Assess growth of each fetus.
  ○ Determine placental location.
  ○ Evaluate amniotic fluid volume.
  ○ Measure cervical length and assess for dilation of the internal os.
- Order glucose screening by 26 weeks due to increased risk of gestational diabetes.

- Assess for preterm labor (PTL) at each visit:
  - Review PTL symptoms carefully at each visit.
  - Perform cervical examination as indicated.
  - Modify work load and/or schedules as indicated.
- Encourage adequate rest with one or several rest periods during each day.
- Screen for preeclampsia:
  - Close observation of blood pressure measurement, weight gain, proteinuria, and edema
  - Assessment for headaches and visual changes
- Fetal surveillance:
  - If twins are concordantly grown:
    - Weekly biophysical profile from week 36-38 until birth
  - If discordant growth:
    - Weekly or twice weekly biophysical profile from identification of discordance until birth
    - Referral for consultation and medical management

Polyhydramnios (Hydramnios)

An excessive amount of amniotic fluid.

Etiology

- Most of unknown etiology
- Multiple pregnancy
- Diabetes
- Erythroblastosis
- Fetal malformations:
  - Gastrointestinal tract—e.g., TE fistula
  - Central nervous system—e.g., anencephaly, meningomyelocele

Complications

- Preterm labor
- Maternal dyspnea and shortness of breath
- Fetal malpresentations
- Abruptio placentae
- Cord prolapse
- Uterine dysfunction during labor
- Immediate postpartum hemorrhage

Signs and Symptoms

- Uterine enlargement, abdominal girth, and fundal height greater than gestational age
- Tense uterine wall causes difficulty in palpitation of fetal outline, large and small parts
- Elicitation of a uterine fluid thrill
- Mechanical problems such as dyspnea, lower extremity and vulvar edema; back pain, heartburn, nausea, and vomiting
- Unstable fetal lie
- Decreased maternal perception of fetal movement

Diagnosis

- Obtain an ultrasound:
  - Assess amniotic fluid index (AFI).
    - AFI > 23 cms = polyhydramnios
  - Screen for fetal anomalies.
  - Identify abnormal placental findings.

Management

- Physician consultation is indicated.
- Screen for gestational diabetes (if 28 week screen normal, rescreen at diagnosis of polyhydramnios).
- Screen for Rh(D) isoimmunization.

- Patient education about:
  - Risks for preterm labor
  - Potential cord prolapse with SROM

Oligohydramnios

Abnormally small amount of amniotic fluid; associated with a marked increase in perinatal mortality.

Etiology

- Uteroplacental insufficiency
- Congenital anomalies (e.g., renal agenesis, Potter's syndrome)
- Viral diseases
- Response to indocin as a tocolytic
- Preterm rupture of membranes
- Postmaturity syndrome

Associated Complications

- Fetal hypoxia
- Meconium-stained fluid and meconium aspiration

Signs and Symptoms

- Lagging fundal height
- "Molding" of the uterus around the fetus
- Fetus easily outlined abdominally
- Fetus not ballotable
- Decreased maternal perception of fetal movement
- Multiple fetal heart rate variable decelerations

Diagnosis

- Ultrasound for:
  - Amniotic fluid index (AFI):
    - AFI ≤ 8 cms = borderline at term

- AFI ≤ 5 cms at term = oligohydramnios
- Only single pocket of fluid ≤ 2cms = oligohydramnios
  - Assessment of fetal growth and anatomy
  - Doppler velocimetry
- Physical examination:
  - Rule out rupture of the membranes.
  - Assess fetal position.
- If viral origin is suspected, perform indicated laboratory studies.

Management

- Collaboration with physician consultation
- Biophysical profile with nonstress test for full evaluation of fetal status
- Assessment of maternal hydration
- Assessment of maternal status, e.g., hypertension, diabetes
- Assessment for readiness for labor
- Conservative management may include bed rest, hydration, good nutrition, monitoring of fetal well-being (fetal movement counts, NSTs, biophysical profile, Doppler velocimetry).
- Consider induction of labor, amnioinfusion, and delivery (see Section 14).

Diabetes in Pregnancy

Pregestational Diabetes

Diagnosis of Diabetes Mellitus antedated the pregnancy

- Type I diabetes:
  - True insulin-dependent diabetes mellitus
  - Typically develops prior to adolescence
  - Usually diagnosed prior to pregnancy

- Type II diabetes:
  - Not necessarily insulin dependent; often controlled with diet, exercise, and oral hypoglycemic agents when not pregnant
  - Usual onset is over age 40, less common in pregnancy
- All pregestational diabetics (Type I or Type II) will require insulin during pregnancy and should have medical management.

Gestational Diabetes Mellitus (GDM)

Onset or first recognition occurs during pregnancy. The overall incidence of GDM in the United States is about 7%. Ethnic groups with an increased prevalence include Hispanic, African, Native American, and South or Eastern Asian or Pacific Island women.

Screening

All recommended screening and diagnostic guidelines in this text are from the American Diabetes Association. They are published in: Gestational diabetes mellitus. Clinical Practice Recommendations 2002: Position Statement. *Diabetes Care, 25(suppl)*, 94–96.

Every pregnant woman should be screened for diabetes; first by history taking and, as indicated, by laboratory testing.

History

Criteria for early screening (at the first prenatal visit or when the risk factor first presents).

- Marked obesity
- History of GDM in a prior pregnancy
- Strong family history of diabetes (parents, siblings, grandparents)

- Previous infant > 4000 grams
- History of previous unexplained stillbirth
- Poor obstetrical history (e.g., spontaneous abortions, congenital anomalies)
- Recurrent glycosuria (two positive tests) in clean-catch specimens, not explained by dietary intake

---

Table 11-17 Women for Whom Glucose Challenge Screening Test Is **NOT** Required

---

Women with no identifiable risk factors by history (**ALL** criteria must be met):
- Age <25 years
- Weight normal before pregnancy
- Member of an ethnic group of low prevalence of GDM (white American or Western European)
- No known diabetes in first-degree relatives
- No history of abnormal glucose tolerance
- No history of poor obstetric outcome

When serum glucose values have shown the following results, the diagnosis of gestational diabetes can be made without further screening.
- Fasting glucose ≥ 126 mg/dl **OR**
- Random (nonfasting) glucose sample is ≥ 200 mg/dl

Routine Laboratory Screening

50 gm oral glucose challenge test (GCT) (see Table 11-18). At 26 to 28 weeks gestation:

- Screen all women with no initial risk.
- Rescreen women who had normal screening results early in pregnancy.
- If the results are normal, no further testing is needed unless new risk factors develop.

Further Screening

If secondary risk factors are identified, consider rescreening when these risk factors are first noted.

- Preeclampsia
- Polyhydramnios
- Macrosomic fetus

Table 11-18   Glucose Challenge Test (GCT)

Procedure:

1. Random test (nonfasting)
2. Oral 50 gram glucose solution taken within 10 minutes
3. No eating, drinking (except water), or smoking during the test period
4. Draw a serum glucose level 1 hour after completing the glucose solution.

Interpretation:

Blood glucose level:

≤139 mg/dl	Normal result, no further screening needed
≥140 mg/dl	Send for 3 hour OGTT*
>200 mg/dl	Diagnosis of GDM is made without further testing

---

*OGTT = Oral glucose tolerance test

Note: Some sites use a threshold of 130 mg/dl or 135 mg/dl. Choose a single standard for the practice or facility.

Table 11-19   Procedure for a Three-Hour Oral Glucose Tolerance Test

---

1. Three days prior to the test, the daily intake of carbohydrates must exceed 150 grams (essential for women with a minimal carbohydrate intake).
2. Perform the test in the morning after an 8 to14-hour fast (except water).

3. Draw a fasting blood glucose level.
4. Administer 100 gms oral glucose mixture, to be ingested within 10 minutes.
5. Note the time the solution was completed.
6. At one, two, and three hours, draw a blood glucose level.
7. No eating or drinking (other than water), no vigorous exercise, and no smoking is permitted during the testing period.

Table 11-20 Diagnostic Criteria for Gestational Diabetes

3-hr, 100 g OGTT

Abnormal, or diagnostic for GDM: two or more of the following plasma glucose values are met or exceeded:

Fasting	95 mg/dL
1 hr	180 mg/dL
2 hr	155 mg/dL
3 hr	140 mg/dL

—OR—

2-hr, 75 g OGTT (an alternative diagnostic test)

Abnormal, or diagnostic for GDM: two or more of the following plasma glucose values are met or exceeded:

Fasting	95 mg/dL
1 hr	180 mg/dL
2 hr	155 mg/dL

—OR—

If the screening GCT glucose value is > 200 mg/dL, then the diagnosis of GDM is made without a 2- or 3-hr OGTT.

Note: When processing the serum samples, the vast majority of laboratories will spin the blood down and use the plasma for evaluation of the glucose levels. Therefore, the values used here reflect the norms for plasma. If the testing is done in an office setting using whole blood samples with a glucometer, the normative values should be approximately 15% lower than listed above for plasma samples.

Source: American Diabetes Association. (2002). Gestational diabetes mellitus. Clinical practice recommendations 2002: Position statement. *Diabetes Care, 25 (suppl.),* 1, S95.

Glucose Management

The goal of management of GDM is to maintain a normal fasting blood sugar. Women with GDM should be managed with:

- Medical nutritional therapy (MNT)
- Routine glucose monitoring
- Home finger stick glucose monitoring:
  - Monitoring in the office or laboratory is an acceptable alternative
  - Urine glucose monitoring is not useful
- Mild to moderate exercise

If a woman is unable to maintain her blood sugar values on medical nutrition therapy (MNT), consult a physician to evaluate her need for insulin.

Target blood glucose values for whole blood with a glucose monitor should be:

Fasting	< 95 mg/dl
1 hour postprandial	< 140 mg/dl
2 hour postprandial	< 120 mg/dl

If a laboratory sample is performed with plasma, the values should be:

Fasting	< 105 mg/dl
1 hour postprandial	< 155 mg/dl
2 hour postprandial	< 130 mg/dl

Antepartum Management

- Observe for common complications of GDM:
  - Macrosomia
  - Polyhydramnios
  - Hypertension or preeclampsia
- Fetal movement counting may be initiated by 34 to 36 weeks for diet-controlled GDM.

- At 40 weeks, a biophysical profile should be performed twice weekly until delivery.
- For women with GDM without complications, await spontaneous labor.
- With history of term stillbirth, induction at 40 weeks should be considered.

Management of Labor

- Diet-controlled GDM is no different than normal labor.
- IV glucose solutions should be avoided.
- Carefully evaluate the estimated fetal weight and progress of labor with a higher level of suspicion for shoulder dystocia.
- Inform pediatrics of GDM status due to risk for neonatal hypoglycemia.

Postpartum Management

- With GDM, no further glucose testing is needed in the immediate postpartum period.
- All GDM women should have a 2- or 3-hour OGTT after their 6-week postpartum visit.
- Women with pregestational diabetes should seek preconception counseling.

Rh(D) Isoimmunization

Most humans have an antigen against erythrocyte surface antigen (D). Those with the antigen are Rh(D)-positive. Those without the Rh factor are termed Rh(D)-negative. Rh(D)-negative women will develop antibodies against the Rh factor if it is introduced into the blood. This can occur with a blood transfusion of Rh(D)-positive blood or in a pregnancy with an Rh(D)-positive fetus if fetal blood enters the maternal circulation. The most common time for feto-maternal hemorrhage is at the time of birth (see Table 11-21).

History

- Previous blood transfusion
- Previous baby needing a blood transfusion
- Stillbirth or neonatal death resulting from causes unknown to the mother
- Rh(D) immune globulin required after previous deliveries or abortions
- Known Rh(D)-negative blood type

Laboratory

Order an ABO type and Rh group for all women at the first prenatal visit.

- If the Rh(D) is positive, no further evaluation is necessary.
- If the Rh(D) is negative, refer to results of the antibody screen.
- A normal antibody screen will be negative.
- If anti D antibodies are present—a titer of greater than 1:4—the woman is Rh(D)-sensitized and referral for medical management is indicated.

Table 11-21 Opportunities for Feto-Maternal Hemorrhage and Dose of Rh(D)-Immune Globulin

Cause of Feto-Maternal Hemorrhage	Dose of Rh(D)-Immune Globulin (RhoGAM)
First trimester	
Abortion (spontaneous or elective)	50 μg
Ectopic pregnancy	50 μg
Chorionic villus sampling	50 μg
Second trimester	
Ectopic pregnancy	300 μg
Amniocentesis	300 μg
Second or third trimester	
Blunt abdominal trauma	300 μg
Fetal death, stillbirth	300 μg
Fetal manipulation—e.g., external cephalic version	
Vaginal or cesarean birth	300 μg
Major hemorrhage—e.g., placental abruption, uterine rupture	20 μg/ml estimated fetal whole blood (refer to Kleihauer-Betke)

Management

For women who are Rh(D)-negative, antibody screen negative:

- Rh(D) immune globulin should be given:
  - Routinely at 28 weeks
  - **AND** as indicated in Table 11-21
- The antibody screen is frequently repeated at 28 weeks prior to the dose of Rh(D)immune globulin.

○ This testing is optional, and the results are not required prior to administration of Rh immune globulin.

Placenta Previa

Definitions

Complete placenta previa	The body of the placenta fills the lower uterine segment, entirely overlying the cervical os.
Partial placenta previa	The placental edge covers (totally or partially) the cervical os.
Marginal previa	The edge of the placenta is near, but not actually over the internal cervical os (see Figure 11-5).

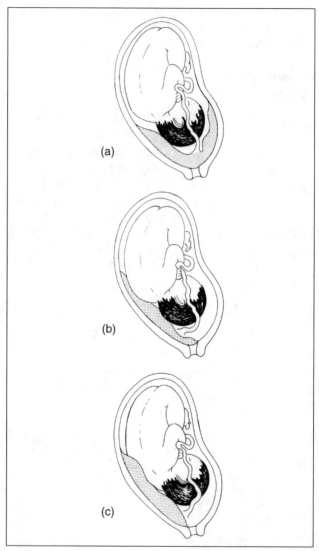

Figure 11-5   Placenta previa: (a) complete; (b) partial; (c) marginal.

Risk Factors

- Multiparity
- Maternal age greater than 35
- Previous placenta previa
- Previous uterine surgery, including cesarean section
- Multiple pregnancy (larger placenta)
- Smoking (possible larger placenta)

Signs and Symptoms

- Painless vaginal bleeding
- Sudden onset of bleeding
- Usually third trimester
- May be associated with uterine irritability
- Malpresentations (breech, transverse lie, floating head)

Diagnosis

- Ultrasound examination
- If a sonogram shows a low-lying placenta prior to 28 weeks, repeat the scan in the third trimester (best 32–34 weeks) after the lower uterine segment has developed.

Management

- If placenta previa is asymptomatic, no intervention is necessary.
- Instruct the woman to call immediately with any evidence of vaginal bleeding.
- Ultrasound at 32–34 weeks should confirm placental location.
- If the placenta is over the cervix at term, vaginal birth is contraindicated.

- If a woman presents with painless vaginal bleeding in the third trimester, *it is imperative that the midwife not perform a vaginal examination until placental position is identified.*
- When bleeding is associated with the placenta previa, management is dictated by the gestational age, severity of bleeding, and fetal status.
- If the bleeding stops and the uterus remains quiet, the woman may be discharged to bed rest at home.
- 24-hour access to emergency transport is required.
- Nothing should be inserted into the vagina (e.g., vaginal therapeutics, douches, penis).
- Sexual stimulation to orgasm is contraindicated.

Abruptio Placentae

Premature separation of the normally implanted placenta is associated with the following conditions:

- Maternal hypertensive disorders
- Advanced maternal age or parity
- Maternal smoking
- Poor maternal nutrition
- Chorioamnionitis
- Maternal blunt abdominal trauma
- History of previous abruptio placentae
- Sudden decrease in uterine volume or size (rupture of the membranes in polyhydramnios or between delivery of babies in multiple gestation)
- External cephalic version
- Cocaine, particularly crack cocaine, usage

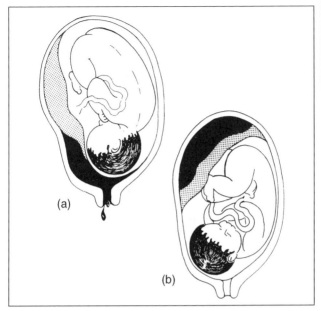

Figure 11-6 Abruptio placentae: (a) marginal separation with obvious bleeding; (b) central separation with concealed bleeding.

Signs and Symptoms

- Depend on the degree of separation. The woman's perception of pain may be out of proportion to what the examiner feels.
- Contractions may be very mild, with generalized back pain and colicky, discoordinate uterine activity alternating with relaxation of the uterus.
- Bleeding may be concealed or obvious.
- Increased uterine tone between contractions.
- Painful localized or generalized uterine tenderness can be present.

- The classic hypertonic, boardlike uterus and uterine rigidity will usually occur only with a large abruption (Grade 2-3).
- The FHR pattern may be normal with a small degree of abruption. A greater degree of separation will produce abnormal FHR patterns with variable or late decelerations, loss of beat-to-beat variability, or a sinusoidal pattern.
- Fetal movements may be decreased or absent for up to 12 hours prior to any obvious signs of an abruption. Or there may be violent fetal movement with a large abruption and massive hemorrhage.
- There may be uterine enlargement with a large concealed hemorrhage and symptoms of maternal shock.
- *Do not think that the blood loss from obvious bleeding is the total actually lost, as there may be concomitant concealed hemorrhage.*

Management of Hemorrhage Due to Placenta Previa or Abruptio Placentae

- Call for help and the physician consultant STAT.
- Start 5% dextrose in Ringer's lactate intravenously with a 16-gauge intracatheter.
- When starting the IV, obtain blood for type and cross-match for four or more units, CBC, platelets, prothrombin, partial prothrombin, fibrinogen, and a tube for clotting time to hang on the wall (see Table 11-22).
- Place the woman in Trendelenburg position.
- Monitor blood pressure, pulse, and fetal heart tones.
- Administer oxygen to the woman.
- Cover the woman with warm blankets.
- Start a second IV. Two intravenous infusion routes are needed: one for electrolyte solutions and the other for blood transfusion.
- Inform the mother and her partner of the emergency nature of treatment as well as possible.need for cesarean birth, blood transfusion, and neonatal resuscitation.
- Have the operating room set up for an emergency cesarean section.
- Insert a Foley catheter to measure output and in preparation for possible surgery.

Table 11-22   Rapid Fibrinogen Assay—Use in the Presence of Hemorrhage for a Rapid Assessment for Coagulation Defect

Draw a red top tube of whole blood.

Tape to the wall; note time of blood draw.

If a clot has not formed in 6 min, or if a clot forms and lyses within 30 min, the fibrinogen level is <150 mg/dl.

Hypertensive Disorders of Pregnancy

Hypertension is the most common medical disorder of pregnancy. The National Institutes of Health, through the National High Blood Pressure Education Program Working Group on High Blood Pressure in Pregnancy, has guidelines for definition and management that are used in this section.

Complications of hypertensive disorders in pregnancy:

Maternal

- Abruptio placentae
- Disseminated intravascular coagulation
- Cerebral hemorrhage
- Hepatic failure
- Acute renal failure

Fetal

- IUGR
- Prematurity
- Fetal death in utero

Definition of Hypertensive Disorders of Pregnancy

Chronic Hypertension

- Observed before pregnancy or by 20 weeks gestation
- High blood pressure is measured as > 140 mm Hg systolic or > 90 mm Hg diastolic.
- If diagnosed during pregnancy but unresolved postpartum, it is chronic hypertension.

Preeclampsia

- A pregnancy-specific syndrome that usually occurs after 20 weeks, except with trophoblastic disease, and can be diagnosed by any of the following criteria:
  - There is gestational blood pressure elevation to ≥ 140 mm Hg systolic or ≥ 90 mm Hg diastolic in a previously normotensive woman, accompanied by proteinuria ≥ 0.3 grams protein in a 24-hour specimen or ≥ 30 mg/dl ($\geq 1+$ reading on dipstick).
  - If gestational hypertension is present without proteinuria, headache, blurred vision, abdominal pain, low platelets, or abnormal liver enzymes suggests the diagnosis of preeclampsia.

Severe Preeclampsia

- Blood pressure ≥ 160 mm Hg systolic or ≥ 110 mm Hg diastolic
- Proteinuria of > 2.0 grams in 24 hours ($2+$ or $3+$ dipstick), occurring for the first time in pregnancy and regresses after delivery
- Serum creatinine increased to > 1.2 mg/dl (unless known to be previously elevated)

- Platelet count < 100,000 cells/ml
- Hepatic enzyme activity elevated (AST, ALT)
- Neurologic symptoms: persistent headache, visual disturbances
- Persistent epigastric pain
- Oliguria ≤ 400 milliliters in 24 hours

Two notable changes have been made from the classic guidelines regarding diagnosis of preeclampsia.

- Edema is no longer considered to be a part of the diagnostic triad for preeclampsia
- Gestational hypertension has been newly stated as being ≥ 140 mm Hg systolic or ≥ 90 mm Hg diastolic after 20 weeks of pregnancy.

Conditions associated with or that predispose to the development of preeclampsia.

- Nulliparity
- Trophoblastic disease (occurs in up to 70% of women with hydatidiform mole)
- Multiple pregnancy, regardless of parity
- Preexisting medical disease:
  ○ Chronic hypertension
  ○ Chronic renal disease
  ○ Pregestational diabetes mellitus
- Family history of preeclampsia or eclampsia
- Previous history of preeclampsia
- Increased risk for multipara with a new sexual partner
- African American or Asian ethnicity

Eclampsia

- Presence of seizure in addition to preeclampsia, if seizures cannot be attributed to another cause

Gestational Hypertension

- Gestational blood pressure elevation to ≥ 140 mm Hg systolic or ≥ 90 mm Hg diastolic
- Previously referred to as pregnancy-induced hypertension
- Onset after 20 weeks without proteinuria or abnormal laboratory findings during pregnancy and returning to normal by 12 weeks postpartum
- Final determination of gestational hypertension versus preeclampsia made only in the postpartum period

Preeclampsia Superimposed on Chronic Hypertension

- Worsens prognosis for mother and fetus
- Any new evidence of proteinuria
- Sudden increase in blood pressure when previously well controlled
- Thrombocytopenia ($> 100,000$ platelets)
- Increase in hepatic enzymes

HELLP (Hemolysis-Elevated Liver Enzymes-Low Platelets) Syndrome

- Controversy as to whether this is a separate syndrome from severe preeclampsia
- Perinatal morbidity similar to severe preeclampsia

History for Hypertension Disorders

- Persistent headaches unresponsive to usual remedies, careful history regarding the headaches and visual disturbances to rule out migraine headaches, need for glasses, and stress.

- Dizziness, blurring of vision, spots before the eyes, or scotomata
- Persistent epigastric pain

Physical Examination

- Blood pressure elevation $\geq$ 140 mm Hg systolic or $\geq$ 90 mm Hg diastolic
- Most accurate blood pressure taken:
  - With an appropriate sized cuff
  - Patient sitting, or lying with left tilt, using right arm approximately at the level of the heart
  - After period of rest
  - Identified on two occasions 4 to 6 hours apart
  - Auscultated to hear last sound for diastolic pressure, not the diminishing sound
- Ophthalmic examination:
  - Papilledema
  - A-V nicking
  - Vessel narrowing
  - Hemorrhagic areas

Laboratory Tests

- Urine for protein followed by 24-hour urine
- Hemoglobin and hematocrit
- Platelet count: if platelets < 100,000 cells/ml, order coagulation studies:
  - Fibrinogen
  - Fibrin split products
  - PT (prothrombin time)
  - PTT (partial prothrombin time)
- Liver function tests
- Renal function tests:
  - 24-hour urine for total protein, creatinine clearance
  - Serum creatinine
  - Serum uric acid

Table 11-23 Interpretation of Laboratory Findings in Preeclampsia

Laboratory Test	Finding	Interpretation	Comment
Hemoglobin and hematocrit	Increased	Hemoconcentration	Fluid moves from intravascular to extra-cellular, causing edema
Platelet count	Decreased	Cause unknown / Reflects severity of preeclampsia	Falling platelets indicate progressive disease <100,000 platelets is severe disease
Serum uric acid	Increased	Decreased renal clearance	Serum uric acid increases as renal excretion of uric acid decreases
BUN	Normal / Increased	Mild preeclampsia / Decrease in renal blood flow and GFR indicates worsening preeclampsia	Doubling of BUN represents 50% reduction in renal blood flow
Serum creatinine	Normal / Increased	Mild preeclampsia / Decrease in renal blood flow and GFR indicates worsening preeclampsia	Doubling of serum creatinine represents 50% reduction in renal blood flow
Creatinine clearance	Decreased	May be normal in mild preeclampsia; decreased in severe preeclampsia	More useful measure than a single serum creatinine value

Laboratory Test	Finding	Interpretation	Comment
Liver function tests	Elevated	Liver cell damage	Serious complication of preeclampsia is subcapsular hemorrhage in the liver
LDH		Indicates severe disease	
AST (SGOT)			
ALT (SGPT)			
Coagulation profile		Abnormal clotting function is indicative of severe disease	
Fibrinogen	Low		
Fibrin split products	Present		
PT	Prolonged		
PPT			
Urine protein (dipstick)	Increased	3+ and 4+ in severe disease	2+ indicates need for 24-hour collection
Urine protein (24-hr)	Increased protein	Renal compromise with increased permeability	300 mg in 24 hr, or 1 g/L in preeclampsia; 5 g/L in 24 hr in severe disease
	Decreased urine volume	Hypovolemia, hypoperfusion, renal compromise	Less than 400–500 mL in 24 hr in severe disease

BUN = Blood urea nitrogen; LDH = lactate dehydrogenase; AST (SGOT) = serum glutamic oxalacetic transaminase; ALT (SGPT) = serum glutamic pyruvic transaminase; PT = prothrombin time; PTT = partial prothrombin time; GFR = glomerular filtration rate

Management

The only cure for preeclampsia is delivery. It is in the mother's best interest to facilitate delivery as soon as possible. However, gestational age may make this a life-threatening risk for the fetus. Therefore, management of preeclampsia is a balancing act between the best interests of mother and infant. If delivery is not indicated for fetal well-being, then the goal of treatment is to mediate maternal condition in order to allow for maturity of the fetus.

When the diagnosis of preeclampsia is made or strongly suspected

- Physician consultation is required.
- Fetal well-being is assessed by biophysical profile. (See Section 10 for discussion of fetal testing with maternal hypertensive disorders.)

If preeclampsia is mild and progressing slowly, the woman may remain at home.

- Modified bed rest
- Home assessment of urine protein
- Frequent office or home visits for assessment of blood pressure and other symptomatology
- Education of woman and family in the signs and symptoms of worsening preeclampsia
- Must be able to access medical attention 24 hours a day
- Must be able to rest and do self-care at home
- She cannot be primarily responsible for child care and care of the home environment
- Ongoing laboratory assessment of hematologic, renal, and hepatic function

If the woman's blood pressure continues to rise, proteinuria progresses, laboratory studies indicate worsening disease, or fetal testing is nonreassuring, hospitalization is required for management of the duration of the pregnancy. The decision to prolong pregnancy must be revisited daily, based on progression of maternal disease and fetal status.

Table 11-24 Indications for Delivery in Preeclampsia

Maternal	Fetal
Gestational age >38 weeks[a]	Severe fetal growth restriction
Platelet count <100,000 cells/mm^3	Nonreassuring fetal testing
Progressive deterioration in hepatic function	Oligohydramnios
Progressive deterioration in renal function	
Suspected abruptio placentae	
Persistent severe headaches or visual changes	
Persistent severe epigastric pain, nausea, or vomiting	

[a]Delivery should be based on maternal and fetal conditions as well as on gestational age.

Source: National High Blood Pressure Education Program Working Group on High Blood Pressure in Pregnancy. (2000). Report of national high blood pressure education program working group on high blood pressure in pregnancy. *Am J Obstet Gynecol, 183*, (1), S1–S22. Reprinted by permission.

Intrapartum

- Dosages and monitoring of magnesium should be managed by the physician.
- Table 11-24 lists indications for delivery based on maternal and fetal risk factors.
- The preferred route of delivery is vaginal in order to avoid the additional stresses and risk of surgery to mother and fetus.

- When the decision is made to deliver, aggressive induction of labor should ensue.
- Epidural anesthesia is the anesthetic of choice for labor or cesarean birth.
- General anesthesia carries increased risks and should be avoided if possible.

Eclampsia

Eclampsia is when preeclampsia progresses to seizures.

- Most common prior to delivery
- May occur up to 10 days postpartum

Premonitory Signs and Symptoms

- Headache
- Visual disturbances
- Epigastric or upper-right quadrant pain
- Restlessness

Emergency Management of an Eclamptic Seizure

- Call for help; notify the physician STAT.
- Observe the seizure, do not attempt to stop it.
- Eclamptic seizures last 30 to 90 seconds, regardless of intervention. Observation is critical to assist with differential diagnosis of the seizure etiology. Eclamptic seizures are generalized tonic-clonic seizures.
- Prevent injury:
  - Put up side rails.
  - Turn the woman on her side to prevent aspiration.
  - Do not restrain the woman except to keep her in bed; forced restraint could result in injury.

- Protect the airway.
- Avoid stimulation of a gag reflex.
- Prepare to administer magnesium sulfate as soon as the seizure is over, or start immediately if the woman has a patent IV. Nothing will stop the current seizure. Magnesium sulfate is the drug of choice to prevent future seizures.

Postseizure Stabilization

- Clear the airway; suction thoroughly.
- Place a soft airway to maintain airway and facilitate suctioning until the woman is conscious.
- Administer oxygen by facemask at 8 liter/min—the woman had no respirations during the seizure.
- Initiate or reestablish electronic fetal monitoring to evaluate fetal status.
- Observe for FHR abnormalities. The fetus may be bradycardic during the hypoxic phase of the seizure, then have a rebound tachycardia, and gradually return to preseizure baseline. A compromised fetus may be unable to tolerate the hypoxic episode, and demonstrate prolonged bradycardia, late decelerations, or sustained severe tachycardia.
- Evaluate contractions and labor status. Contractions usually increase in frequency and intensity for up to 15 minutes following a seizure. If the woman was in active labor when the seizure occurred, her labor may now progress rapidly.
- Examine the woman for injury.
- Document the course of events including timing, specific occurrences associated with the seizure, any interventions, maternal and fetal vital signs prior to and following the seizure, who was notified, and what follow-up actions were taken.

- Refer to medical management, and provide for
  intensive care to help prevent complications such
  as intracranial hemorrhage, pulmonary edema,
  renal damage, and detached retina.
- Expedite delivery based primarily on maternal
  indications. The mother's condition must be sta-
  bilized before induction or cesarean section can
  be considered. When the woman is stable, fetal
  indications for delivery may be considered.
- Management of a woman with eclampsia must be
  by the obstetrician–gynecologist.

Fetal Death

Pregnancy loss in the first half of pregnancy is considered
to be a spontaneous or missed abortion. After the expected age of viability (22 to 24 weeks), it is classified as
a fetal death.

Signs and Symptoms

- Cessation of uterine growth or decrease in uter-
  ine size—fundal height stationary or decreasing
  over time
- Cessation of fetal movement
- Cessation of fetal heart tones—e.g., FHT not
  heard with an electronic monitor
- Cessation of maternal weight gain or decrease in
  weight
- Retrogressive breast changes
- Collapsed fetal skull felt upon examination
- Sonographic signs:
  ○ No heart movement
  ○ No fetal movement
  ○ Overriding skull bones

- Radiologic signs (x-ray ordered if ultrasonography is not available):
  - Spalding's sign—overlapping of the skull bones
  - Exaggerated curvature of the fetal spine
  - Gas formation in the circulatory system of the fetus

Management

- Consult with the physician.
- Decision to induce labor or wait for spontaneous labor depends on:
  - Woman's preference
  - Cervical status
  - Medical issues, e.g., DIC
- Expectant management:
  - Await the onset of labor
  - Monitor coagulation studies
  - Monitor woman's coping
- Emotional support is extremely important.
- Assist the family in decisions regarding autopsy and burial.

References

American Academy of Pediatrics. (2000). Parvovirus. B19 In *AAP 2000 red book: Report on the committee of infectious diseases* (25th ed.). Elk Grove Village, IL: AAP.

American College of Obstetricians and Gynecologists. (1999). Prevention of Rh(D) alloimmunization. *ACOG Prac Bull, May,* 4.

American College of Obstetrics and Gynecology. (2002). Thyroid disease in pregnancy: Clinical management guideline #37. *Obstet Gynecol, 5,* 878–879.

American Diabetes Association. (2002). Gestational diabetes mellitus. Clinical practice recommendations 2002: Position statement. *Diabetes Care, 25(suppl),* 94–96.

American Diabetes Association. (2002). Evidence-based nutrition principles and recommendations for the treatment and prevention of diabetes and related complications. *Diabetes Care.* January, *25(suppl)*, 50–60.

Beckles, G.L.A., & Thompson-Reid, P.E., (Eds.) (2001). *Diabetes and women's health across life stages: A public health perspective.* Atlanta, GA: Centers for Disease Control and Prevention.

Centers for Disease Control and Prevention. (2002). Prevention of perinatal group B streptococcus disease. *MMWR Morb Mortal Wkly Rep, 51(RRII)*, 1–22.

Centers for Disease Control and Prevention. (1998). Measles, mumps, and rubella—Vaccine use and strategies for elimination of measles, rubella, and congenital rubella syndrome and control of mumps: Recommendations of the Advisory Committee on Immunization Practices (ACIP). *MMWR Morb Mortal Wkly Rep, 47*(RR-8).

Centers for Disease Control and Prevention. (2001). Notice to readers: Revised ACIP recommendation for avoiding pregnancy after receiving a rubella-containing vaccine. *MMWR Morb Mortal Wkly Rep, 50*, 1117.

Centers for Disease Control and Prevention, National Center for Infectious Diseases. Cytomegalovirus (CMV) infection page. (2002). Available at: http://www.cdc.gov/ncidod/diseases/cmv. htm. Accessed October 26.

Centers for Disease Control and Prevention. (2000). Preventing toxoplasmosis. *MMWR Morb Mortal Wkly Rep, 49* (RR-2), 57–75.

Centers for Disease Control and Prevention. (2002). National immunization program—Varicella. In *Epidemiology and prevention of vaccine-preventable diseases* (7th ed.). Atlanta, GA: CDC.

Dajani, A.S., Taubert, K.A., & Wilson, W., et al. (1997). Prevention of bacterial endocarditis: Recommendations by the American Heart Association. *JAMA, 227*, 1794–1801.

Gaytant, M.A., Steegers, E.A., Semmekrot, B.A., et al. (2002). Congenital cytomegalovirus infection: Review of the epidemiology and outcome. *Obstet Gynecol Surv, 57*, 245–256.

Gei, A.F., & Hankins, G.D.V. (2001). Cardiac disease and pregnancy. *Obstet Gynecol Clin, 28*, 465–512.

Landon, M.B., Catalano, P.M., & Gabbe, S.G. (2002). Diabetes mellitus. In Gabbe, S.G., Niebyl, J.R., & Simpson, J.L. *Obstetrics: Normal and problem pregnancies* (4th ed.). New York: Churchill Livingstone.

Mestman, J.H. (2002). Endocrine diseases in pregnancy. In Gabbe, S.G., Niebyl, J.R., & Simpson, J.L. *Obstetrics: Normal and problem pregnancies* (4th ed.). New York: Churchill Livingstone.

National Center for HIV, STD, and TB Prevention. (2002). *Core curriculum on tuberculosis: What the clinician should know* (4th ed.). Online version of core curriculum on tuberculosis. Available from http://www.cdc.gov/nchstp/tb/pubs/corecurr. Accessed August 13.

National High Blood Pressure Education Program Working Group on High Blood Pressure in Pregnancy. (2000). Report of National High Blood Pressure Education Program Working Group on High Blood Pressure in Pregnancy. *Am J Obstet Gynecol, 183*, S1–S22.

American Diabetes Association. (2002). Gestational diabetes mellitus. Clinical practice recommendations 2002: Position statement. *Diabetes Care, 25(suppl)*, 94–96.

US Department of Health and Human Services, US preventive services task force. (1996). Screening for Rh(D) incompatibility. *Guide to clinical preventive services* (2nd ed.). Washington, DC: Office of Disease Prevention and Health Promotion.

SECTION 12

Birth in the Home and in the Birth Center

Birth is profoundly affected by the environment in which it takes place. Ideally, every laboring woman and the team that supports and facilitates her efforts to birth work together in an environment that is the most comfortable and safe for the birthing mother. For many women, families, and providers, that safe, comfortable place to birth is in the home or birth center.

Midwives working in the home or birth center have an opportunity to develop the hands-on, low-tech skills that are a hallmark of midwifery. The women are true partners with their midwives to create the process of care.

Characteristics of Birth Center and Home Birth

1. Centrality of the birthing woman is clearly recognized as essential.
2. Consumers are healthy women who are:
   a. Experiencing normal pregnancy
   b. Actively working to promote their own health
   c. Taking a partnership role in decision making
3. Environments are optimal for normal birth
4. Midwife and family have increased authority.
5. Safety is preserved by adherence to essential principles.
6. Complex technologies are kept at a distance.
7. Practices are often owned by midwives.
8. Independence in midwifery practice is fostered.

   9. Bureaucracy is minimized.
   10. Family participation is accommodated.

Safety Characteristics

A wealth of data exists describing safe, healthy outcomes in home and birth center births. Studies show that planned home and birth center births for healthy women with a normal pregnancy are as safe as birth in the hospital with lower rates of obstetrical interventions.

In order to preserve safety at home and in the birth center, it is necessary to adhere to the following essential principles:

- The woman must be committed to actively engage in health promotion.
- The place of birth must be planned before the onset of labor. This includes that the mother's health and the pregnancy are normal when labor begins and preparations for support are in place.
- The attendant must be skilled, able to screen appropriately, provide vigilant care, and manage emergency complications.
- There is a system for access to medical consultation, hospitalization, and emergency transport.

Table 12-1 Influences on Birth Site Selection

	Hospital	Birth Center	Home Birth
1. Normalcy of the pregnancy		X	X
2. Prepregnancy medical history	X	X	X
3. Physical and laboratory findings	X	X	X
4. Decreased chance of infection		X	X
5. Extended time for prenatal visits		X	X
6. Education is core component	sometimes	X	X
7. Low-tech, high touch environment	sometimes	X	X
8. Minimal interruption in activities of daily living			X
9. Support for unmedicated birth maximized		X	X
10. Culturally sensitive environment	sometimes	X	X
11. Qualifications of provider	X	X	X
12. Relationship with provider	X	X	X
13. Previous hospital experience	X	X	X
14. Preferences of family members	X	X	X
15. No separation from baby	sometimes	X	X
16. Children can be included	sometimes	X	X
17. No limitation on persons attending birth	sometimes	X	X

	Hospital	Birth Center	Home Birth
18. Feeling that home environment is unsatisfactory	X	X	
19. Family not responsible for clean-up	X	X	
20. Society's expected birth site	X		
21. Considered safer by general population	X	X	
22. Medication for pain relief available	X	sometimes	
23. Complex technology on site	X		
24. Birth treated as a medical event	X		
25. Managers complicated pregnancy	X		
26. Transport necessary for high-tech interventions		X	X
27. Small intimate environment		X	X
28. Familiar environment	sometimes	X	X
29. Minimal bureaucracy		X	X
30. Cost effective	sometimes	X	X
31. Insurance company limitations	X	X	X
32. Birth takes place outside the hospital		X	X
33. Out-of-hospital alternative for families geographically too far for home birth		X	
34. No trip to or from birth place			X

Source: From BirthCare & Women's Health, Ltd., Alexandria, VA. (2001). Reprinted by permission.

Informed Consent

The midwife and the mother should review and sign an informed consent document detailing the following points:

- Advantages and disadvantages of the decision to give birth out-of-hospital attended by a midwife
- Qualifications of the midwife
- Mother's consent to examination and treatment
- Responsibilities of mother and midwife
- Possible complications of child birth
- Definition of common terms
- Emergency equipment the midwife brings to the home or has at the birth center
- Agreement to hospital transfer if indicated according to the midwife's professional judgment

Shared Responsibility

When a woman plans to birth in the home or the birth center, it is easier to see the connection between her actions and outcomes. She understands that she has responsibilities and that her actions can make a difference.

Midwife Responsibilities

- Explain working in a midwife/client partnership
- Outline responsibilities of the midwife to clarify the mother's expectations
- Provide education, guidance, and health care, with particular emphasis on signs of normalcy and/or signs of deviation from normal
- Discuss the role of the primary support partner
- Make 24-hour midwifery services available
- Describe referral and transport services
- Review resources to cover remuneration to both midwife and consultant in case of transfer

Client Responsibilities

- Participate in basic health promotion including good nutrition, adequate rest and exercise, stress reduction, keeping scheduled appointments, and avoiding drugs, alcohol, and cigarettes.
- Ensure participation of a support partner to take responsibility to be available during pregnancy, labor and birth, and postpartum.
- Provide an adult other than the primary support partner to provide care for children at the birth.
- Prepare for breastfeeding.
- Gather birth supplies.
- Attend childbirth education classes.
- Tour the hospital.
- Arrange for a pediatric health care provider.
- Meet with the physician consultant during the pregnancy if indicated.
- Establish with the midwife a written payment plan including insurance information and a schedule for payments.

Table 12-2 Indications for a Change in Birth Site from Home or Birth Center to Hospital

---

1. Severe chronic hypertension and/or preeclampsia requiring management with medication
2. Current mental illness that the midwife deems would have a harmful effect on the perinatal course
3. Thromboembolic event requiring heparin
4. Current substance abuse including alcohol, cigarettes, and other drugs
5. Insulin-dependent diabetes
6. Clinically significant blood antibodies during current pregnancy
7. Two or more cesarean sections

8. No documented prenatal care
9. Medical indication for induction of labor
10. Placenta previa at term
11. Active preterm labor that cannot be stopped
12. Postdates greater than 42 weeks' gestation
13. Nonreassuring fetal surveillance results
14. Active herpes lesions of cervix, vagina, introitus, labia, or anus during labor
15. Multiple gestation diagnosed before or during labor
16. Persistent noncephalic presentation during labor
17. Febrile condition in labor with or without spontaneous rupture of membranes that does not resolve with hydration
18. Evidence of chorioamnionitis
19. Evidence of fetal intolerance of labor
20. Thick meconium stained amniotic fluid
21. Irresponsible attitude or action of parents
22. Unsafe home or location for birth

Note: The above list is not all-inclusive, and the midwife's clinical judgment may determine that additional conditions indicate a hospital birth. It must also be noted that there are recognized religious communities such as the Amish or Plain people who claim religious exemptions, choosing to give birth in the home or birth center setting even though they have conditions such as breech presentation or multiple gestation. The midwives caring for these women are responsible for acquiring the clinical skills necessary to manage these conditions, for obtaining informed consent from the mother, and for having a consultation agreement in place.

Source: From BirthCare & Women's Health, Ltd., Alexandria, VA. (2001). Reprinted by permission.

References

Varney, H., Kriebs, J.M., & Gegor, C.L. (2003). *Varney's midwifery* (4th ed.). Sudbury, MA: Jones and Bartlett Publishers.

World Health Organization Maternal and Newborn Health/ Safe Motherhood Unit. (1996). Geneva: World Health Organization.

SECTION 13

Care of the Woman at Birth: Intrapartum and Immediate Postpartum Care

Signs of Impending Labor

Lightening, which occurs approximately two weeks before labor, is the descent of the presenting part of the baby into the true pelvis, and is characterized by:

- Decreased shortness of breath
- Increased urinary pressure and frequency
- Pelvic pressure
- Increased edema due to venous stasis
- Cervical ripening
- Increased frequency and strength of irregular contractions
- Loss of mucus plug

Maternal Physiologic Changes in Labor

Table 13-1 Maternal Physiologic Changes in Labor

Physiological Change

Blood Pressure

Rises during contractions with the systolic rising an average of 15 (10–20) mm Hg and the diastolic rising an average of 5–10 mm Hg

Between contractions, the blood pressure returns to its prelabor levels.

A shift of the woman from a supine to a lateral position eliminates the change in blood pressure during a contraction.

Pain, fear, and apprehension may further raise the blood pressure.

Metabolism

During labor, both aerobic and anaerobic carbohydrate metabolism steadily rises. These increases are due largely to anxiety and to skeletal muscle activity.

The increased metabolic activity is reflected by an increase in body temperature, pulse, respirations, cardiac output, and fluid loss.

Temperature

Slightly elevated throughout labor; highest during and immediately after delivery

To be considered normal, this elevation should not exceed 1 to 2°F (0.5 to 1°C). It reflects the increase in metabolism that occurs during labor.

Pulse (Cardiac Rate)

Marked change during contractions with an increase during the increment, a decrease during the acme to a rate lower than that between contractions, and an increase during the decrement to the rate usual for the woman between contractions.

The marked decrease during the acme of the uterine contraction does not occur if the woman is in a lateral rather than a supine position.

The pulse rate between contractions is slightly higher than during the immediate prelabor period. This reflects the increase in metabolism that occurs during labor.

Respirations

A slight increase in respiratory rate is normal during labor and reflects the increase in metabolism that is occurring.

Prolonged hyperventilation is abnormal and may result in alkalosis.

Renal Changes

Polyuria is frequent during labor. It may be the result of a further increased cardiac output during labor and probable increase in glomerular filtration rate and renal plasma flow. Polyuria is less pronounced in the supine position, which has the effect of decreasing urine flow during pregnancy.

Slight proteinuria (trace, 1+) is common in a third to half of women in labor.

Proteinuria 2+ and above is abnormal.

Gastrointestinal Changes

Gastric motility and absorption of solid food are severely reduced. This, combined with a further decrease in the secretion of gastric juice during labor, brings digestion to a virtual standstill and yields a significantly prolonged gastric emptying time. Liquids are not affected and leave the stomach in the usual amount of time. Food ingested during the immediate prelabor period or the prodromal or latent phase of labor will most likely remain in the stomach throughout labor.

Nausea and vomiting are not uncommon during the transition phase marking the end of the first stage of labor.

Hematologic Changes

Hemoglobin increases an average of 1.2 gm/100 mL during labor, returning to prelabor levels the first postpartum day in the absence of abnormal blood loss.

Blood coagulation time decreases and there is a further increase in plasma fibrinogen during labor.

The white blood cell count progressively increases throughout the first stage of labor by about 5000 to an average total WBC count of 15,000 at the time of complete dilatation. There is no further increase after this.

Blood sugar decreases during labor, dropping markedly in prolonged and difficult labors, most likely as a result of the increase in activity of the uterine and skeletal muscles.

SECTION 13

Diagnosis of Labor

- Labor is defined as uterine contractions, increasing in frequency, length and intensity, and leading to cervical change.
- False labor consists of short, irregular contractions; the pattern does not change over time or with activity and produces no cervical change.
- Prolonged prodromal labor is the condition in which regular contractions persist and may intensify over time with minimal cervical change. This condition can be managed with rest, as for prolonged latent phase labor.

Admission Evaluation

History

Chief complaint (labor, ruptured membranes, etc.)
HPI

- Maternal age
- Gravity, parity
- Gestational age
- Estimated date of birth and method by which determined
- Membranes status
- Bleeding
- Pain/contractions
- Fetal activity
- Recent food or fluid intake
- Other complaints as described by the woman

The following items can be obtained from the prenatal record when available, and reviewed as necessary with the laboring woman:

- Demographic information
- Allergies

- PFSH for relevant findings, e.g., asthma, diabetes, prior abdominal surgery
- Social history for relevant findings, e.g., family support, substance abuse, education
- GynH for relevant findings, e.g., recurrent STDs, infertility
- Prior obstetric history
  - Gravity, parity
  - Route of births
  - Weight of prior infants
  - Complications of prior pregnancies
- Current pregnancy history
  - Timing of initial visit, total visits, pattern of visits
  - Weight gain, height, blood pressure range
  - Fetal growth curve
  - Any abnormalities noted during visits
  - Complications of pregnancy
  - Laboratory values

Physical Examination

In addition to a standard medical examination, the following obstetric examination should be performed:

- Abdominally
  - Fetal heart tones
  - Fundal height
  - Lie, presentation, and position of the fetus within the uterus
  - Estimated fetal weight
  - Contraction pattern and intensity
  - Uterine tone
- Pelvic
  - Vaginal discharge
  - Status of membranes by observation, nitrazine, fern test

- If membranes ruptured, color and quantity of amniotic fluid
- Cervical position, effacement, and dilation
- Fetal lie, station, presentation, position
- Synclitism/asynclitism
- Molding/caput
- Bloody show
- Tissue integrity and muscle strength
- Presence of varicosities or lesions
- Clinical pelvimetry
- Extremities
  - Edema
  - Varicosities
  - Reflexes, clonus
  - Pain

Testing

The number and types of laboratory tests performed when a woman is in labor vary with the setting of birth—both geographic and facility. The following pertain primarily to the hospital setting:

CBC or hemoglobin/hematocrit/platelets
Blood type, Rh factor, and antibody screen
RPR/VDRL
Urinalysis

Additional tests, depending on status of prenatal care, maternal indications, and local custom, may include:

Urine culture
Gonorrhea/chlamydia test
Group B streptococcus (if not previously done)
Herpes culture (for known positive women)
HIV/HbSag

None of these in the second list need be ordered indiscriminately. In most cases, prenatal testing will be available and adequate.

An ultrasound can be performed if necessary to verify fetal viability, number, lie, presentation or position, adequacy of amniotic fluid, placental location, or for a biophysical profile. Admission monitoring of the fetus is found in the section on monitoring during labor.

Assessment of Ruptured Membranes

- Visible pool or drainage of fluid which is clearly not urine
- Vaginal pooling in the posterior fornix, particularly if fluid can be seen coming from the cervical os with Valsalva maneuver
- Nitrazine-positive specimen from either of the above (pH ~ 7.0)
- Fern positive test—plated and dried before examination

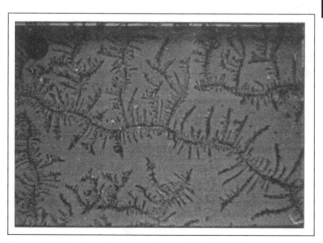

Figure 13-1   Fern pattern of amniotic fluid. *Source:* Reproduced with permission by the College of American Pathologists.

Dilation and Effacement

Dilation of the cervix is assessed at the internal os. It is arbitrarily described in centimeters, with 10 cm being the definition of fully dilated.

Healthy women with cervical dilation less than 4 cm do not generally require admission to the place of birth for observation. Among exceptions to this rule one might include those with a history of fast labor, prolonged prodrome with maternal exhaustion, maternal indications such as diabetes, fetal indications such as low BPS or decreased amniotic fluid, multiple gestations, and in some institutions, rupture of the membranes.

On average, the cervix protrudes into the vagina 4 cm. Effacement may be described as a percentage, with 100% being paper thin, or in centimeters. When describing effacement in centimeters, it is important to remember that the internal length of the cervix can be significantly longer than the externally palpable portion.

Station

Station is assessed in relation to the ischial spines. It is measured from the leading edge of the presenting part. When significant molding or caput has developed, station becomes more difficult to appreciate.

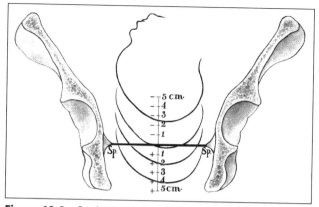

Figure 13-2   Station, or level of descent, of the head of the fetus through the pelvis. The location of the forward leading edge (lowest part of the head) is designated in centimeters above or below the place of the interspinous line. *Source:* From Greenhill, J. P., & Friedman, E. A. (1974). *Biological principles and modern practice of obstetrics.* Philadelphia, PA: Saunders. Reproduced by permission.

Bishop Scoring

Table 13-2   The Bishop Scoring System

Point Value	0	1	2	3
Dilatation (cm)	0	1–2	3–4	>5
Effacement (%)	0–30	40–50	60–70	>80
Station	−3	−2	−1/0	+1/+2
Consistency	Firm	Medium	Soft	
Position	Posterior	Midposition	Anterior	

Source: Adapted from Bishop, E. H. (1964). Pelvic scoring for elective induction. *Obstet. Gynecol, 24,* (2), 267.

Determining Lie, Presentation, Position, and Variety

Lie

The relationship of the long axis of the fetal body to the maternal abdomen, described as longitudinal, transverse, and oblique

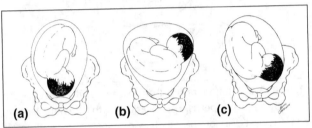

Figure 13-3   Lies: (a) longitudinal; (b) transverse; (c) oblique.

Attitude

Characteristic posture of the fetus

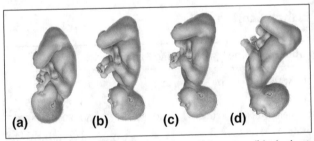

Figure 13-4   Attitude of the fetus in (a) vertex, (b) sinciput, (c) brow, and (d) face presentations.

Presentation

The presenting part is the first portion of the fetus to enter the pelvis and is either cephalic, breech, or shoulder.

Table 13-3 Possible Fetal Relationships to the Maternal Pelvis for Each Lie and Presentation

Lie	Presentation	Arbitrarily Chosen Point on the Fetus	Designation for Position (left or right side) and Variety (anterior, transverse, or posterior portion of the mother's pelvis)
Longitudinal	Cephalic		
	Vertex	Occiput	ROA LOA
			ROT LOT
			ROP LOP
	Sinciput	Sinciput (bregma, anterior fontanel)	Sinciput and brow presentations usually convert to either a vertex or a face presentation.
	Brow	Brow	
	Face	Mentum (chin)	RMA LMA
			RMT LMT
			RMP LMP
	Breech		
	Frank	Sacrum	RSA LSA
			RST LST
			RSP LSP

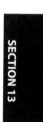

Lie	Presentation	Arbitrarily Chosen Point on the Fetus	Designation for Position (left or right side) and Variety (anterior, transverse, or posterior portion of the mother's pelvis)	
	Full/Complete	Sacrum	Same as frank presentation	
	Footing	Sacrum	Same as frank presentation	
Transverse	Shoulder	Acromion	RAA	LAA
			RAP	LAP
			A transverse variety is not possible.	
Oblique			With an oblique lie, the midwife will feel nothing at the inlet. There is no presentation, position, or variety associated with an oblique lie, which is usually a transitory condition.	

Position

The relationship of an arbitrarily chosen point on the fetus to the maternal abdomen—left or right

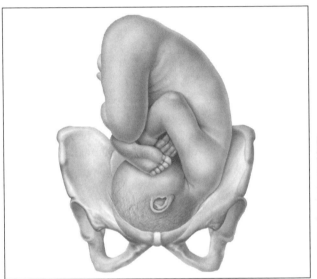

Figure 13-5 Left occiput transverse (LOT).

Variety

The relationship of an arbitrarily chosen point on the fetus to the maternal pelvis—anterior, transverse, posterior

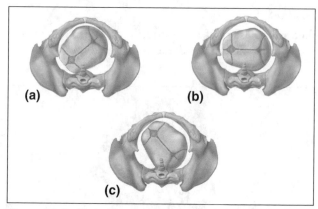

Figure 13-6 Varieties of the cephalic left occipital position, view from below: (a) left occipital anterior (LOA); (b) left occipital transverse (LOT); (c) left occipital posterior (LOP).

The Fetal Head

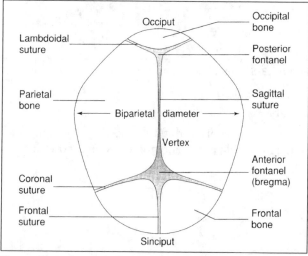

Figure 13-7 Fetal skull: landmarks, bones, fontanels, sutures, and biparietal diameter.

Synclitism/Asynclitism

Entering the pelvis, the fetal head commonly presents in the transverse. Synclitism is determined by the relationship of the sagittal suture to the symphysis and sacrum. The shift from posterior to anterior asynclitism assists the fetal head in descending. Conversely, the fetal head that enters the pelvis with anterior asynclitism experiences more difficulty adapting itself to the pelvis as it descends.

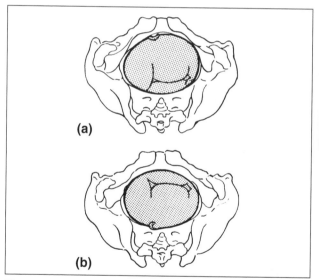

Figure 13-8   Left occiput transverse (LOT).

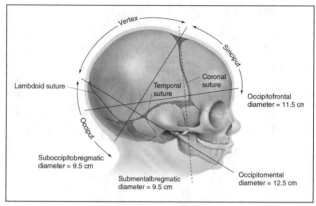

Figure 13-9 Diameters of the fetal head.

Molding

The overriding of fetal skull bones to permit adaptation to the pelvis in labor

Caput Succedaneum

Generalized edema developing over the dependent aspect of the presenting fetal head

Cephalhematoma

Bleeding beneath the periosteum, does not cross sutures

Mechanisms of Labor

The cardinal movements of labor for a cephalic presentation:

- Engagement—BPD passes the pelvic inlet
- Descent throughout
- Flexion
- Internal rotation

- Birth of the head by extension
- Restitution—The first 45° of rotation after the delivery of the head, which returns the head to a right angle with the shoulders
- External rotation
- Birth of the shoulders and body by lateral flexion via the curve of Carus

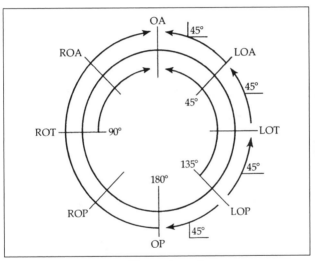

Figure 13-10 Degrees of internal rotation.

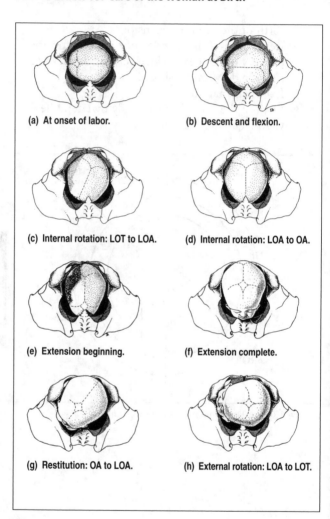

Figure 13-11 LOT to OA mechanisms of labor. *Source:* From Oxorn, H. (1986). *Oxorn-foote human labor and birth* (5th ed.). Norwalk, CT: Appleton-Century-Crofts, p. 159. Reproduced by permission.

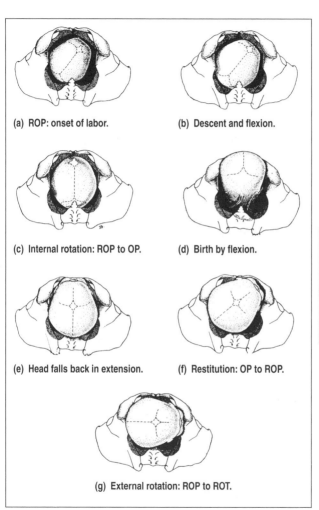

(a) ROP: onset of labor.

(b) Descent and flexion.

(c) Internal rotation: ROP to OP.

(d) Birth by flexion.

(e) Head falls back in extension.

(f) Restitution: OP to ROP.

(g) External rotation: ROP to ROT.

Figure 13-12 ROP to OP short arc rotation mechanisms of labor. *Source:* From Oxorn, H. (1986). *Oxorn-foote human labor and birth* (5th ed.). Norwalk, CT: Appleton-Century-Crofts, p. 173. Reproduced by permission.

SECTION 13

General Course of Labor

Table 13-4   Length of Normal Active Labor for Nulliparas

Author	Mean (hours)	Upper Limit[a] (hours)
Friedman (1956; 1967)	4.9	11.7
(Measured from 3–4 cm to 10 cm)		
Kilpatrick and Laros (1989)		
(Measured from regular, painful contractions q 3–5 min by history to 10 cm)		
No conduction anesthesia	8.1	16.6
With conduction anesthesia[b]	10.2	19.0
Albers, Schiff, and Gorwoda (1996)	7.7	19.4
(Measured from 4 cm to 10 cm)		
Albers (1999)	7.7	17.5
(Measured from 4 cm to 10 cm)		

[a]Mean plus two standard deviations (95th percentile)
[b]Conduction anesthesia: 95% epidurals; 5% saddle blocks

Table 13-5   Length of Normal Active Labor for Multiparas

Author	Mean (hours)	Upper Limit[a] (hours)
Friedman (1956; 1967)	2.2	5.2
(Measured from 3–4 cm to 10 cm)		
Kilpatrick and Laros (1989)		
(Measured from regular, painful contractions q 3–5 min by history to 10 cm)		
No conduction anesthesia	5.7	12.5
With conduction anesthesia[b]	7.4	14.9

Albers, Schiff, and Gorwoda (1996)	5.7	13.7
(Measured from 4 cm to 10 cm)		
Albers (1999)	5.6	13.8
(Measured from 4 cm to 10 cm)		

[a]Mean plus two standard deviations (95th percentile)

[b]Conduction anesthesia: 95% epidurals; 5% saddle blocks

Management Decisions in Labor

Each of these varies with the site of birth, the woman's preferences, the midwife's practice, and other factors. In the home or birth center, some of these decisions have been made as the family plans their birth, simply by their choice of birth site. In the hospital setting, policies vary. Families who have been encouraged during the antenatal period to plan their birth, have discussed the plan with their clinician, and have had their questions answered, will feel more comfortable in any setting.

1. Availability of food, and acceptability of eating and drinking in labor
2. Need for intravenous access
3. Limitations the woman may have in positioning or ambulation
4. Frequency of assessing vital signs
5. Method of assessing fetal status
6. Identification and role of the woman's significant others
7. How frequently vaginal examinations are to be performed
8. When and whether to rupture membranes artificially
9. Medication availability, route of administration, and timing
10. Availability of and desire for epidural anesthesia
11. When to prepare for birth
12. Whether and when physician consultation or collaboration is necessary

Characteristics of the Fetal Heart Rate

Description of the FHR requires both qualitative and quantitative assessment of:

- Baseline rate
- Baseline FHR variability
- Presence of accelerations
- Periodic or episodic decelerations
- Changes or trends over time

Baseline

Mean FHR in 5-beat increments, for at least 2 consecutive minutes of a 10-minute window, excluding periodic or episodic changes, marked variability, and segments of baseline differing by greater than 25 beats per minute (bpm). The normal baseline range is 110–160 bpm. The average changes with gestational age.

20 weeks—155
33 weeks—144
40 weeks—140

Variability

Fluctuations of ≥ 2 cycles/minute, irregular in amplitude and frequency, measured peak to trough. FHR variability is quantified as:

- Absent: Amplitude range undetectable
- Minimal: > Undetectable ≤ 5 bpm
- Moderate: > 5 bpm ≤ 25 bpm
- Marked: > 25 bpm

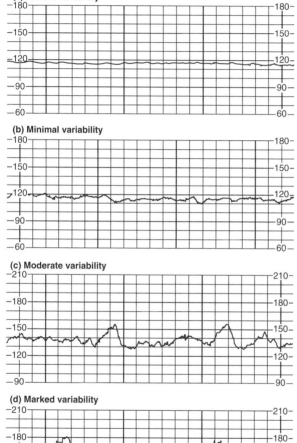

Figure 13-13 Range of FHR variability.

FHR variability is an indicator of CNS maturity and integrity. Decreased variability without decelerations of the fetal heart is rarely associated with hypoxia.

Causes of FHR variability:

- Gestational age
- Fetal behavioral state
- Fetal oxygenation
- Fetal anomalies affecting brain development or function
- Maternal medication

Alterations in Baseline FHR
Tachycardia

Sustained baseline FHR > 160 bpm for > 10 minutes

Causes of tachycardia:

- Fetal
  - Prematurity
  - Congenital anomaly
  - Fetal anemia
- Maternal
  - Fever
  - Medication, e.g., terbutaline, hydralazine
  - Dehydration
  - Hyperthyroidism

Bradycardia

Sustained baseline FHR < 110 bpm for > 10 minutes; if > 80 bpm and with adequate variability, rarely associated with acidemia

Causes of bradycardia:

- Fetal
  - Prolapsed cord
  - Hypoxemia

- ○ Vagal stimulation
- ○ Cardiac anomalies
- Maternal
  - ○ Hypothermia
  - ○ Medications, e.g., propanolol, anesthetics

Assessment

- Duration
- Presence or absence of variability
- Late or prolonged variable decelerations
- Time to delivery
- Presence of prolapsed cord

Periodic changes are those associated with contractions. Episodic changes are those not associated with contractions.

Accelerations

- Increase in FHR above baseline, with onset to peak in < 30 seconds
- Peak is ≥ 15 bpm
- Lasts ≥ 15 seconds and < 2 minutes
- Prior to 32 weeks, 10 bpm × 10 seconds
- These changes are
  - ○ Often coupled with fetal movement
  - ○ Reassuring as to fetal oxygenation and neurologic integrity

Accelerations lasting > 2 minutes and < 10 minutes are considered prolonged.

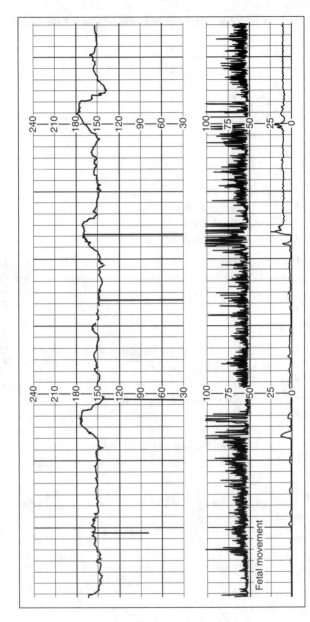

Figure 13-14 Accelerations of the fetal heart rate. Note the correlation with fetal movement.

Decelerations

Early Decelerations

- Physiologic
- Head compression during a contraction →
  decreased cerebral blood flow → hypoxia/
  hypercapnia → hypertension → baroreceptor
  response → parasympathetic stimulated
  bradycardia
- Nadir reached in ≥ 30 seconds
- Follows pattern of contraction, with onset, nadir
  and resolution matching onset, peak and completion of the contraction

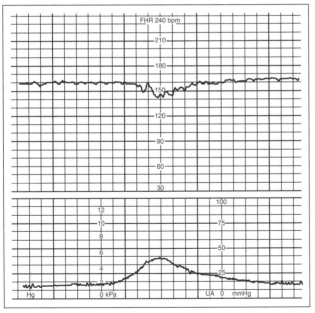

Figure 13-15   Early decelerations. Note that the onset and
nadir are consistent with the peak of the contraction.

Variable Decelerations

- Acute compression of umbilical cord, or fetal head with vagal stimulation → decreased blood flow → fetal hypotension → sympathetic stimulation → release of catecholamines
- Inconsistent onset in contraction pattern
- Irregular in depth and length
- Rapid descent and return of FHR, reaching nadir in < 30 seconds
- Decrease is ≥ 15 bpm from baseline, ≥ 15 seconds and < 2 minutes in length
- May see accelerations preceding and following deceleration
- The duration and depth of decelerations over time define significance

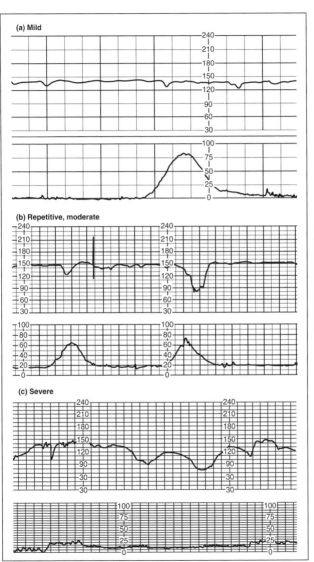

Figure 13-16 Variable decelerations.

Late Decelerations

- Reflect fetal hypoxia
- Initiated near contraction peak with gradual onset (start to nadir $\geq$ 30 seconds)
- Reach lowest point usually within 90 seconds
- Onset, nadir, and resolution lag behind contraction
- Repetitive and persistent *not* an isolated event
- Pattern reflects pattern of contraction

Reflex Late Decelerations

- Caused by acute insult (e.g., maternal hypotension) producing CNS hypoxia when fetus generally has adequate oxygen stores

Nonreflex Late Decelerations

- Generally caused by decreased oxygenation due to decreased placental reserve, thus decreased cardiac function
- Can occur in association with preeclampsia, fetal growth retardation

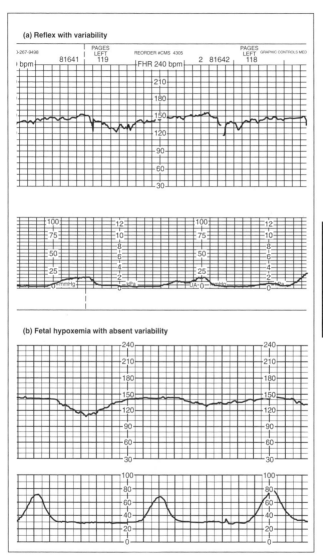

Figure 13-17   Late decelerations.

Nonreassuring Deceleration Patterns

- Are followed by loss of variability, or associated with increasing tachycardia
- Return to baseline slowly in variable decelerations
- Are persistent and late in timing

Recurrent Decelerations

Defined as occurring with more than 50% of the contractions in any 20-minute segment

Prolonged Decelerations

- NICHD—A term used to describe decelerations greater than 15 bpm, lasting ≥ 2 minutes and < 10 minutes
- In contrast, the ACOG definition is 90 seconds duration, with abrupt onset and isolated appearance
- Can be produced by any mechanism that produces transient fetal hypoxia
- May be followed by tachycardia and loss of variability as fetus compensates
- Significance is indicated by frequency, severity, fetal compensation with return to normal pattern

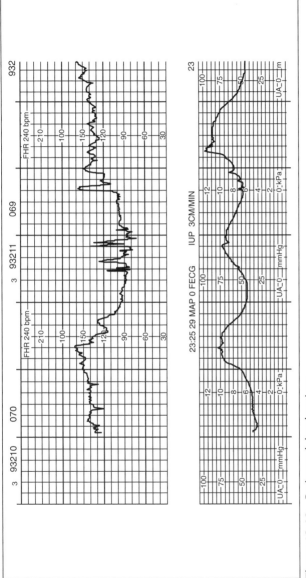

Figure 13-18 Prolonged decelerations.

Sinusoidal Patterns

- Undulating, repetitive, uniform FHR changes unrelated to contractions or fetal activity
- Amplitude of < 15 bpm above and below baseline, lasting at least 10 minutes
- Always nonreassuring
- Associated with
  - Chronic fetal anemia
  - Occasionally, severe fetal hypoxia with acidosis
- Pseudosinusoidal patterns can be associated with maternal medication

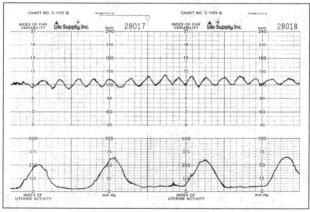

Figure 13-19   Sinusoidal pattern. Courtesy of Nancy McCluggage, CNM, MA.

Wandering Baseline

A late manifestation of progressive fetal hypoxia, always ominous. Cannot determine baseline, FHR range usually 110-160 bpm. Loss of variability.

Monitoring the Fetal Heart in Labor

The functions of monitoring the fetal heart during labor are to assess oxygenation of the fetus and to prevent asphyxia.

Admission Tracings

Often required in hospital setting prior to the institution of intermittent monitoring. Multiple studies have demonstrated no benefit, and a possible increase in the risk of operative delivery.

Intermittent Monitoring

Intermittent auscultation of the fetal heart in labor is an effective means of monitoring the healthy, low-risk woman while increasing her ability to choose her own activity level and position in labor. A fetoscope, hand held Doppler, or even an electronic monitor can be used.

SECTION 13

Table 13-6   Guidelines for Intermittent Auscultation

Minimum Frequency of Auscultation

Without risk factors:

    q 30 min in active phase

    q 15 min in 2nd stage

With risk factors:

    q 15 min in active phase after a contraction

    q 5 min in 2nd stage

After establishment of a baseline and regular rhythm, listen for

    30 sec minimum after a contraction.

Also auscultate prior to:

    AROM

    Ambulation

    Immersion in water or shower

    Administration of analgesics/anesthesia

Minimum Frequency of Auscultation

Assess and document FHR following:

   ROM

   Recognition of abnormal uterine contraction patterns

   Expulsion of an enema

   Vaginal examination

   Ambulation

   Evaluation of analgesia and/or anesthesia

Table 13-7   Benefits and Limitations of Intermittent Auscultation

Benefits

Neonatal outcomes are comparable to those with EFM.

Cesarean birth rates are lower.

Technique is noninvasive.

Woman can move freely.

The FHR can be assessed if the woman is immersed in water.

The equipment is less costly than EFM equipment.

Hands-on, individualized care must be provided.

Limitations

The use of a fetoscope may limit the ability to hear the FHR
   (e.g., in cases of maternal obesity or increased amniotic fluid).

FHR variability cannot be detected.

Periodicity of FHR decelerations (variable, late, early) cannot be
   determined.

There is no permanent visual record of the data.

There is a potential need to increase or to realign staff to meet
   the 1:1 nurse-to-patient ratio that is recommended based on
   RCTs that compare auscultation and EFM.

Some women may feel auscultation is more intrusive.

Intermittent monitoring is not the appropriate method of fetal assessment in labor when:

- The mother has received IV pain medication.
- Labor is being induced or augmented with continually administered medications.
- Fetal growth retardation, preeclampsia, or other conditions increase the risk of fetal compromise.
- Auscultation is not clearly audible or cannot be distinguished clearly from the maternal pulse.

Continuous Electronic Fetal Monitoring

Table 13-8   Benefits and Limitations of EFM

Benefits

Recorded data provide for collaborative decision making and education.

Continuous recording is perceived by nursing administrators to decrease need for 1:1 nursing care.

It is an excellent predictor of fetal well-being.

Recorded strip demonstrates FHR and contractions simultaneously.

Some women are reassured with use of high tech.

May offer assistance with coaching to identify onset of contractions.

Limitations

Increased cesarean sections (which then includes increased rates of general anesthesia and infection).

Interrater reliability is poor.

Prevents normal movement, walking during labor.

Creates false sense of security.

There is no consensus on guidelines for interpretation of FHRs.

There is no agreement regarding need for or timing of intervention.

SECTION 13

Terminology is varied and not precise.

Cannot be used in water.

There is increased operative vaginal delivery (forceps and vacuum assist).

Uses expensive equipment.

There is a high false-positive rate for suspected fetal compromise.

Source: Adapted from Schmidt, J. V. (2000). History and development of fetal heart rate assessment a composite. *JOGGN, 29,* (3), 295–305.

Internal fetal heart rate monitoring is recommended when:

The external tracing is not interpretable
The tracing is nonreassuring and delivery is remote

Intrauterine pressure catheters:

Allow assessment of uterine resting tone and contraction strength through Montevideo units
Provide for amnioinfusion

Montevideo units provide a method of determining the adequacy of labor forces.

- Using an IUPC, calculate the difference in mmHg between resting tone and contraction peak.
- Sum all contractions for a 10-minute window.
- Labor is adequate if the average for each 10-minute period is 200 MVU or greater.

Management of Nonreassuring Tracings

These are newly developing patterns in a fetus that has had a reassuring pattern. Communicate with the woman and her family by explaining what is going on, why you are intervening, what the risk is, what can be done.

- Consider whether a cause can be identified which does not increase the risk of fetal hypoxia, such as maternal medication, fetal sleep cycle— do not delay intervention while doing so
- Reposition in side-lying position
- Assess hydration, increase fluids
- Check fetal scalp stimulation, scalp blood sample, or VAS
- Consider EFM if using auscultation
- Consider internal scalp electrode if using EFM
- Notify consultant if no improvement or inadequate improvement

If the pattern is persistent or severe:

- Notify the consultant immediately
- Examine for rapid labor progress or fetal descent, check fetal scalp stimulation, check for prolapsed cord, consider ISE
- Estimate time to vaginal birth based on examination
- Increase IV hydration, without glucose
- Discontinue oxytoxics
- Give terbutaline if indicated for tachysystole or titanic contraction
- Start O_2 by facemask at 8–10 L/min
- Consider amnioinfusion, if the pattern is amenable to that intervention
- Prepare for cesarean if condition worsens

Amnioinfusion

Reasons for use:

- Dilution and removal of meconium in amniotic fluid
- Alleviation of cord compression

Assessment of Acid-Base Balance

Fetal scalp stimulation—15-second rub or pinch of fetal scalp. A positive response of 15 bpm rise in FHR for 15 seconds indicates fetal blood pH $\geq$ 7.20. A negative response is not a good predictor of fetal hypoxia.

Vibroacoustic stimulation—A 3–5-second sound stimulus on maternal abdomen over fetal head. Accelerations with stimulation are associated with pH $\geq$ 7.25.

Fetal scalp sampling—A blood sample taken from the presenting part

- pH > 7.25 reassuring; repeat every 30 minutes until delivery or resolution of nonreassuring tracing
- $\geq$ 7.20 needs repeat in 5 minutes
- < 7.20 requires intervention to deliver

Umbilical Cord Gas Values

Table 13-9   Normal Blood Gas Values of Umbilical Artery and Vein

	Mean Value	Normal Range
Artery		
pH	7.27	7.15 to 7.38
PCO_2	50	35 to 70
Bicarbonate	23	17 to 28
Base excess	−3.6	−2.0 to −9.0
Vein		
pH	7.34	7.20 to 7.41
PCO_2	40	33 to 50
Bicarbonate	21	15 to 26
Base excess	−2.6	−1.0 to −8.0

Source: From Garite, T. J. (2002). Intrapartum fetal evaluation. In Gabbe, S. G., Niebyl, J. R., and Simpson, J. L. (Eds.) *Obstetrics: Normal and problem pregnancies* (4th ed.). New York: Churchill Livingstone, p. 425. Reprinted by permission.

Documentation of Assessment for Fetal Well-being in Labor

- Rate
- Baseline
- Variability
- Accelerations
- Decelerations—type, pattern, depth, duration
- Contraction pattern
- Contraction intensity

Pain Relief in Labor

Techniques for Supportive Care in Labor

Repositioning
Change in activity level
Water—shower or tub
Relaxation techniques—music, exercises, meditation
Controlled breathing techniques
Promoting rest
Maintaining privacy
Explanations of what is happening—validation of
   her experience
Touch—massage technique, back rub, effleurage,
   leaning into a partner
Cool washcloths
Maintaining cleanliness—includes mouth care
Birthing balls or stools, squat bars
Increasing hydration and maintaining an empty
   bladder
Supporting her support people in helping her cope

Table 13-10   Dosing Ranges

Drug	Single Dose and Route	General Timing
Demerol	50 mg IM	Active labor
	12.5–25 mg IV	Active labor
Nubain	10–20 mg SQ or IM or IV	Active labor
Morphine	10–15 mg IM or IV	Prodromal labor or prolonged latent phase
		Hypertonic uterine dysfunction
Phenergan	25–50 mg IM or IV	Early or active labor, or both
Stadol	1–2 mg IM or IV	Active labor
Vistaril	50 mg IM	Early or active labor, or both
Seconal/	100 mg po	False labor
Nembutal	100 mg IM	Early labor

Epidural Anesthesia

Indications for epidural:

- Relief of pain for active labor and for birth
- Cesarean delivery
- Avoidance of general anesthesia during operative procedures
- Need to decrease maternal expulsive efforts
- Decreased fear for some women
- Rest in protracted or difficult labor

Contraindications for epidural:

- Patient refusal
- Patient inability to cooperate
- Skin or soft tissue infection at insertion site
- Coagulopathy

- Uncorrected maternal hypovolemia
- Lack of trained provider to administer anesthesia

Conditions for which consultation is recommended if epidural is a consideration:

- Spinal cord abnormalities, such as spina bifida, scoliosis
- Prior back surgery
- Arthritis affecting the spine
- Preexisting tracheostomy
- Neuromuscular or neurologic disease
- Cardiac disease
- Significant pulmonary disease
- Obesity
- Low platelet count, current anticoagulation therapy
- Preexisting coagulopathy
- Prior anesthesia complications
- Family history of significant anesthesia complications
- Allergy to anesthetics
- Suspected difficult airway
- Patient anxiety

Side effects and complications of epidural:

- Itching
- Nausea/vomiting
- Transient hypotension
- Maternal fever
- Bladder distension
- Postdural puncture headache
- Pain at insertion site
- Very rarely: spinal cord injury 0.00001%, total spinal anesthesia 0.03%, drug toxicity 0.01%

Hand Maneuvers for Birth

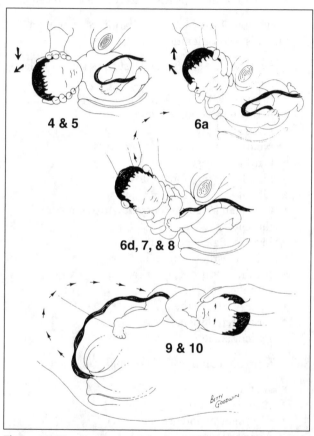

Figure 13-20   Hand maneuvers for the birth of a baby in occipital anterior position with the mother in dorsal position. Numbers correspond with the numbered paragraphs in the narrative text on the hand maneuvers and their rationale, found in Chapter 71 of *Varney's Midwifery*, 4th edition.

Other Anesthetic Techniques for Labor/Delivery/Repair

- Local 1% lidocaine injection
- Pudendal block
- Paracervical block

Third Stage of Labor

Signs of placental separation:

- Uterus rises into abdomen and becomes globular
- Spurt of vaginal bleeding

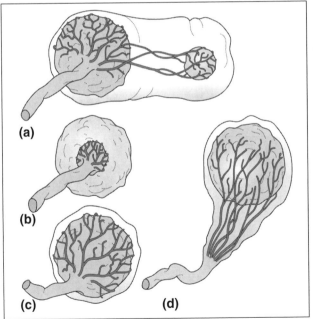

Figure 13-21 Placental abnormalities; (a) succenturiate lobe, (b) circumvallate placenta, (c) marginal cord insertion (battle-dore), (d) velamentous cord insertion.

- Lengthening of umbilical cord

Placental inspection:

- Verify number of vessels—2 arteries, 1 vein
- Verify membranes are complete
- Inspect maternal side for completeness, calcifications, infarcts, tumors or cysts, edema, color, multiple placenta
- Inspect fetal side for cord insertion, cysts, meconium staining

References

Varney, H. B., Kriebs, J. M., & Gegor, C. L. (2003). *Varney's midwifery* (4th ed.). Sudbury, MA: Jones and Bartlett Publishers. Chapters 26–28, 63–75.

SECTION 14

Intrapartum and Immediate Postpartum Complications

Vaginal Birth after Cesarean Section (VBAC)

Vaginal birth after one or more previous cesarean sections (VBAC) is an area of great controversy. While the old adage, "Once a cesarean, always a cesarean" is no longer considered quality care, there is concern for the woman laboring with a previous uterine incision. The absolute risk of a uterine rupture with an attempted VBAC is argued in the literature. Some of this information is summarized in Table 14-1.

Table 14-1 Risk Factors for Uterine Rupture with VBAC

Risk Factors	Potential for Uterine Rupture (number/1000 women)
Spontaneous onset of labor	5.2/1000
vs	vs
Repeat cesarean section without labor	1.6/1000 women

Risk Factors	Potential for Uterine Rupture (number/1000 women)
Induction of labor without prostaglandins	7.7/1000 women
vs	vs
Induction with prostaglandins	24.5/1000 women
Low segment transverse incision	1.9/1000–8/1000
vs	vs
Classical vertical uterine incision	120/1000
Single-layer uterine closing	Double-layer uterine closing may be stronger and have less ruptures than single layer
vs	
Double-layer uterine closing	
Gestational age < 28 weeks without labor	Lower segment undeveloped, so any incision is into the contractile uterine segment

Types of Uterine Rupture from Previous Uterine Scar

- Catastrophic—separation of old incision for most of its length with significant bleeding, rupture of fetal membranes , and all or part of the fetus extruded into the peritoneal cavity
- A traumatic dehiscence (window) in which separation of old incision does not involve entire length, membranes do not rupture, fetus remains in utero, bleeding is minimal or absent

Maternal Increased Morbidity and Mortality Associated with a Repeat Cesarean

- Anesthesia risks
- Inadvertent injury to bowel or bladder

- Hemorrhage
- Wound infection
- Increased newborn respiratory problems

Factors Associated with Higher Success Rate for VBAC

- Nonrepetitive indications (e.g., malpresentation, fetal distress, preeclampsia)
- Spontaneous onset of labor
- Normal progression of labor
- History of previous VBAC

Factors Associated with Repeat Cesarean Section after a Trial of Labor

- Possible recurrent indications for the previous cesarean (e.g., CPD, failure to progress, labor dystocia)
- Use of induction or augmentation
- No prior vaginal birth
- Nonreassuring fetal heart tones on initial labor assessment

First OB Visit for Woman with Previous Cesarean Section

History

- Gestational age at time of cesarean birth
- Type of uterine incision
- Reason for cesarean birth
- Length of labor
- Cervical dilation at the time of cesarean birth

Physical Exam

- Abdominal scar (describe)

Pelvic Examination

- Clinical pelvimetry
- Nulliparous cervix and vaginal introitus if all previous babies have been delivered by cesarean birth

Cesarean Incisions

The abdominal incision is not always the same as the uterine incision

The operative report is the only definitive information regarding the location of the uterine incision, the type of incision and type of closure used. The operative report usually has information regarding the indication for cesarean and the course of labor that may be helpful in decision making.

Management Options

- For a previous classical cesarean section
  - Repeat cesarean birth before the onset of labor
- For a previous low transverse or low vertical
  - Scheduled, elective repeat cesarean birth
  - Elective repeat cesarean birth after the onset of labor
  - Trial of labor for a vaginal birth

Informed Consent

All women who had an incision in the lower uterine segment and have no contraindications should be encouraged to attempt vaginal birth. Available options should be reviewed with the woman and the risks and benefits of a repeat cesarean section versus VBAC should be discussed. Documentation of this discussion should be recorded in the chart. Part of informed consent is that morbidity has been found to be higher in women who attempt VBAC and labor but deliver again by cesarean section than in either women who attempt VBAC and birth vaginally (lowest risk) or women who have an elective repeat cesarean birth.

Midwifery Support

VBAC candidates may require special support:

- Referral to VBAC course or support group
- Exploration of issues of body image, fear of failure, and self-image
- Comparison of the woman's recollection of her labor and reason for the prior cesarean section with her medical records in order to discuss any lack of knowledge or misperception that would lead to unrealistic concerns on her part.

Management of Care of the Woman Planning VBAC

Management of care in labor and for birth is the same as for any woman in labor, except for:

- Monitoring the fetal heart every 15 minutes during the first stage and every 5 minutes in second stage if not using continuous electronic fetal monitoring (the first indication of uterine rupture usually is fetal bradycardia)
- Cautious use of oxytocin for induction or augmentation
- Prostaglandins should not be used for ripening the cervix and misoprostol (Cytotec) is contraindicated.

Uterine Dehiscence or Rupture

See discussion of uterine rupture later in this section.

Management of Third Stage

- Increased incidence of placental implantation over the uterine scar
- Increased incidence of placenta accreta
- In the case of retained placenta, call for assistance from the consulting physician before attempting manual removal of the placenta.

Induction of Labor

Indications for Induction of Labor

Indications include but are not limited to:

- Nonreassuring antepartum fetal testing (see Section 10)
- Oligohydramnios
- Worsening preeclampsia at term
- Insulin-dependent diabetes
- IUGR at term
- History of a previous term stillbirth
- True postdates pregnancy

Contraindications to Induction of Labor

- Preterm (<37 weeks) unless medically indicated
- Placenta previa
- Transverse lie or breech other than complete breech presentation
- Any suspicion of abruptio placenta
- History of classical cesarean section or myomectomy entering the uterine cavity

Table 14-2 The Bishop Scoring System

Point Value	0	1	2	3
Dilatation (cm)	0	1–2	3–4	>5
Effacement (%)	0–30	40–50	60–70	>80
Station	−3	−2	−1/0	+1/+2
Consistency	Firm	Medium	Soft	
Position	Posterior	Midposition	Anterior	

Source: Adapted from Bishop, E. H. (1964). Pelvic scoring for elective induction. *Obstet. Gynecol, 24,* (2), 267.

Table 14-3 Hormonal Methods for Induction of Labor

1. Oxytocin (Pitocin) administered intravenously (FDA approved for induction of labor)
2. Prostaglandins
   a. Misoprostol
      (1) Brand name Cytotec: A synthetic PGE1 analogue tablet administered intravaginally (FDA approved for peptic ulcer prevention, *not induction*)
   b. Dinoprostone
      (1) Brand name Cervidil: A synthetic PGE2 preparation available as controlled release 10-mg vaginal insert (FDA approved for induction of labor)
      (2) Brand name Prepidil: A synthetic PGE2 preparation available in 0.5-mg gel form and administered intracervically (FDA approved for induction of labor)
3. Mifepristone (RU 486, a progesterone receptor antagonist) (FDA approved as a first trimester abortifacient, *not induction*) available in 200 mg tablet to be taken orally

---

Table 14-4   Nonhormonal Methods for Induction of Labor

---

1. Membrane stripping or sweeping
2. Artificial rupture of the membranes (AROM)
3. Breast pump or nipple stimulation
4. Ingestion of castor oil
5. Foley bulb or balloon catheter
6. Sexual activity
7. Herbal preparations

Postdates Pregnancy

Probably the most common indication for which midwives induce labor is for pregnancies persisting past 40 weeks. The true definition of postdates is a pregnancy which endures longer than 42 completed weeks since the LMP.

- Reliable diagnosis of postdate pregnancy remains a challenge.
- There is no consensus on the clinically appropriate time to suspend anticipatory management in favor of an effort to initiate birth.
- There are no clear evidence-based guidelines for the induction of labor in the uncomplicated postdate pregnancy.

Table 14-5   Anticipatory Management of a Woman with a Pregnancy Between 40 and 42 Weeks

---

1. Review EDB with woman as the midpoint in a 4-week range (40+ weeks).
2. Review postdate management plan with woman; carefully document mutual acceptance of the plan (40+ weeks).

3. Initiate nonstress test (NST) twice weekly, starting by 41 weeks, continuing until birth.
4. Initiate amniotic fluid volume (AFV) twice weekly, starting by 41 weeks, continuing until birth.
5. Initiate full biophysical profile and consult with a physician for nonreactive NST or low AFV.
6. Consult with a physician (providing documentation) for any pregnancy reaching 42 weeks.
7. If the pregnancy continues to 42 weeks and dates are reliable, begin active management per protocol.

Table 14-6   Active Management of Postdate Pregnancy

1. Midwife follows steps 1 through 6 in Table 14-5, as needed.
2. Woman may self-administer castor oil after 40+ weeks when the cervix is ripe, according to woman and midwife preference.
3. Midwife may sweep membranes after 41+ weeks, according to woman and midwife preference.
4. Midwife may administer prostaglandin gel (Prepidil) or insert (Cervidil) if cervix is unripe, in anticipation of induction, between 41 and 42 weeks.
5. Midwife may schedule pitocin induction of labor if 42 weeks is reached, according to woman, midwife, and consulting physician preference.
6. Midwife should not allow pregnancy to extend beyond 42 completed weeks (300 days) if dates are reliable.

Note: Prostaglandins and oxytocin are never administered simultanously.

Preterm Labor and Birth

Preterm labor and birth are:

- 12% of US births
- Second leading cause of neonatal mortality (after birth defects)
- 75% of perinatal deaths
- Up to 50% of infant neurological handicaps

It can be difficult to distinguish from the reported history of birth weight and months of gestation whether a previous infant was preterm or growth retarded. Therefore, an attempt should be made to obtain the medical records for any woman who had a previous infant weighing less than 2,500 grams or who delivered prior to 36 weeks of gestation.

The signs and symptoms of preterm labor should be included as a routine part of the woman's prenatal education beginning around 20 to 24 weeks of gestation.

Table 14-7   Predisposing Risk Factors for Preterm Labor

Risk Factors	Comments
Low socioeconomic status	
Nonwhite race	
Poor nutritional status	• Low prepregnancy weight • Weight gain of less than 10 pounds by 20 weeks • Weight loss • Inadequate protein and caloric intake
Previous history of a preterm labor or birth	One previous preterm birth = 20% to 40% risk of recurrence Risk ↑ or ↓ with subsequent preterm or full-term births, respectively

One or more spontaneous second trimester abortions	
Short interval between pregnancies	Rawlings, et al found the pregnancy interval associated with preterm labor to be: • Black women: <9 months • White women: <3 months
Multiple gestation	10% of preterm births are multiple gestations
Substance abuse	• Cigarettes • Alcohol • Illicit drugs, particularly cocaine
Inadequate prenatal care	Registered >24 weeks and/or ≤3 prenatal visits
Uterine anomalies	
Incompetent cervix	
DES exposure in utero	
Urinary tract infection	
Hemoglobinopathies	• Sickle cell anemia • G6PD
Genital tract colonization and infection	• Group B streptococci • Ureaplasma urealyticum • Mycoplasma hominis • Bacterial vaginosis • Bacteroides species • Neisseria gonorrhoeae • Chlamydia trachomatis • Trichomonas vaginalis
Premature rupture of the membranes	
Chorioamnionitis	

Risk Factors	Comments
Severe physical violence during pregnancy	
Abruptio placentae or placenta previa	
Fetal death	
Polyhydramnios	

Table 14-8   Signs and Symptoms of Preterm Labor

- Painful menstrual-like cramps (possible confusion with round ligament pain)
- Dull low backache (distinguished from the common low backache of pregnancy)
- Suprapubic pain or pressure (possible confusion with symptoms of urinary tract infection)
- Sensation of pelvic pressure or heaviness
- Change in character or amount of vaginal discharge (thicker, thinner, watery, bloody, brown, colorless)
- Diarrhea
- Unpalpated uterine contractions (painful or painless) perceived more often than every 10 minutes for 1 hour or more and not relieved by lying down
- Premature rupture of the membranes

Screening for Preterm Labor

Evaluation of the woman with one previous preterm labor/birth and no signs or symptoms of preterm labor this pregnancy:

- Monthly screening for asymptomatic bacteriuria
- Treatment of any vaginal and cervical infections

- Diet history and appropriate nutritional counseling
- Reinforcement of the signs and symptoms of preterm labor
- Counseling, if necessary, regarding cigarette, drug, and alcohol use
- Encouragement to communicate personal stress, to obtain appropriate help with stress reduction

Screening for a woman with two or more previous premature labors/births or a current multiple gestation with no signs/symptoms of preterm labor should include all of the above and the following:

- Vaginal examination every two weeks starting at 24 weeks gestation for changes in cervical position, consistency, effacement, dilatation, and for station of the presenting part
- Change and/or reduction in workload if the woman's job involves heavy lifting, pushing or pulling, long hours, rotating shifts, or a lengthy commute
- Use of condoms during sexual intercourse to prevent STDs and to prevent prostaglandin in the semen from causing uterine irritability
- Avoidance of nipple/breast stimulation to prevent uterine contractions

Assessing Preterm Labor

A woman with signs and symptoms of preterm labor, with or without any predisposing factors, should be seen immediately. Following assessment, if the woman is in preterm labor, notify the consulting physician.

History

- Confirmation of gestational age
- Signs and symptoms of preterm labor

SECTION 14

- Signs and symptoms of urinary tract infection
- Signs and symptoms of vaginitis/cervicitis/sexually transmitted diseases
- Signs and symptoms of viral or bacterial infection
- Signs and symptoms of premature rupture of membranes

Physical Examination

- Vital signs (especially temperature and pulse)
- Evaluation of gestational age
- Evaluation of contractions
- Evaluation of fetal heart rate and pattern
- Abdominal palpation for presentation, position, multiple gestation, estimated fetal weight, and assessment of abdominal pain
- Costovertebral angle (CVA) tenderness
- Assessment of low back pain and suprapubic pain

Pelvic Examination

- Speculum examination to assess for vaginitis or cervicitis, sexually transmitted diseases, premature rupture of the membranes, bloody show, meconium
- Digital examination to evaluate for cervical changes and the station of the presenting part (a digital exam is not done if premature rupture of membranes is diagnosed upon speculum examination)

Laboratory Tests

- Microscopic urinalysis
- Urine culture and sensitivity, if indicated

- Wet mount for bacterial vaginosis and trichomonas vaginalis
- Cultures for Group B streptococcus and any genital lesions
- Specimen for gonorrhea and chlamydia diagnostic testing as clinically appropriate
- Complete blood count (CBC) and differential (if the woman has signs and symptoms of infection)
- Fern test
- Nitrazine test

Assessment of the Fetus

Assessment of the fetus is by external electronic fetal monitoring (see Section 10). A very preterm fetus is so mobile in utero that it may be difficult to monitor. The baseline fetal heart rate is higher in earlier gestation and should be ascertained before any tocolytic agents are given; tachycardia is a frequent side effect of the commonly used beta-adrenergic agonist, terbutaline.

Diagnosis of Preterm Labor

A diagnosis of preterm labor is made between 20 and 37 weeks gestation when the woman is having uterine contractions (usual frequency of 5 to 8 minutes apart) and she exhibits:

(1) Ruptured membranes *or*
(2) Intact membranes *and*
   a. Progressive cervical change, *or*
   b. ≥2 centimeters dilatation, *or*
   c. A positive fetal fibronectin (fFn) test

SECTION 14

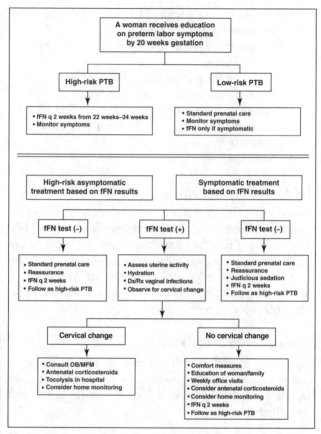

Figure 14-1 Algorithm for use of fetal fibronectin in the identification and management of preterm labor.

Source: Reedy, N.J. (2004). Implementation of midwifery guidelines for the diagnosis and management of preterm labor. Paper presented at the American College of Nurse Midwives, May 31: New Orleans, Louisiana.

(PTB = preterm birth)

Fetal Fibronectin (fFn)

It is often difficult to determine which women are having uterine irritability and which are truly demonstrating symptoms of preterm labor. A negative fFn offers a 99.2% certainty that delivery will not occur within two weeks.

Midwifery Management of Women in Preterm Labor

- Is conducted in collaboration with the consulting physician in the hospital
- Should include knowledge of the level of care immediately available and the length of time needed to transport to a tertiary hospital for access to a neonatal intensive care unit

Management of women with signs and symptoms suggesting preterm labor includes:

- Bed rest in a side-lying position
- External fetal heart and uterine contractility monitoring
- If the membranes are intact, monitoring with vaginal examinations (preferably by the same examiner) for cervical change

Women who do not meet criteria for the diagnosis of preterm labor may be sent home. Consider the following instructions:

- Limit activity—curtail working hours in a non-strenuous and nonstressful job or take a leave of absence from a strenuous or stressful job; do no heavy housework.
- Arrange for someone to help with household and child care responsibilities.
- Engage in no sexual activity prior to reevaluation in one week.

- Resumption of sexual activity depends on uterine activity and the presence of any predisposing factors to preterm labor.
- If sexual activity is subsequently resumed, use condoms.
- If resumption of sexual activity causes an increase or recurrence of uterine contractions, abstain from sexual intercourse or other sexual activity that leads to orgasm in the woman.
- Return for prenatal care and reevaluation for preterm labor in 1 week.
- Continue instructions on nutrition, recognizing signs and symptoms of preterm labor, stress reduction, and use of cigarettes, drugs, and alcohol.

Tocolysis

Candidates for tocolysis:

- Meet the definition of preterm labor
- Are less than 4 centimeters dilated
- Are less than 34 weeks gestation

Tocolysis is the use of medication to inhibit uterine contractions. These drugs are extremely toxic and may produce dangerous side effects in both the mother and the fetus (see Table 14-9). The most commonly used drugs are the beta-adrenergic agonists (betamimetics) terbutaline, and magnesium sulfate. Indomethacin is the most widely used of the prostaglandin synthesis inhibitors and is more effective at inhibiting uterine contractions than any of the betamimetic drugs.

Studies show that, at best, tocolysis prolongs a pregnancy for the short term—24 to 48 hours, and in some instances 3 to 7 days.

Table 14-9 Side Effects of Tocolytic Agents

Maternal Side Effects	Beta-adrenergic Agonists (ritodrine, terbutatine)	Magnesium Sulfate	Prostaglandin Inhibitor (indomethacin)	Calcium Channel Blockers (nifedipine, nicardipine)
Nausea; nausea/vomiting		X	X	X
Headache		X	X	X
Diarrhea			X	
Facial flushing				X
Vasodilation				X
Visual changes		X		
Weakness		X		
Lethargy		X		
Tachycardia	X			
Anxiety/jitteriness	X			
Hyperglycemia	X			
Hypokalemia	X			
Increased systolic blood pressure	X			

	Beta-adrenergic Agonists (ritodrine, terbutatine)	Magnesium Sulfate	Prostaglandin Inhibitor (indomethacin)	Calcium Channel Blockers (nifedipine, nicardipine)
Decreased diastolic blood pressure	X			
Decreased coronary artery perfusion	X			
Decreased peripheral resistance				X
Pulmonary edema	X			
Fluid retention	X			
Peptic ulcer			X	
Paralytic ileus	X			
Urinary retention		X		
Severe allergic reaction			X	
Thrombocytopenia			X	
Hepatotoxicity				X
Respiratory depression/distress	X	X		
Pulmonary embolus	X			
Cardiac arrest		X		
Death	X	X		

Fetal/Neonatal Side Effects

Tachycardia	X	
Hypoglycemia	X	
Hyperinsulinemia	X	
Hydrops	X	
Hypotonia	X	
Drowsiness	X	
Bony abnormalities	X	
Congenital rickets	X	
Decreased uteroplacental blood flow		X
Oligohydramnios	X	
Decreased renal function	X	
Premature closure of the ductus arteriosus	X	

Source: Wheeler, D. (1994). Preterm birth prevention. *Journal of Nurse-Midwifery, 39* (suppl. 2), 76S–78S. Used with permission from the American College of Nurse-Midwives.

SECTION 14

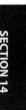

Antenatal Corticosteroid Therapy (ACT)

According to the National Institutes of Health Consensus Statement of "The Effect of Antenatal Steroids for Fetal Maturation on Perinatal Outcomes," ACT has been shown to reduce the incidence and severity of respiratory distress syndrome, intraventricular hemorrhage, and neonatal mortality when administered between 24 and 34 weeks gestation to women at risk for preterm birth within 7 days. Optimal benefits begin 24 hours after initiation of therapy and last 7 days. The corticosteroids used most often and their dosages for therapy are as follows:

- Betamethasone 12mg IM given in two doses 24 hours apart, *or*
- Dexamethasone 6mg IM given in four doses 12 hours apart

Higher or more frequent doses or repeated weekly courses of corticosteroids do not increase the benefits of antenatal therapy or reduce composite morbidity compared to a single course but do increase the risk of adverse short- and long-term neurologic damage, including risk factors for cerebral palsy.

Midwifery Management of Progressive Preterm Labor

Midwifery management of progressive preterm labor to birth is conducted only in collaboration with the consulting physician. Every decision should have the goal of avoiding fetal asphyxia and trauma.

Table 14-10 Midwifery Management of Progressive Preterm Labor: Decisions and Rationale

Management Decision	Rationale/Comments
Decide on the route of birth	This decision is based on the fetal presentation and gestational age.
Decide on the type of analgesia and anesthesia	Narcotics, ataractics, and sedatives should not be used prior to delivery. Pudendal block or local infiltration should be used for episiotomy and repair; or, if necessary, a woman may have an epidural for comfort and control. Maternal hypotension from epidural anesthesia can be lessened by adequate preloading with crystalloid intravenous fluids. If the woman received one of the betamimetic drugs for tocolysis, the increased risk for pulmonary edema must be kept in mind.
Monitor the fetus for signs of infection	A preterm baby has less reserve to tolerate labor. Carefully monitor for tachycardia as a sign of intrauterine infection, especially if the membranes are ruptured or if the fetus is still under the effect of a betamimetic drug.
Consider use of internal vs external fetal monitoring	The preterm fetus has wider fontanels and a different skull bone density and consistency than a term fetus. The decision to use internal fetal monitoring must be based on a real need for internal electronic fetal monitoring and on gestational age.

Management Decision

Decide whether an episiotomy is needed

Neonatologist to be notified and present for the birth

Consider the benefit of delayed cord clamping vs the need to hand the baby over to neonatal specialists.

Make provisions for keeping the baby warm and for transporting the baby if necessary if the birth did not take place in a level III (tertiary) facility.

Rationale/Comments

The need for an episiotomy depends on the estimated fetal weight and the relaxation of the woman's perineum. Arrange for the pediatrician.

A workable compromise is to hold the baby in a warm blanket below the level of the introitus (this speeds the transfer of fetal blood from the placenta to the infant) for 30 to 45 seconds before cutting the cord.

Neonatal mortality is reduced if birth takes place in a level III hospital. If at all possible, it is better to transport the mother if this can be done safely prior to birth than to transport the baby after birth.

Premature Rupture of the Membranes

Related Terms

Premature Rupture of Membranes (PROM)	Rupture of the membranes prior to the onset of labor regardless of gestational age
Preterm Premature Rupture of the Membranes (PPROM)	Rupture of membranes prior to term
Prolonged rupture of membranes	Rupture of membranes more than 24 hours before birth
Latent period	Time from rupture of membranes to onset of labor
Amnionitis	Inflammation of the amnion
Chorioamnionitis	Inflammation of the chorion in addition to the amnion

Risk Factors for PROM

- Incompetent cervix
- Polyhydramnios
- Fetal malpresentation
- Multiple gestation
- Vaginal/cervical infection (e.g., bacterial vaginosis, Trichomonas, chlamydia, gonorrhea, Group B streptococcus)
- Occupational fatigue in nulliparous women

Possible Complications from PROM

- Preterm labor and birth
- Amnionitis and chorioamnionitis
- Prolapsed umbilical cord
- Oligohydramnios

SECTION 14

Diagnosis of PROM

History

- Amount of fluid loss: rupture of the membranes (ROM) may cause a large gush of fluid or a small, continuous discharge
- Inability to control leakage with Kegel exercises: differentiates PROM from urinary incontinence
- Time of rupture
- Color of fluid: clear or cloudy; if meconium stained: yellow or green
- Odor of fluid: a distinct musty odor, different from urine
- Last sexual intercourse: semen expelled from the vagina can be mistaken for amniotic fluid

Physical Examination

- Abdominal palpation to ascertain amniotic fluid volume. With frank ROM it is sometimes possible to detect the decrease in fluid because of increased molding of the uterus and abdominal wall around the fetus and decreased ballottability
- Sterile speculum examination
  - Inspect the external genitalia for signs of fluid.
  - Visualize cervix for flow of fluid from the os.
  - Visualize pooling of amniotic fluid.
  - Have the woman bear down, exert gentle fundal pressure or elevate presenting part abdominally to allow fluid to pass.
  - Observe any fluid for the presence of lanugo or vernix caseosa.
  - Visualize the cervix to estimate dilatation if no digital vaginal examination is done.
  - Visualize the cervix for prolapsed cord or fetal extremities.

Laboratory Tests

- Positive fern test
- Positive nitrazine paper test
- Ultrasound for oligohydramnios if preceding measures give an unclear picture (be certain to rule out other causes of oligohydramnios.)
- Specimen for Group B streptococcus (GBS) culture
- Herpes culture, if indicated

Diagnosis of ROM, Additional Notes

- Fern test is more reliable than the nitrazine paper test because substances other than amniotic fluid have a neutral pH ($\sim$7.0)
  - Cervical mucus
  - Vaginal discharge caused by bacterial vaginosis or trichomonas
  - Blood
  - Urine
  - Semen
  - Glove powder
- The earlier an examination is performed after rupture occurs, the easier it is to diagnose ruptured membranes. When more than 6 to 12 hours pass, many of the diagnostic observations become unreliable because of lack of fluid.
- Observation of fluid coming from the cervical os is diagnostic of ruptured membranes.
- In the absence of direct visualization of fluid from the os, a history strongly suggestive of rupture in conjunction with a positive fern test is diagnostic.

Table 14-11   Procedure for Performing a Fern Test

During the sterile speculum examination:

Use a sterile cotton swab to obtain a specimen from:

the posterior vaginal fornix, *or*

fluid exuding from the cervical os

Be careful not to get into or touch the os itself as cervical mucus will also fern.

Smear the specimen on a microscope slide.

Allow to dry thoroughly for at least 10 minutes.

Inspect the slide under a microscope for a fern pattern.

See illustration of ferning in Section 13, Figure 13-1, page 373.

Management of PROM

Onset of labor after PROM:

- 80–85% of women of all gestational ages will be in labor within 24 hours.
- 10% will be in labor within 72 hours.
- 5% will have a latent period longer than 72 hours.

In term pregnancies (≥37 weeks):

- The infection rate in the first 24 hours ranges from 1.6–29% depending on race, socioeconomic factors, receipt of prenatal care, and gestational age.
- There is an increased incidence of fever if the latent period is more than 24 hours.
- If the latent period is more than 72 hours, there is a significant increase in perinatal mortality.

In preterm pregnancies (<37 weeks):

- Infection rates vary according to gestational age.
- Risks of infection associated with prematurity are much greater than the risk of infection following PROM at term.

Common management options:

- Delivery within 24 hours of PROM
- Expectant management

Delivery Within 24 hours of PROM

- Due to increased risk of infection after 24 hours
- The cesarean rate for women at term who are induced to deliver within 24 hours is 30–50%.
- If the plan is to induce labor to deliver within the first 24 hours after rupture, the digital examination can be done at the time of induction.
- 12 hours can be allowed for the onset of spontaneous labor before oxytocin induction is started.
- During these 12 hours, other methods of inducing labor may be used such as
  - Castor oil (2 oz)
  - Nipple stimulation
  - Rupture of forewaters
- If the cervix is not ripe, preinduction cervical ripening may be indicated.
- Discuss the situation with the consulting physician.

Expectant Management

- Await the onset of spontaneous labor while observing closely for signs and symptoms of chorioamnionitis.

SECTION 14

- An initial digital exam for cervical dilatation is unnecessary, as knowledge of the cervical findings is irrelevant to the management plan.
- Administration of antibiotics when PROM lasts a week or more is associated with prolonging pregnancy and a reduction in clinical chorioamnionitis and neonatal sepsis.
- Obtain vaginal and rectal specimens for GBS culture if not already done in this pregnancy. Repeat in four weeks if birth has not yet occurred.

Expectant Management at Home

Expectant management at home is appropriate when:

- Gestational age ≥36 weeks
- Not in labor, with plan to await the onset of spontaneous labor
- No compounding medical or obstetrical risk factors including
  - Malpresentation
  - Unengaged cephalic presentation
- The woman is able to
  - Take her own temperature
  - Read a thermometer
  - Understand and implement pelvic rest
  - Use a telephone
  - Readily access transportation
  - Have someone with her for support

Frequency of Digital Pelvic Exams

- The incidence of chorioamnionitis increases in direct relationship to the number of pelvic examinations performed.

- Palpation of forewaters does not preclude the existence of ruptured membranes with a high leak.
- A digital examination during the initial examination may only expose the woman to an unnecessary increase in the risk of infection.

Management of Labor and Birth with PROM

Management of labor and birth with PROM is the same as any labor, with these additions:

- Temperature and pulse q 2 hours
- Hourly fetal heart rate checks as long as within normal prior to onset of labor
- Avoid unnecessary vaginal examinations
- When performing a vaginal exam, note the following
  - If the vaginal walls are unusually warm (hot) to touch
  - Odor of the discharge or fluid
  - Color of the discharge or fluid
- Maintain adequate maternal hydration
- Obtain cultures of the maternal and fetal sides of the placenta as well as gastric aspirate of the neonate.
- Method of birth (vaginal or cesarean section) depends on gestational age, presentation, and the severity of the chorioamnionitis.
- Pediatric presence at the birth depends on length of time of PROM, presence of infection, gestational age, and institutional protocols.

Table 14-12 Surveillance for Chorioamnionitis for Expectant Management of Women with PROM Without Labor at 36 Weeks Gestation or More

Management Action	Rationale
Maternal temperature and pulse q 4 h	Slowly rising temperature may indicate infection. Initiate active management to move to delivery before reaching true febrile morbidity.
After initial EFM, check FHTs q 4 h while in the hospital	Fetal tachycardia (>160 bpm) is a good indication of possible chorioamnionitis.
Nonstress tests (NSTs) and/or biophysical profiles (BPP) every two days to weekly to assess fetal well-being	Identify oligohydramnios, cord compression from oligohydramnios, and predict possible or subclinical chorioamnionitis.
Evaluate daily for uterine tenderness (can be done by the woman)	Uterine tenderness prior to delivery is difficult to rely on, because it is variable and may mimic uterine contractions.
White blood cell count (WBC) with differential daily or every other day	Elevated maternal WBC, especially when accompanied by a shift to the left in bands, indicates an infectious process.
Do not perform a vaginal examination unless it is truly indicated for management decisions	Risk of chorioamnionitis multiplies with vaginal examination.
Observe pelvic precautions—no vaginal therapeutics, no douches, no sexual intercourse	Risk of chorioamnionitis increases with anything introduced into the vagina.
If signs or symptoms of chorioamnionitis develop, consultation is indicated	Immediate consultation is indicated for induction of labor and delivery.

Diagnosis of Chorioamnionitis

Presumptive: PROM with a temperature of ≥38°C
(100.4°F)
Definitive: Foul smelling and/or purulent amniotic fluid

Group B Streptococcus: Indications for Prophylaxis

Preterm GBS Prophylaxis

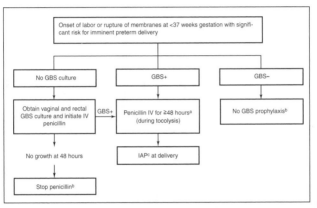

Figure 14-2 Threatened preterm delivery algorithm for prevention of Group B strep.

Source: Centers for Disease Control and Prevention. (2002). Prevention of perinatal group B streptococcal disease. *Morb Mortal Wkly Rep, 51,* (RR-11):12.

[a]Penicillin should be continued for a total of at least 48 hours, unless delivery occurs sooner. At the physician's discretion, antibiotic prophylaxis may be continued beyond 48 hours in a GBS culture-positive woman if delivery has not yet occurred. For women who are GBS culture positive, antibiotic prophylaxis should be reinitiated when labor likely to proceed to delivery occurs or recurs.

[b]If delivery has not occurred within 4 weeks, a vaginal and rectal GBS screening culture should be repeated and the patient should be managed as described, based on the result of the repeat culture.

[c]Intrapartum antibiotic prophylaxis.

Term Pregnancy Group B Streptococcus: Indications for Prophylaxis

Table 14-13 Recommended Regimens for Intrapartum Antimicrobial Prophylaxis for Perinatal GBS Disease Prevention[a]

Recommended	Penicillin G, 5 million units IV initial dose, then 2.5 million units IV every 4 hours until delivery
Alternative	Ampicillin, 2 g IV initial dose, then 1 g IV every 4 hours until delivery
If penicillin allergic[b]	
Patients not at high risk for anaphylaxis	Cefazolin, 2 g IV initial dose, then 1 g IV every 8 hours until delivery
Patients at high risk for anaphylaxis[c]	
GBS susceptible to clindamycin and erythromycin[d]	Clindamycin, 900 mg IV every 8 hours until delivery OR Erythromycin, 500 mg IV every 6 hours until delivery

| GBS resistant to clindamycin or erythromycin or susceptibility unknown | Vancomycin,[e] 1 g IV every 12 hours until delivery |

[a]Broader-spectrum agents, including an agent active against GBS, may be necessary for treatment of chorioamnionitis.

[b]History of penicillin allergy should be assessed to determine whether a high risk for anaphylaxis is present. Penicillin-allergic patients at high risk for anaphylaxis are those who have experienced immediate hypersensitivity to penicillin including a history of penicillin-related anaphylaxis; other high-risk patients are those with asthma or other diseases that would make anaphylaxis more dangerous or difficult to treat, such as persons being treated with beta-adrenergic-blocking agents.

[c]If laboratory facilities are adequate, clindamycin and erythromycin susceptibility testing should be performed on prenatal GBS isolates from penicillin-allergic women at high risk for anaphylaxis.

[d]Resistance to erythromycin is often but not always associated with clindamycin resistance. If a strain is resistant to erythromycin but appears susceptible to clindamycin, it may still have inducible resistance to clindamycin.

[e]Cefazolin is preferred over vancomycin for women with a history of penicillin allergy other than immediate hypersensitivity reactions, and pharmacologic data suggest it achieves effective intra-amniotic concentrations. Vancomycin should be reserved for penicillin-allergic women at high risk for anaphylaxis.

Source: Centers for Disease Control and Prevention. (2002). Prevention of perinatal group B streptococcal disease. *Morb Mortal Wkly Rep, 4,* (RR-11) 10.

Cord Prolapse

- Obstetric emergency requiring prompt diagnosis
- The danger is fetal hypoxia resulting from compression of the cord between the presenting part and the pelvis.
- Route of delivery is cesarean section

Definitions

- Frank cord prolapse: the cord slips through the cervix, allowing compression of the cord by the presenting part.
- Occult cord prolapse: the cord slips down alongside the presenting part but does not protrude through the cervix. Diagnosis is more difficult but can be a cause of prolonged fetal heart rate deceleration or bradycardia.

Diagnosis

- When membranes rupture, check the fetal heart tones.
- If fetal bradycardia, prolonged deceleration, or sudden onset of deep variable decelerations, perform a vaginal examination to palpate for a prolapsed cord.
- If summoned because "something came out between her legs," vaginal examination will differentiate a cord from a mucus plug, a prolapsed foot, or a prolapsed arm.

Table 14-14 Potential Precipitating Causes of Cord Prolapse

Spontaneous rupture of the membranes in the presence of an incomplete application of the fetal presenting part to the cervix, allowing the cord to pass through the cervical opening such as:

Unengaged fetal head or breech
Breech presentation
Compound presentation
Transverse lie
Small fetus (<2000 grams)
Second-born twin

An excessively long umbilical cord

Administration and expulsion of an enema with ruptured membranes

Amniotomy with an unengaged presenting part

Vaginal examination causing inadvertent rupture of the membranes in the presence of tense, bulging membranes and an unengaged presenting part

Displacement of the vertex during fetal assessment or obstetric manipulation (e.g., attempted external cephalic version, fetal scalp electrode application, intrauterine pressure catheter insertion, manual rotation of the head, placement of forceps other than outlet forceps)

Table 14-15   Management of Prolapsed Umbilical Cord

Place your entire hand into the woman's vagina and hold the presenting part up off the umbilical cord at the pelvic inlet.

Do not attempt to replace the cord—you won't be able to replace it; manipulation may cause cord spasm and/or further cord compression.

Inform the woman of what has happened and elicit her cooperation.

Summon help to the bedside. (Warn the woman and, if necessary, yell to get attention and bring people to help.)

Direct others to:
- Call the consulting physician STAT.
- Call for pediatric resuscitation staff.
- Call for surgical staff STAT.
- Call for anesthesia physician STAT.
- Prepare the woman for surgery STAT.

Direct others to get the woman into a position in which gravity will aid in keeping the baby away from the pelvic inlet and pressing on the cord: knee-chest or Trendelenburg position.

If the cord is protruding from the vagina, direct others to wrap it loosely with gauze soaked with warm normal saline.

Do not rely on cord pulsations to be an accurate (reassuring or nonreassuring) indicator of fetal life or well-being.

Fetal well-being can be assessed with doppler, electronic fetal monitoring (external or internal) or ultrasound to detect fetal heart movement. (Do not remove your hand from the vagina to place an internal fetal monitor.)

Direct others to prepare for an emergency cesarean section.

Do not under any circumstances remove your hand from the woman's vagina or from the presenting part until the baby is delivered (usually by cesarean section).

Cephalopelvic Disproportion (CPD)

If disproportion between the size of the fetus and the maternal pelvis exists, then the fetus is unable to descend through the pelvis to deliver vaginally. This may be related to the fetal weight, the diameters of the fetal head, or the specific position the head is presenting to negotiate the pelvis. The determination of CPD is relative and often difficult to assess. Evaluation of the bony pelvis and fetal head diameters is in Section 13. No single finding determines pelvic adequacy or inadequacy. Rather, the total pelvis (its measurements, architecture, shape, and various dimensions) should be taken into account in relation to the fetus (its size, presentation, position, variety, and normality).

Table 14-16 Indicators of Possible CPD

Excessively large fetus (macrosomia or fetus >1 lb heavier than largest previous baby)

The woman's general body type and specific characteristics
- Shoulders wider than hips
- Short, square stature
- Short, broad hands and feet
- Small shoe size

History of pelvic fracture

Spinal deformity, for example, scoliosis or kyphosis (note posture)

Unilateral or bilateral lameness (observe for limp and for marked lordosis)

Other orthopedic deformities—for example, rickets, pinned hip

Platypelloid pelvis

Fetal malpresentation or malposition

Dysfunctional labor, such as failure to progress or uterine dysfunction

Previous cesarean for failure to progress or failure to descend

---

The only true test for CPD is a trial of labor. All women who have failure to progress or an arrest of labor should be evaluated for CPD. Suspected CPD and uterine dysfunction must be managed in a timely fashion with physician consultation due to these possible related outcomes:

- Fetal damage, e.g., fetal intraventricular hemorrhage
- Fetal or neonatal death
- Intrauterine infection
- Uterine rupture
- Maternal death

Management of Suspected CPD

- Careful evaluation of the woman's pelvis, contractions, and fetal well-being
- Provide a trial of labor
- Maximize maternal pelvic space with positioning that matches this particular pelvic architecture with the way this particular fetus is coming through the pelvis
- Avoid maternal exhaustion
- Careful monitoring of fetal well-being
- Consultation with the physician to identify need for cesarean section if there is evidence of
  - Fetal intolerance of labor
  - Failure to progress
  - Arrested active phase of labor

○ Deep transverse arrest
○ Hypotonic uterine dysfunction (despite efforts to strengthen contractions)

Deep Transverse Arrest

Deep transverse arrest is associated with platypelloid and android pelvic types. The flat posterior pelvic configuration of these pelves inhibits the mechanism of labor of internal rotation that brings the sagittal suture from being in the transverse diameter to being in the antero-posterior diameter of the mother's pelvis.

Deep transverse arrest should be considered when there is:

- Prolonged second stage
- Fetal sagittal suture in the transverse diameter of the pelvis
- Second stage hypotonic uterine dysfunction
- Extensive molding of the fetal head
- Formation of considerable caput succedaneum
- Lack of descent of the fetal head

Means to avoid deep transverse arrest :

- Have the woman assume positions that promote pushing (e.g., squatting, kneeling)
- Provide for good maternal hydration when entering second stage
- Avoid maternal exhaustion from pushing; encourage woman to push only with the peak of the contraction or when strong urge to push

Management of Deep Transverse Arrest

- Carefully monitor the progress of labor
- Ascertain true engagement abdominally with Leopold's fourth maneuver

- Vaginally evaluate degree of molding and caput
- Improve uterine activity with oxytocin
- Correct maternal exhaustion
- Physician consultation for use of oxytocin, need for operative birth (forceps, vacuum, cesarean)

Dysfunctional Labor Progress

Uterine dysfunction is identified as a prolongation of any phase or stage of labor by a lack of progress in cervical dilatation or in descent of the presenting part. Intensity of uterine contractions can be measured by abdominal palpation and cervical examination to determine progress. This can also be done with an intrauterine pressure catheter (IUPC) to measure the frequency and pressure of contractions.

Dysfunctional Labor with Hypotonic Contractions

- May not be painful
- Normal gradient pattern of contractions (greatest in the fundus and decreasing to weakest in the lower uterine segment and cervix)
- Poor tone or intensity of contractions (<15 mm/Hg of pressure in each contraction or <200 Montevideo units in a 10 minute period when measured with an IUPC), which is inadequate pressure to dilate the cervix
- Normal labor progress until active phase or to second stage, then slowed dramatically or stopped
- Prolonged labor, increasing the risk of maternal exhaustion, hemorrhage, and, if the membranes are ruptured, intrauterine infection
- Usually tolerated by the fetus unless the condition is prolonged and/or intrauterine infection develops

Assessment

When evaluating the woman for hypotonic uterine dysfunction, assess:

- Frequency, length, interval, intensity of contractions and any changes in pattern
- Maternal exhaustion
- Maternal environment for any stress factors
- Fetal well-being
- Presentation, position, engagement, and station
- Caput, flexion, asynclitism, pelvic adequacy, potential for CPD
- Progress of labor: effacement, dilatation, descent

Management Options

In collaboration with the consulting physician, the management options can be used singly or in combination:

- Modify the environment to decrease maternal stress
- Correct maternal exhaustion and dehydration
- Discuss any underlying fears or concerns for the mother, her baby or the delivery
- Provide epidural anesthesia for relief of pain or release from tension or fear
- Facilitate ambulation and use of shower or tub
- Give an enema
- Rupture the membranes
- Nipple stimulation
- Oxytocin stimulation

Hypertonic Uterine Dysfunction

Contractions have a distorted gradient pattern (midportion of the uterus contracting more forcefully than the fundus and with areas of hypertonicity throughout the uterus)

SECTION 14

which may lead to maternal exhaustion and fetal intolerance of labor. Occurs early in labor during latent phase.

Signs and Symptoms of Hypertonic Uterine Dysfunction

- Usually occurs in primigravidas
- Contractions excessively painful for the period of labor and the severity of the contractions by palpation
- Occurs early in labor during the latent phase
- Contractions frequent and irregular in tonicity
- Lack of progress in dilatation and descent

Management of Hypertonic Uterine Contractions

- Collaborate with the consulting physician
- Assess for other pathology, e.g., placental abruption
- Assess maternal and fetal well-being
- Stop the discoordinate labor
- Induce an obstetric rest, usually with morphine

Most women will awaken in normal, coordinated labor.

Maternal Exhaustion (Maternal Distress: Ketoacidosis)

Signs and Symptoms

- Weakness, apathy, anxiety
- Prolonged labor
- Dehydration (dry lips and mouth, parched throat)
- Restlessness
- Rising pulse
- Elevated temperature
- Circumoral pallor

- Vomiting
- Concentrated urine (elevated specific gravity)
- Urine ketones

Management

- Prevention is best
- Correction of fluid/electrolyte imbalance
- Consultation regarding abnormal length of phases of labor

Uterine Rupture

Uterine rupture, a rare event, encompasses injuries to or defects of the uterus occurring either before or during the present pregnancy. The 5–50% maternal mortality and 50% fetal mortality associated with dramatic rupture demand rapid recognition of the signs and symptoms of uterine rupture and the immediate emergency steps.

Common Causes

- Previous surgery in the uterine fundus or corpus
  - Classical cesarean section
  - Previous removal of intrauterine myomata that invaded the myometrium
- Injudicious use of oxytocin or prostaglandins induction or augmentation of labor, especially with
  - High parity
  - Induction of labor for VBAC
  - Single-layer closure of a previous low segment incision for cesarean section
- Abnormal presentations, especially in the thin lower uterine segment of a grand multipara

Signs and Symptoms

- May be either dramatic or quiet
- Change in the fetal heart rate pattern
- Fetal bradycardia, abrupt and persistent (may be the only indication of uterine rupture)
  - Recurrent late decelerations not relieved by repositioning, stopping oxytocin, or administering oxygen
  - The most ominous pattern is recurrent late decelerations followed by prolonged decelerations and terminal bradycardia

Dramatic Rupture Signs

- Sharp, shooting pain in the lower abdomen at the height of a severe contraction
- Persistent uterine contractions usually do not stop
- Vaginal bleeding slight or hemorrhagic
- Abdominal palpation changes from previous findings
  - Presenting part may be movable above the pelvic inlet
  - Dramatic repositioning or relocation of the fetus in the mother's abdomen with corresponding loss of station
  - Fetal parts may be more easily palpated than before
- Fetal movements becoming violent and then reduced to no fetal movements
- A round, firm (contracted) uterus felt beside the fetus (the fetus is felt outside of the uterus)
- Possibly signs and symptoms of shock—elevated pulse (rapid and thready); decreased blood pressure; pallor, cold, clammy skin, apprehensiveness,

feeling of impending doom or death, air hunger (shortness of breath), restlessness; and visual disturbances

Quiet Rupture Signs

- May have vomiting
- Increased tenderness over the abdomen
- Hypotonic uterine contractions
- Lack of further progress in labor
- Feeling of faintness
- Hematuria
- Vaginal bleeding
- Some pain
- Signs of progressive shock
- Fetal heart tones may be lost

Epidurals

Epidurals may be used, as pain is not a common sign of uterine rupture.

Additional Information

- Signs and symptoms may mimic amniotic fluid or pulmonary embolus
- Possible codiagnosis is abruptio placentae

Management

- Notify the consulting physician and pediatrics STAT
- Start two intravenous infusion routes with 16-gauge intracatheters: one for electrolyte solutions (e.g., lactated Ringer's solution) and the other for blood transfusion (keep the infusion line open with normal saline until the blood is obtained)

- Notify the blood bank
  - Need for a STAT blood transfusion
  - Estimated number of units needed
  - Probable need for fresh frozen plasma
- Administer oxygen
- Make all preparations for immediate abdominal surgery (laparotomy and possible hysterectomy)
- Inform the woman and her family of the emergency and elicit their full cooperation

Shoulder Dystocia

Possible Predictors of Shoulder Dystocia

While not predictable, some findings are correlated with the possibility of shoulder dystocia. If any of the following are present, shoulder dystocia should be considered in the management plan for the birth.

- Large fetus, as determined by palpation or ultrasound diagnosis of macrosomia. Birth weight alone is not predictive for shoulder dystocia; 50%–60% of shoulder dystocias occur in infants weighing less than 4,000 grams.
- Maternal diabetes, particularly gestational or Type II, class A diabetes
- Postdates
- Obstetric history of large babies
- Family history of large siblings
- Maternal obesity
- Varney's predictive factor of an estimated fetal weight 1 lb or more greater than the woman's largest previous baby
- Obstetric history of a difficult delivery or previous shoulder dystocia

- Cephalopelvic disproportion
  - Pelvic shape that shortens the anterior-posterior diameters
  - Deformed pelvis (e.g., the result of an accident or rickets)
- Desultory active phase of the first stage of labor
- Protracted second stage of labor
- Indication for midpelvic rotation and/or delivery with either forceps or vacuum extractor (This is the predictive factor that most likely will be combined with a large fetus, prolonged second stage of labor, and cephalopelvic disproportion, and that most strongly indicates consideration of a cesarean section with the physician.)

Management of Shoulder Dystocia

When shoulder dystocia is identified, take the following steps to manage the emergency situation. The first six steps occur concurrently; the rest occur according to clinician decision making.

- Stay calm. You know what to do and will effectively manage this situation.
- Request that the consulting physician be called immediately if not already alerted.
- Request readiness for a full-scale newborn resuscitation effort.
- Request readiness for an immediate postpartum hemorrhage.
- Briefly tell the mother there is a problem with delivery of the baby's shoulders and elicit her cooperation. Tell her *not* to push now.
- Place the woman in exaggerated lithotomy position with her buttocks at the edge of or overhanging the bed (McRoberts maneuver). The knee-chest position is the same as the exaggerated lithotomy position, only upside down.

- Check the position of the shoulders. Rotate them into one of the oblique diameters of the pelvis if they are in either the transverse or anteroposterior diameter of the mother's pelvis. *Again, instruct the mother not to push.* To rotate the shoulders, place all of the fingers of one of your hands on one side of the baby's chest (e.g., right side) and all of the fingers of your other hand on the baby's back on the opposite side (left side) and then press with the amount of force necessary to move the baby. It is important to use your entire hand for maximum strength. ***Under no circumstances make the mistake of thinking that moving the head will move the shoulders.***
- Have someone else apply suprapubic pressure while you exert your usual downward and outward pressure on the side of the baby's head. Pressure on the baby's head should be firm but not excessive. Suprapubic pressure is most effective if the person applying it stands on a footstool in order to get greater force behind the downward push. This person places both hands palm down, one on top of the other, in the abdominal midline just above the symphysis pubis and then pushes straight downward into the lower abdomen. Suprapubic pressure can be directed to adduct the shoulders to a lesser bisacromial diameter and help them move from their anteroposterior position above the symphysis pubis to an oblique diameter. You need to instruct the person applying suprapubic pressure as to the position of the baby and which way to direct the pressure so that it is applied against the back of the shoulder and then laterally and downward.

- *Under no circumstances should you allow fundal pressure to be given.*
- If the baby has not delivered, take the time (approximately 40 to 45 seconds) to give yourself every piece of knowledge, advantage, and bit of room to deliver the shoulders.
  - Catheterize the woman to empty her bladder.
  - Ascertain the need to cut or enlarge the episiotomy. This decision requires clinical judgment and depends on the tightness or laxity of the woman's perineum and the ease with which you can insert your hands for necessary manipulations.
  - Do a vaginal examination to rule out other causes of labor dystocia after the head is born.
    - Short umbilical cord (relative or absolute)
    - Enlargement of the thorax or abdomen of the fetus such as might be caused by tumors, gross deformities, or severe edema
    - Locked twins or conjoined twins
    - Bandl's retraction ring
- If the labor dystocia is diagnosed as resulting from shoulder dystocia, attempt again to deliver the baby with McRoberts and directed suprapubic pressure while you observe for birth of the anterior shoulder and continue attempts to move the shoulder to an oblique position. The baby will have delivered after this step if the condition was a moderate shoulder dystocia.
- If the baby has not delivered, perform the corkscrew maneuver, utilizing the screw principle of Woods. Place your hands in the same manner as you did for rotation of the shoulders previously. Rotate the baby 180°, thereby substituting the

posterior shoulder for the anterior shoulder. Always rotate the body of the baby so that the back is rotated anteriorly (back up). This means that you alternately rotate the baby 180° clockwise and then 180° counterclockwise (or vice versa) until the baby is screwed out, but without being twisted upon itself. It also means that as you begin the maneuver your hand on the baby's back will be on the anterior shoulder pushing forward and down, and your hand on the baby's chest will be pushing backward toward the posterior shoulder and up.

- If the baby still has not delivered, deliver the posterior arm. Delivery of the posterior arm is accomplished by placing your entire hand deep into the vagina behind the posterior shoulder. Following the arm down from the shoulder, find the elbow and lower arm. If the arm is extended, press in the antecubital space to cause the arm to flex, or if the arm is jammed, splint the lower arm down from the elbow and sweep it up and across the baby's abdomen and chest in its normal range of motion until you can grasp the baby's hand and deliver the entire arm. In doing this maneuver, ***resist any temptation to hook your fingers under the baby's axilla or into the armpit.***

- Attempt to deliver the baby now by the combination of McRoberts and suprapubic pressure. If the baby has not delivered, rotate the baby's body 180°. This will substitute the now delivered posterior shoulder for the anterior shoulder. If the baby has not been delivered, the condition is a severe shoulder dystocia.

- In an exceptionally rare situation (which the majority of midwives will not see in an entire career), the baby will not have delivered and you then proceed to the next step, to break the baby's clavicle. The anterior clavicle is broken first in order to collapse the anterior shoulder and dislodge it from behind the symphysis pubis. The danger in breaking the clavicle is the possibility of puncturing the underlying lung with the broken ends of the bone, causing pneumothorax or injuring the subclavian vessels.
- In rare situations, the final step would be to use the Zavanelli maneuver to replace the head back into the vagina followed by delivery of the baby by cesarean section. To replace the head, reverse the mechanisms of labor and depress the posterior vaginal wall while supporting the head. While the Zavanelli maneuver has been successful in some cases, it is not always easy to perform. The Zavanelli maneuver is a final option, unless you found an obstructive tumor on vaginal examination, in which case you would go directly to the Zavanelli maneuver, as it is not possible to deliver the baby vaginally.

Documentation of Shoulder Dystocia

After the birth is completed and mother and infant are recovering, it is important to document in a detailed and comprehensive manner. Review the chart, the fetal monitoring strips, your previous documentation, and the nurse's documentation of labor and delivery events so you have a clear picture of the course of the labor and birth. Then consider the following data points to determine if

SECTION 14

they are already in the chart or if this information needs to be added. Be certain to note the time of your entry and identify any notes which are late entries.

- 28 week glucose test results
- Diagnosis of gestational diabetes if appropriate
- Maternal height and weight
- Estimated fetal weight on admission
- Total weight gain in pregnancy
- Fetal position on admission and as labor progresses
- Progress in labor
- Basis for the diagnosis of shoulder dystocia
- Time when obstetrician and pediatrics were called
- Who was called and their response (e.g., OB consultant, anesthesia, pediatrics, OR team, nursing staff)
- Steps taken, in sequence and approximate time for each as well as progress made (McRoberts, suprapubic pressure, rotation of shoulders, wood screw maneuver, delivery of posterior arm, fracture of clavicle)
- Episiotomy if done (if not, you may want to state why)
- Time of birth of head, then time for birth of the body
- Apgar scores
- Assessment by pediatric team
- Fetal weight
- Cord blood gases
- Response by mother and family members
- All professionals involved
- Documentation of all consultations throughout the admission, labor, and birth

Delivery of the Infant with a Face Presentation

Many babies with face presentations begin labor in a brow presentation and convert to a face presentation during descent.

The diagnosis of a face presentation is based on the following:

- Abdominal palpation (Leopold's third and fourth maneuvers): with hyperextension of the head, the occiput becomes the cephalic prominence, is easily palpable, and is located on the same side of the mother's abdomen as the hyperextended "hollowed" or arched back; the head may feel larger than you would anticipate as compared to a well-flexed head.
- Pelvic examination: you may be unable to identify both fontanels clearly or may feel only the anterior fontanel if the baby is in a hyperextended presentation. With a brow presentation, you will feel the brow and possibly the anterior fontanel, but no other common identifying landmarks. In a face presentation, you will be able to feel the baby's eyes, nose, mouth, and chin, although initially the presenting part may feel soft and lumpy, similar to a breech presentation. On further examination and palpation, the landmarks of the face become evident.

Once a face presentation is diagnosed, be cautious with vaginal examinations and do not apply an internal electrode in order to avoid damage to the infant's face or eyes.

Mechanisms of Labor for a Face Presentation

1. Extension: the arbitrarily chosen point on the fetus used to determine the position in a face presentation is the chin (mentum), which is palpable because the head is extended rather than flexed.

SECTION 14

2. Engagement: engagement takes place when the trachelobregmatic (submental bregmatic) diameter (9.5 cm) has passed through the pelvic inlet. Approximately 70% of all face presentations engage as either mentum anterior or mentum transverse varieties, and 30% engage as a posterior variety. The axis of the face (midchin to midbrow, bisecting the nose) is used as the fetal diameter in relation to the mother's pelvis in determining in which oblique diameter of the pelvis engagement takes place.

3. Descent occurs throughout: further extension occurs when resistance is encountered and the brow and occiput are forced toward the back of the baby while the chin becomes the lowermost part of the presenting part and leads the way in descent through the mother's pelvis.

4. Internal rotation: usually occurs late in labor when descent enables the entire face to be well applied to the pelvic floor. Rotation of the chin is either anterior or posterior as follows:

   a. Rotation of the chin anteriorly (Figure 14-3):
      45° for RMA and LMA to MA
      90° for RMT and LMT to MA
      135° for RMP and LMP to MA
   b. Rotation of the chin posteriorly:
      45° for RMP and LMP to MP

   If the chin rotates posteriorly into a mentum posterior position, the mechanisms of labor cease at this point because the baby cannot deliver vaginally from this position (Figure 14-4). The fetal neck is only about half as long as the length of the sacrum. Therefore it is not possible for the chin to escape from the vaginal floor over the perineum, allowing the remainder of the head to be born by flexion.

The midwife must recognize this condition immediately before impaction of the head takes place
which has an extremely poor prognosis for the
fetus. Delivery is by cesarean section.

5. Birth of the head: when the chin rotates to
mentum anterior, birth of the head is by a double
mechanism of extension followed by flexion.
Extension is maintained until the chin is born by
escaping beneath the symphysis pubis. The submental area beneath the chin impinges beneath the
symphysis pubis and becomes the 45° pivotal point
for the delivery of the rest of the head by flexion.
The rest of the head is born sequentially starting
with the mouth, then the nose, eyes, brow, anterior
fontanel, and posterior fontanel, and ending with
the occiput as the head flexes.

6. Restitution: takes place 45° in the direction from
which the head rotated during internal rotation.
For example, if internal rotation was from RMT to
MA, then restitution is 45° to the RMA (or LOP)
position.

7. External rotation: takes place another 45° in the
same direction as restitution, for example, to the
RMT (or LOT) position.

8. Birth of the shoulders and body: occurs by lateral
flexion via the curve of Carus.

In Figure 14-3, note engagement in ROP, descent
throughout, internal rotation of 135° to mentum anterior, and birth of the head first by extension and then by
flexion.

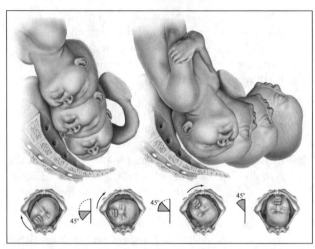

Figure 14-3 Mechanisms of labor for a baby in right mento-posterior position.

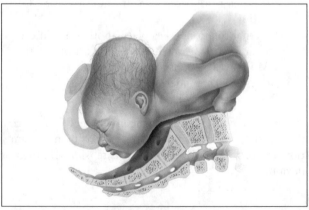

Figure 14-4 Face presentation with chin directly posterior (MP). Unless rotation to mentum anterior (MA) occurs, vaginal birth is not possible.

Management of a Face Presentation

1. Recognize that the position is a face presentation and notify the consulting physician of this malpresentation.
2. Reevaluate the adequacy of the pelvis and consult with the physician if there is a question of possible cephalopelvic disproportion.
3. Closely monitor the mechanism of labor of internal rotation. The midwife must immediately inform the physician if rotation is to a direct mentum posterior position.
4. For delivery of the head:
   a. It may be necessary to apply pressure on the fetal brow to maintain extension until the chin is born. This is done by pressing on the posterior perineal body as the vaginal orifice distends. Protect your gloved hand from contamination from the rectum during this maneuver by covering it with a towel.
   b. Control the head, thereby allowing the gradual flexion and birth of the remainder of the head. Most face presentations deliver spontaneously with little need for extensive hand maneuvers.
5. Delivery of the shoulders and body is the same as for other cephalic presentations.
6. Request pediatric attendance at the delivery. If there is extensive edema of the neck (trachea), nose, and mouth, respiratory function may be compromised.
7. Reassure parents, family, and significant others that the position of the head and neck of the baby (neck extended, head fallen backwards), the long molded head, and the extensive swelling and distortion of the features of the face will improve noticeably in a day or two and completely disappear in a few days.

Delivery of an Infant in a Breech Presentation

In recent years, studies have demonstrated a decrease in perinatal and neonatal mortality and neonatal morbidity with a cesarean delivery in the place of a vaginal breech birth. The American College of Obstetricians and Gynecologists has issued a report stating that: "Patients with persistent breech presentation at term in a singleton gestation should undergo planned cesarean delivery." Although only a few women at term with breech presentation will have a planned vaginal birth, a midwife may be confronted with delivery of a breech presentation for women with no prenatal care who present in late active labor, women who make an informed choice for vaginal birth, or women for whom the second twin is in a nonvertex presentation. In these situations, the midwife must know how to manage the delivery of a baby with a breech presentation.

An anticipated birth of a breech presentation by a midwife should always involve close collaboration with, and immediate availability of, the consulting physician due to potential problems such as difficulty in delivery of the after-coming head and need for extensive resuscitation measures for the newborn.

Before the actual delivery begins, the following should have taken place:

- Careful abdominal examination, sonography, or x-ray to rule out hyperextension of the head, hydrocephalus, or a footling or kneeling breech
- Complete cervical dilatation
- Elimination of any question about the adequacy of the pelvis
- Emptying the bladder
- Cutting an episiotomy if needed
- Determination of effective maternal pushing effort

- Preparations for a full-scale newborn resuscitation effort
- Positioning the woman with plenty of room for lateral flexion and downward traction, in lithotomy position, in stirrups or at the edge of a bed
- Notifying the consulting physician who should either be present or immediately available

If this is an in-hospital emergency situation with a woman who has not been seen before and has not previously been examined, the first action should be to inform the nursing staff of the situation and request that a STAT call be placed to the consulting physician, anesthesia personnel, and the pediatric team.

Table 14-17 Correlation of Mechanisms of Labor and Hand Maneuvers for Delivery of a Breech Presentation

Mechanism of Labor	Hand Maneuvers
1. Descent occurs throughout.	**1, 2, 3.** Normally you will not need to intervene in the first three mechanisms of labor. In the event that the breech does not descend, cephalopelvic disproportion and hydrocephalus must be ruled out. It is possible, however, that failure to descend may be due to a splinting effect caused when it is a frank breech and the extension of the legs across the baby's abdomen prevents the fetus from maneuvering and arrests progress. In such an event, use of the Pinard maneuver will break up the breech and enable you to bring down the feet and legs, thereby changing a frank breech presentation to a footling breech presentation. This is done as follows:
2. Engagement of the hips takes place in an RSA position with the sacrum in the left anterior portion of the mother's pelvis and the bitrochanteric diameter in the right oblique diameter of the mother's pelvis.	**a.** With your vaginal hand (left hand if the baby is in a left sacrum position, right hand if the baby is in a right sacrum position) follow the posterior side of a thigh up from the buttocks to the popliteal fossa behind the knee. Your thumb will be on the anterior side of the thigh.
3. Internal rotation of the buttocks 45° from RSA to RST. This brings the anterior hip, which descended more rapidly than the posterior hip and initiated internal rotation when it encountered resistance from the pelvic floor, 45° forward (anterior)	**b.** Move the leg laterally away from the midline and the baby's body while pressing in the popliteal fossa. This will cause the leg to flex at the knee, thereby bringing the foot, which was at the level of the baby's face and out of reach, down to where you can grasp it.

to underneath the pubic arch. The bitrochanteric diameter is now in the anteroposterior diameter of the mother's pelvis.

4. Birth of the buttocks by lateral flexion. When born spontaneously, the posterior hip is born first; the anterior hip impinges beneath the symphysis pubis and serves as the pivoting point for the lateral flexion necessary for the posterior hip to follow the curve of Carus to birth. The baby's body then straightens out as the anterior hip is born.

The legs and feet usually follow the birth of the breech and are also born spontaneously.

c. Bring the leg down by drawing it across the baby's abdomen in its natural range of motion and down for its delivery.

d. Repeat for the other thigh, leg, and foot.

4. You should deliberately avoid using any hand maneuvers at this point—keep your hands off the baby. The one exception is if the baby is in a frank breech presentation and the extended legs prevent the necessary lateral flexion for birth of the buttocks. In such an event, the Pinard maneuver is used for delivery of the feet and legs and then the buttocks.

The legs and feet may not be born spontaneously if it is a frank breech presentation. In such an event, the Pinard maneuver will cause delivery of the legs and feet. Because 70% of breech deliveries are frank breech presentations, it is important to know how to do Pinard's maneuver inasmuch as it is the solution for three possible times of arrest during descent and

Mechanism of Labor	Hand Maneuvers

5. (a) External rotation of the buttocks 45° from RST to RSA and (b) engagement of the shoulders with the bisacromial diameter in the right oblique diameter of the mother's pelvis (the same as for the engagement of the buttocks). These two mechanisms occur simultaneously, with the external rotation of the buttocks being visible evidence of the entry of the shoulders into the true pelvis as the body untwists and aligns itself with the descending shoulders. Descent of the shoulders after their engagement is rapid.	delivery of the buttocks. However, prior to using this maneuver to deliver the buttocks, legs, and feet (e.g., during descent), you must clearly rule out cephalopelvis disproportion.
	
	5. Continue a hands-off approach. The rationale for this management is as follows:
	  a. There is no need to facilitate the progress of the mechanisms of labor until the baby is born up to the umbilicus. After that, the remainder of the baby needs to be born in 3 to 5 minutes to avoid any anoxia from compression of the umbilical cord against the pelvic brim.
	  b. Traction exerted on the baby prior to birth up to the umbilicus may cause (1) the arms to fly up in a reflex action, thereby extending them above, over, or behind the head and causing later difficulties in the delivery, and/or (2) the head to deflex, which may cause dangerous problems with birth of the head.
	  c. Natural progress using the bulk of the breech maintains cervical dilatation and lessens the possibility that the cervix may clamp around the baby's head or neck.
	    It is a good time to request a warm towel to use next.
	    When the baby is born up to the umbilicus you do two things:
	  d. Pull down a good-sized loop of umbilical cord to prevent stress on its insertion in the umbilicus during the rest of the delivery.

e. Place the warm towel around the baby from just below the umbilicus down. This helps keep the baby warm and gives you a nonslippery hold on the baby, which is essential both for safety and to allow you to exert the traction now needed.

6. Internal rotation of the shoulders 45°, bring the bisacromial diameter of the fetus from the right oblique diameter to the antero-posterior diameter of the mother's pelvis. This is evidenced externally when the delivered body also rotates and the sacrum returns to an RST position from an RSA position.

7. Birth of the shoulders by lateral flexion. When born spontaneously, the anterior shoulder impinges beneath the symphysis pubis and serves as the pivotal

6. After birth of the umbilicus, you exert downward and outward traction while facilitating internal rotation of the shoulders by rotating the body so the sacrum again rotates from RSA to RST. To do this safely without injury to internal organs or structures (e.g., kidneys, adrenal glands) resulting from the pressure you apply in order to exert traction, the placement of your hands on bone is vitally important.

   a. Grasp the baby on its hips with your thumbs on either sacroiliac region and your fingers on the corresponding iliac crests.

   b. Continue this traction until you can see not only the lower half of the scapula of the anterior shoulder but *also its corresponding axilla.*

7. It does not matter which shoulder is delivered first. The following methodology is in accord with the mechanisms of labor:

   a. Grasp the feet of the baby in one hand with your index finger between the legs and your middle finger and thumb each encircling a leg.

   b. Holding the baby by its feet, exert upward traction for the entire body

Mechanism of Labor

point for the lateral flexion necessary for delivery of the posterior shoulder via the curve of Carus. Birth of the anterior shoulder then follows as the body straightens out.

Hand Maneuvers

and draw the baby's abdomen toward the mother's inner thigh. Be careful to keep the back from turning upward so that the head will enter the pelvis in the transverse diameter.

c. This draws the posterior shoulder over the perineum to birth, followed by the arm and hand of the same side.

d. If necessary, such as when the arm has become extended, deliver the arm first, as follows:

   (1) Insert the fingers of your vaginal hand (in this instance of the baby's sacrum being to the right, you would be holding the baby's feet with your right hand and your left hand would be the vaginal hand) and follow the humerus of the posterior arm until you feel the elbow.

   (2) Use these fingers now as a splint for the arm and sweep it across the baby's chest downward to delivery.

e. Now exert downward traction on the baby for delivery of the anterior shoulder, arm, and hand. To exert this downward traction, again place your hands on the baby's hips as you did in Step 6 .

f. Again, if necessary, such as when the arm has become extended, deliver the arm first, as described in Step 7d.

g. If there is a nuchal arm (the arm is extended from the shoulder but flexed at the elbow so that the lower arm is wedged behind the head), attempts to deliver it the same way as for extended arms as in Steps 7d and 7f will not work. Delivery of a nuchal arm is as follows:

(1) Grasp the baby by placing your hands on the baby's hips as you did for Step 6.

(2) Rotate the baby's body 90–180° in the direction in which the hand behind the head is pointing until the arm is dislodged from behind the head. This is accomplished by the friction of the body rotating against the vaginal outlet in a direction that forces the elbow toward the face and places the arm in a position from which it can now be delivered.

(3) Deliver the arm as for an extended arm as described in Step 7d.

(4) If both arms are nuchal arms, then repeat this process for the other arm, rotating the baby in the direction indicated, after delivery of the first arm.

h. If all else fails (a rate circumstance), break the arm by hooking a finger over it and pulling on it. Such trauma is indicated when weighed against the baby's life. Such a fracture usually heals well without deformity.

Mechanism of Labor

8. Engagement of the head takes place with the sagittal suture in either the transverse or left oblique diameter of the mother's pelvis and the occiput in the right side of the pelvis. The head enters the pelvis as the shoulders near the outlet and may engage prior to or after internal rotation of the shoulders—which explains why engagement is in either the transverse or oblique diameter of the pelvic inlet.

9. Internal rotation of the head 45° or 90°, bringing the sagittal suture from the left oblique or transverse diameter, respectively, into the anteroposterior

Hand Maneuvers

8. Suprapubic pressure should be applied to maintain the normal flexion of the baby's head. You need to request that someone else apply the pressure because your hands are well occupied with delivery of the shoulders. Suprapubic pressure is continued until the head is born.

9. Facilitate rotation of the head to an occiput anterior position:

   a. Grasp the baby by placing your hands on the baby's hips as you did for Step 6.

   b. Monitor the rotation of the head by observing the external rotation of the body.

diameter of the mother's pelvis with the occiput directly anterior and the brow in the hollow of the sacrum of the mother's pelvis. This rotation is evidenced externally because the delivered body also rotates, thereby bringing the bisacromial diameter of the shoulders into the horizontal plane of the mother and the sacrum into a direct anterior position (e.g., the back of the baby is upward and the baby is facing down).

10. Birth of the head by flexion.

c. *Do not allow the head to rotate to an occiput posterior position* as evidenced by rotation of the back posteriorly. If this rare event should begin to occur, counteract by rotating the baby so its back is anterior. Rotation of the head posteriorly so that the occiput is posterior and the chin is facing the symphysis pubis makes delivery of the head extremely difficult and dangerous. Fortunately this posterior rotation is quite rare.

10. It is vital to keep the head flexed at this time by continuing suprapubic pressure and by using the Mauriceau-Smellie-Veit maneuver. This maneuver is performed as follows:

a. One hand is introduced into the vagina palmar side up beneath the baby's face.

Hand Maneuvers

   (1) Place the index finger of this hand in the baby's mouth and press the back of the finger against the maxilla (upper jaw bone), e.g., against the roof of the mouth.

   (2) This finger is used to help keep the head in flexion and should never be used for traction.

   (3) Take care not to allow the finger to slip and apply pressure and/or traction against the mandible (lower jaw bone) and the base of the tongue, as this could cause serious injury.

   (4) Use the rest of this hand to support the body of the baby, which is positioned astride your arm.

b. Your other hand is placed on the baby's upper back with your index finger hooked over one shoulder on one side of the neck and your middle finger hooked over the other shoulder on the other side of the neck.

   (1) This hand will be used for exerting traction.

   (2) Place your hooking fingers as far as possible away from the neck to avoid pressure on the cervical or brachial nerve plexuses.

   (3) Grasp the shoulders with your thumb and remaining fingers.

c. Modifications of the Mauriceau-Smellie-Veit maneuver include the following:

(1) Placement of the index and fourth fingers of the lower hand on the upper jaw (malar bones) on either side of the nose with the middle finger in the baby's mouth. Another alternative is to put the index and fourth finger on the infraorbital ridge and the middle finger in the mouth, but you must be *extremely* careful not to misplace your fingers and damage the baby's eyes. These modifications allow you to exert traction with your lower hand.

(2) Extension of one or two fingers (index or index and middle fingers) of the upper hand up the back of the baby's neck under the symphysis pubis and up the occiput, thereby splinting the baby's neck, keeping the head from extending, and facilitating flexion.

d. Apply downward and outward traction with your hand on the baby's shoulders until you can see the suboccipital region (hair line) under the symphysis pubis.

e. Now apply upward traction while elevating the body of the baby so that the chin, mouth, nose, eyes, brow, anterior fontanel, posterior fontanel, and occiput follow the curve of Carus and are born in sequence as the head remains flexed for birth.

f. Birth of the head is controlled by the pressure of your hands. If this step proceeds too fast and the head pops out, intracranial damage may result; and if it is too slow, hypoxia becomes a concern.

Delivery of a Multiple Gestation

This is a high risk pregnancy and is therefore inappropriate for independent midwifery management. Midwifery management of the labor and delivery of a woman with a multiple gestation should be performed only in the hospital in collaboration with a consulting obstetrician to allow for assistance with malpresentation of the second twin, delay in resumption of labor for delivery of the second twin, neonatal resuscitation, prematurity, and/or immediate postpartal hemorrhage, or for cesarean section for unanticipated nonreassuring fetal heart rate patterns. Midwives may also find themselves confronted with an emergency birth of multiple gestation infants, when she or he must know how to effect safe delivery of all viable fetuses.

Steps for Assisting the Labor and Birth of a Woman with Multiple Gestation

Antepartum Considerations

Thorough 1st and 2nd trimester sonogram to determine accurate dating and chorionicity, rule out major structural anomalies, and assess fetal growth for size and concordance. See Section 11 for AP management of multiple gestations.

Intrapartum—Labor Considerations

- Only twins with twin A in vertex presentation are appropriate for consideration for vaginal birth.
- The consulting obstetrician should be notified and readily available at the time of admission for labor.
- Ultrasound evaluation of fetal position on admission is required.

- If the twins are preterm, an EFW is indicated. If either twin is <1500 gms, refer; Cesarean section should be considered.
- Both twins must be continuously electronically monitored throughout labor.
- IV access with a patent heparin lock or infusing IV fluids is required.
- Blood type and antibody screen are required, and cross-match should be strongly considered.
- Minimize use of depressant analgesic or sedative type medications. Ataractics (e.g., Vistaril or Phenergan) as well as epidural anesthesia may be used effectively.

Preparation of Space, Equipment, Staff

- Nursing personnel must be notified in advance to prepare multiples of equipment, supplies, and paperwork.
- Electronic fetal monitoring equipment to monitor both twins simultaneously must be set up (this may be one monitor with twin capability or two separate monitors).
- The delivery room must be prepared for the birth, with readiness for possible emergency cesarean section.
- Ultrasound equipment should be available in the delivery room to track the position of the second twin.
- Preparation for full-scale resuscitation should be completed prior to the birth.
- Preparation should be made for potential immediate postpartum hemorrhage.

SECTION 14

Conduct of the Birth

- The presentation and position of all babies should be known prior to the start of the birth.
- The consulting obstetrician should be notified and present at the start of the birth.
- Anesthesia personnel should be notified and on standby.
- Pediatric staff should be notified and at least one person per infant who is skilled in newborn resuscitation should be present for the birth.
- Ability to perform an emergency cesarean birth for the second twin is necessary and therefore requires that the birth be performed in the delivery (operating) room as opposed to a birthing suite without operative capability.
- Lithotomy position allows room for any necessary manipulations.
- The bladder should be empty at the start of the birth.
- An episiotomy can be cut at any time during the birth if determined to be necessary. Need for an episiotomy depends on the estimated fetal weights, the anticipated need for manipulation if there are fetal malpresentations, and the relaxation of the perineum. If an episiotomy is to be performed, choose the type of incision that will allow the most room for manipulative maneuvers and, in the event of small size or prematurity, reduce the risk of intracranial damage.
- The first twin is delivered in accord with its presentation and position. Clamp and cut the cord and pass the baby to the awaiting pediatric team and return your attention to the second twin.

- Have an assistant direct the second twin into position abdominally under ultrasound guidance as you deliver the first twin.
- The fetal heart rate should be closely monitored and the vagina constantly scrutinized for any sign of bleeding (indicating placental separation) or evidence of prolapse of the second cord, while waiting for labor to resume.
- As long as the fetal status is reassuring and there is no bleeding, haste is not indicated.
- The usual time for the second twin to be born is between 3 and 15 minutes after delivery of the first twin, which allows the baby to come through the just fully dilated cervix before it starts to close again.
- If the second twin is vertex, anticipate a second vaginal birth. If the second twin is in a position other than vertex, plans are made with the physician regarding the consideration of a spontaneous breech birth, a breech extraction, external cephalic version or cesarean section.
- Once the presenting part is fixed into the pelvis, consider rupturing the membranes. Leave your hand in the vagina to ascertain whether the cord has prolapsed. There is less chance of a prolapsed cord if the membranes are ruptured with no pressure (contractions or fundal) behind them and if they are leaked rather than torn. If labor has not resumed up to this point, rupturing the membranes may stimulate contractions to resume.
- If contractions still have not resumed, Pitocin augmentation may be initiated.
- Birth of the second twin is conducted as usual.
- Immediate postpartum hemorrhage is common.

Retained Placenta

A retained placenta has not fully separated and creates no visible hemorrhage. For the placenta to be considered retained, the time between the birth of the baby and the delivery of the placenta is more than 30 minutes, after which physician consultation is required. If bleeding increases, then more rapid intervention may be indicated. Natural interventions include:

- Putting the baby to breast
- Nipple stimulation
- Having the woman assume a squatting position
- Ensuring an empty bladder

While awaiting spontaneous separation and birth of the placenta:

- Monitor vital signs
- Check for visible external bleeding, and hidden internal bleeding (increased fundal height)
- Notify the consulting physician of the situation

If the placenta still has not delivered in 30 minutes, consider manual removal. This should be done in-hospital, necessitating transfer of the woman if she is in an out-of-hospital setting. Placenta accreta should be considered when the placenta does not spontaneously deliver within a reasonable period of time or when a plane of cleavage is not evident upon attempted manual removal.

Manual Removal of the Placenta

Table 14-18 Manual Removal of the Placenta

Indications
- Delivery of the retained placenta
- Management of a third-stage hemorrhage

Preparation

- Call for physician consultation.
- The woman should have a patent IV.
- Analgesia or anesthesia is preferred, as this can be extremely painful.
- The bladder should be empty.
- Use of an elbow length glove is preferred, but not required over the surgical gown.

Procedure

- The entire hand (including the thumb) is placed inside the uterus by following the cord to the placenta.
- The second hand grasps the uterus (fundus) externally through the abdominal wall to:
  1. Control mobility of the uterus
  2. Keep the fundus as contracted and thick as possible
  3. Facilitate placental separation and reduce the risk of perforation of the uterus by the internal hand
- When you locate the placenta, quickly feel the entire fetal surface of the placenta to obtain an anatomical perception of the size of the placenta and where the cord is inserted.
- Sweep the margin of the placenta to find any area of separation to get a starting point in the right plane for separating the placenta from the uterus.
- Place the back of your internal hand against the uterine wall.
- Insinuate your fingers between the placenta and the uterus to establish a line of cleavage.
- Sweep your hand back and forth from side to side, cutting through the decidua with the outer edge of your little finger, fingertips, and first finger.
- You will perceive a spongy feeling with a definite give to it as the placenta separates from the uterus. You may need to turn your hand over in order to separate the anterior portion of the placenta. This leaves the back of your hand still against the uterine wall.

- The entire placenta should be in the palm of your hand before you bring it out. Be certain the placenta is totally separated before bringing it out so as not to invert the uterus when you remove your hand (and the placenta).
- Bring the entire placenta out at once; don't pull on just a piece, as that piece will simply tear from the rest of the placenta and make assessment of the placenta difficult and potentially inaccurate. Bring the placenta out slowly as your external hand continues to keep the uterus contracted as it empties.
- The membranes may need to be teased out, which is done the same way as for any delivery of the placenta and membranes.
- Make sure the uterus is contracted and immediately inspect the placenta, membranes, and cord.

Uterine exploration
- **Advantage:** adds assurance that all of the placenta and membranes have indeed been removed
- **Disadvantage:** repeated intrauterine manipulation may increase the risk of infection, trauma, and uterine rupture.
- **Required:** when the placenta comes out in pieces or is not intact on inspection

Medications
- IV oxytocin is given after the placenta is delivered and exploration of the uterus (if done) is complete to ensure contraction of a now traumatized and possibly exhausted uterus.
- Antibiotic coverage may be used if the placental removal was traumatic, the placenta was removed in pieces, multiple insertions of the examining hand into the uterus were used and/or if there was chorioamnionitis.

Postpartum (Third-Stage) Hemorrhage (PPH)

Early PPH is bleeding greater than 500 ml within the first 24 hours following birth. It is the third most common cause of maternal mortality in the United States.

General Management

PPH can progress very quickly resulting in a significant maternal blood loss. Regardless of the cause, proceed with the following steps as soon as PPH is suspected:

- Have the nurse or birth assistant call the consulting physician STAT.
- Initiate transfer if out of hospital.
- Catheterize the woman unless you are sure that her bladder is empty.
- Make certain there is a patent IV with a 16- or 18-gauge needle and Ringer's lactate solution running.
- Draw a type and cross-match if not already available.
- Closely monitor maternal blood pressure and pulse.
- If the blood loss is not stopped prior to loss of 1,000 ml of blood, order 2 to 4 units of packed red blood cells.

Management of Early Postpartum Hemorrhage by Specific Cause

Table 14-19 Management Related to Cause of Early Postpartum Hemorrhage

Cause	Management
Cause Uterine atony—most common cause Risk factors: • Overdistension of the uterus (e.g., macrosomia, polyhydramnios, multiple gestation) • Rapid or prolonged labor, use of oxytocin, chorioamnionitis • Tocolytics • General anesthesia • Retained placenta or placental fragments	**Management** • Thoroughly massage the uterus. Massage at this time may complete placental separation. This action, with a well-contracted uterus, is combined with controlled cord traction so when separation is complete, delivery of the placenta occurs immediately. • Once the placenta is delivered, perform bimanual massage of the the uterus in order to dislodge clots and to stimulate uterine contractility. • If atony persists, use of a uterotonic medication is indicated. Refer to Table 14.20. • If atony still persists, uterine curettage may be indicated to remove retained products of conception. By this time, referral to the physician is required.
Uterine atony due to incomplete separation of the placenta	If uterine massage is not effective, manual removal of the placenta may be indicated. See Table 14.18 for this procedure.

Uterine atony due to placenta accreta, increta, percreta

Lacerations:
- Perineal, vaginal sulcus, or cervical

Uterine rupture or dehiscence

Risk factors:
- Previous cesarean section, repair of cornual ectopic pregnancy or myomectomy
- Hyperstimulation of the uterus, CPD
- Cocaine use

If manual removal of the placenta is not successful, abnormal placentation must be strongly considered and the patient emergently referred to the physician for evaluation and possible hysterectomy.

- If the uterine fundus is found to be contracted, the midwife must then critically evaluate the woman for lacerations and proceed to repair same with physician consult, assistance, or referral as indicated.

- Hematomas may also form and be unrecognized until the woman complains of severe pain or her vital signs deteriorate. Rapid assessment and referral are required.

Referral to MD for:
- Emergency cesarean birth if the woman is undelivered
- If delivered, consideration of abdominal exploration, uterine repair or hysterectomy

Cause

Uterine inversion

- Complete—when the uterus turns inside out and is exposed through the cervix and vaginal introitus
- Incomplete—the uterine fundus inverts into the body of the uterus and may extend to the cervix
- Prolapsed—the fundus extrudes beyond the vulva

Coagulopathy
Risk factors:

- Severe preeclampsia, HELLP syndrome
- Abruptio placentae
- Idiopathic thrombocytopenia
- Amniotic fluid embolism
- Inherited coagulopathies

Management

This emergency must be identified rapidly.

- If possible, replace the uterus with the placenta attached in order to minimize bleeding, See Figure 14-5.
- If the cervix has contracted around the uterus, uterine relaxing agents must be used.
- Once replaced, reinitiate uterine contractile agents.
- MD referral is required; however, the midwife must know the emergent steps to minimize blood loss.

Management based on cause of coagulopathy.
Referral to MD is required.

Uterotonics

Table 14-20   Uterotonics for Control
of Postpartum Hemorrhage

Medication	Route/Dosage	Contraindications
Oxytocin (Pitocin)	10 units IM or 10–40 units/1000cc IV fluid	
Methylergonovine maleate (Methergine)	0.2 mg/mL IM or IV 0.2 mg/tablet po q 2–4 h prn	Hypertension or preeclampsia
15-methyl-prostaglandin F_{2a} (Hemabate)	250 mcg IM into the myometrium	Asthma, active cardiac, pulmonary or renal disease
Dinoprostone (Prostin/15M)	0.25 mg/ml pr	Asthma
Misoprostol (Cytotec)	400–600 po or pr	

Placenta Accreta

Placenta accreta is a rare, abnormal, partial or total adherence of the placenta to the uterine wall.

Placenta accreta	The placenta adheres directly to the myometrium with either defective decidua or no decidua in between.
Placenta increta	The chorionic villi extend through the myometrium to penetrate the uterine wall.
Placenta percreta	The chorionic villi invade through the entire uterine wall to the serosa.

Risk Factors

- Placenta previa
- A previous cesarean section scar
- Unexplained elevated MSAFP

Clinical Management

- Diagnosis is suspected when the placenta's adherence is discovered during attempted manual removal.
- Do not continue to attempt to remove the placenta manually if it is difficult.
- Call for immediate assistance from the consulting MD, the anesthesiologist, and nursing staff.
- Follow the steps above for general management of postpartum hemorrhage.
- Advise the woman that there is a serious complication and her participation is needed.
- Definitive diagnosis is made by pathology of the placenta and uterus if hysterectomy has occurred.

Uterine Inversion

The uterus literally turns inside out.

Incomplete = The fundus protrudes through the cervical os.

Complete = The fundus descends to immediately within the vaginal introitus.

Prolapsed = The fundus extrudes beyond the vulva.

In the first two positions, the fundus, on vaginal examination, feels like a soft tumor filling the cervical or vaginal orifice. Abdominally, a funnel-like depression may be felt instead of the fundus. (See Figure 14–5.)

Risk Factors

- Uterine atony or uncontracted uterus
- A patulous, dilated cervix
- Fundal pressure after the birth
- Traction caused by pulling on the umbilical cord or placenta

Clinical Management

Follow the steps in Table 14-19. Specific steps for repositioning the inverted uterus are in Table 14-21.

Table 14-21   Procedure for Repositioning the Inverted Uterus

---

- Manual repositioning can be done if inversion is diagnosed and the manipulation is performed immediately.
- Repositioning of the uterus is done with the placenta still attached.

Procedure:

- Place one entire hand in the vagina, fingertips around the circumference of the junction where the uterus has turned on itself with the inverted fundus in the palm of the hand.
- Apply pressure with the palm of the hand on the fundus and fingertips on the uterine walls.
- "Walk" the fingertips up the uterine walls as the fundus is repositioned.
- Be cautious not to puncture or rupture the soft uterine wall.
- Lift the uterus high out of the pelvis, above the level of the umbilicus, and hold there for several minutes. This puts tension on the uterine ligaments, which keeps the uterus reinverted.
- This procedure is usually quite painful, and deep anesthesia or an intravenous uterine relaxant (e.g., magnesium sulfate, halogenated anesthetic agents, terbutaline) is desirable.

SECTION 14

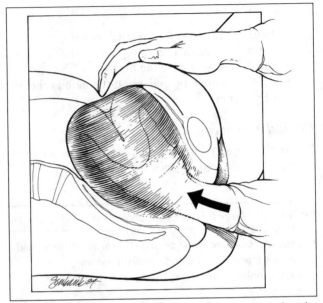

Figure 14-5 Repositioning the inverted uterus. Note that the abdominal hand feels a funnel-like depression instead of the fundus.

Source: Gabbe, S. G., Niebyl, J., & Simpson, J. L. (1991). *Obstetrics: normal and problem pregnancies* (2nd ed.). New York: Churchill.

References

Alexander, J. M., McIntire, D. D., & Leveno, K. J. (2000). Forty weeks and beyond: Pregnancy outcomes by week of gestation. *Obstet Gynecol, 96,* 291–294.

American College of Obstetricians and Gynecologists. (1997). ACOG practice patterns. *Management of Postterm Pregnancy.* Washington, DC: ACOG. No. 6.

American College of Obstetricians and Gynecologists. (1995). Induction and augmentation of labor. Washington, DC: ACOG. ACOG Technical Bulletin No. 217.

American College of Obstetricians and Gynecologists. (1999). Induction of labor. Washington, DC: ACOG. Practice Bulletin No. 10.

American College of Obstetricians and Gynecologists. (1999). Induction of labor with misoprostol. Washington, DC: ACOG. Committee Opinion 228.

American College of Obstetricians and Gynecologists. (1998). Monitoring during induction of labor with dinoprostone. Washington, DC: ACOG. Committee Opinion 209.

American College of Obstetricians and Gynecologists. (1998). Postpartum hemorrhage. Washington, DC: ACOG. ACOG Educational Bulletin No. 243.

American College of Obstetricians and Gynecologists. (2000). Response to searle's drug warning on misoprostol. Washington, DC: ACOG. Committee Opinion 228.

American College of Obstetricians and Gynecologists, Committee on Obstetric Practice. (1994). Vaginal delivery after a previous cesarean birth. Washington, DC: ACOG. ACOG Committee Opinion No. 143.

Bujold, E., Bujold, C., Hamilton, E. F., Harel, F., & Gauthier, R. J. (2002). The impact of a single-layer or double-layer closure on uterine rupture. *Am J Obstet Gynecol, 186*, 1326–1330.

Dove, D. & Johnson, P. (1999). Oral evening primrose oil: its effect on length of pregnancy and selected intrapartum outcomes in low-risk nulliparous women. *J Nurse-Midwifery, 44*, 320–324.

Gherman, R. B. & Goodwin, T. M. (1998). Shoulder dystocia. *Curr Opinion Obstet Gynecol, 10*, 459–463.

Irion, O. & Boulvain, M. (2000). Induction of labour for suspected fetal macrosomia. *Cochrane Review.* No. 4.

Lyndon-Rochelle, M., Holt, V., Easterling, T., & Martin, D. (2001). Risk of uterine rupture during labor among women with a prior cesarean delivery. *N Engl J Med, 345*, 3–8.

National Institute of Child Health and Human Development, Network of Maternal-Fetal Medicine. (1994). Trial of induction of labor versus expectant management in postterm pregnancy. *Am J Obstet Gynecol, 170*, 716–723.

National Institutes of Health. (1994). *The effect of antenatal steroids for fetal maturation on perinatal outcomes.* Washington, DC: NIH. Consensus Statement, 1–118.

Newman, R. B., Goldenberg, R. L., Moawad, A. H., et al. (2001). Occupational fatigue and preterm premature rupture of membranes. *Am J Obstet Gynecol, 184,* 438–446.

Rawlings, J. S., Rawlings, V. B. & Read, J. A. (1995). Prevalence of low birth weight and preterm delivery in relation to the interval between pregnancies among white and black women. *N Engl J Med, 332,* 69–74.

Rosen, M. G., Dickinson, J. C. & Westhoff, C. L. (1991). Vaginal birth after cesarean: a meta-analysis of morbidity and mortality. *Obstet Gynecol, 77,* 465–470.

Ryo, E., Kozuma, S., Sultana, J., et al. (1999). Fetal size as a determinant of obstetrical outcome of post-term pregnancy. *Gynecol Obstet Invest, 47,* 172–176.

Sciscione, A. C., Nguyen, L., Manley, J., et al. (2001). A randomized comparison of transcervical foley catheter to intravaginal misoprostol for preinduction cervical ripening. *Obstet Gynecol, 97,* 603–607.

Summers, L. (1997). Methods of cervical ripening and labor induction. *J Nurse-Midwifery, 42,* 71–85.

Varney, H., Kriebs, J. M. & Gegor, C. L. (2004). *Varney's Midwifery* (4th ed.). Sudbury, MA: Jones and Bartlett Publishers. Chapter 5.

Wing, D. & Paul, R. (1999). Vaginal birth after cesarean section: Selection and management. *Clin Obstet Gynecol, 42,* 836–848.

Zelop, C., Shipp, T. D., Repke, J. T., et al. (2000). The effect of previous vaginal delivery on the risk of uterine rupture during a subsequent trial of labor. *Am J Obstet Gynecol, 183,* 1184–1186.

Postpartum Period

The Normal Puerperium

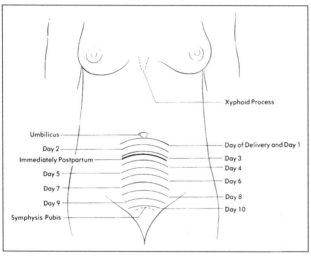

Figure 15-1 Fundal height assessment and normal involution.

During the first hours after birth, the uterus may be displaced upward and sometimes toward the right by the bladder. The bladder should be emptied prior to assessing fundal height. The uterus will shrink by half within 1 week, and return to normal by 8 weeks postpartum.

Immediately after birth, finding the uterine fundus above the umbilicus requires assessment and intervention; common conditions producing this effect include:

- Uterine atony with associated bleeding or retention of clots and blood
- Distended bladder, inability to void

Assessment of the New Mother

Review of Records

- Prenatal and birth history
- Length of time since birth
- Plan of care/orders
- Vital signs
- Medication use
- Laboratory/procedure results
- Progress notes

Issues Specific to the Early Postpartum Assessment

- Recollection of birth experience
- Appetite
- Ambulation
- Bowel and bladder function
- Pain/physical discomfort
- General mood
- Response to new baby
- Infant feeding method and success
- Mother's questions or concerns

Physical Assessment Specific to the Early Postpartum

- Breasts and nipples (regardless of feeding method)
- Abdomen (diastasis, uterine involution, bladder)

- Perineum (edema, inflammation, bruising, hematoma, wound separation, status of repair, infectious discharge, hemorrhoids)
- Lochia (color, amount, odor)
- Extremities (edema, reflexes, calf pain, heat, varicosities, Homan's sign)

Other aspects of the physical exam are performed as needed, including:

- Throat
- Cardiac
- Respiratory
- CVA tenderness
- Vital signs if not current in chart

Common Orders in the Early Postpartum

- Diet and activity level
- Intravenous management (in or out, why)
- Bladder management if not voiding, including catheterization
- Bowel management if significant laceration or episiotomy
- Pain medications
- Sleep aid
- Laxatives
- Vitamins/iron
- Rubella vaccine if not immune
- Rh immune globulin if Rh− mother with Rh+ infant
- Methergine series/pitocin drip if inadequate uterine contractility

Teaching Topics

- Self-care, activity level
- Relief for common discomforts

- Nutrition
- Breast care
- Normal bowel and bladder function
- Infant care
- Infant feeding
- Breastfeeding assistance
- Postpartum blues and depression

Postpartum Complications

Morbidity

Temperature > 100.4°F on any 2 of the first 10 days postpartum, excluding the first 24 hours
  Differential diagnosis:

- Maternal dehydration
- Mastitis
- Urinary tract infection
- Upper respiratory infection

Infection

Bacterial infection of the genital tract during or following birth

Signs and Symptoms

- Temperature > 100.4°F
- Malaise
- Malodorous lochia
- Pain at site of infection

Treatment

As organisms may be genital, colorectal, or environmental (hands, droplet, etc.), cultures followed by broad spectrum antibiotics will produce the best effect.

Infected Genital Trauma
Signs and Symptoms

- Localized pain
- Fever
- Localized edema
- Inflamed edges of repair/laceration
- Purulent discharge
- Wound separation

Treatment

- Remove stitches from affected area
- Open and debride wound
- Broad spectrum antibiotics

As organisms may be genital, colorectal, or environmental (hands, droplet, etc.), cultures followed by broad spectrum antibiotics will produce the best effect.

Endometritis
Signs and Symptoms

- Persistently elevated fever above 100.4°F
- Tachycardia
- Chills
- Uterine tenderness extending laterally
- Pelvic pain with bimanual examination
- Subinvolution
- Abdominal distension
- Lochia may be scanty and odorless or heavy, seropurulent and malodorous
- Onset depends on the organism; GBS typically earlier
- Elevated white blood cell count

Treatment

Mild endometritis is sometimes treated with oral therapy; however, significant disease mandates hospital admission for IV therapy. Prior to initiating outpatient therapy, the midwife should consult with her physician colleague regarding symptoms and treatment.

Any suspicion of worsening infection, unexplained symptoms, or acute pain mandates immediate physician consultation and referral. Sequelae of unrecognized or inadequately treated infection include salpingitis, septic thrombophlebitis, peritonitis, and/or necrotizing fasciitis.

Hematoma

Signs and Symptoms

- Commonly on vulva or in the vagina
- Acute pain
- Tense, fluctuant swelling
- Bruised appearance of the tissue

Broad ligament hematomas, requiring immediate physician consultation, are characterized by:

- Lateral uterine pain, extending into the flank
- Painful swelling on high rectal exam
- Lateral ridge above pelvic brim
- Abdominal distension

Subinvolution

Failure of the uterus to effectively contract during the postpartum period

Causes

- Retained fragments of placenta or membranes
- Myomata
- Infection (early postpartum)

Signs and Symptoms

- Unresolved increased or persistent lochia
- Boggy uterine fundus
- Uterus elevated above expected location

Treatment

- Methylergonavine 0.2 mg every 4 hours for 6 doses
- Antibiotics as required for infectious cause

Delayed Hemorrhage

Excessive bleeding occuring after the first 24 hours postpartum

Causes

- Subinvolution
- Retained placental fragments/membranes
- Undiagnosed laceration
- Hematoma

Signs and Symptoms

- Bleeding
- Symptomatic anemia
- In extreme cases, shock

Treatment

- Physician consultation
- Uterotonic drugs for atony or retained fragments (see Section 14)
- Repair of laceration, as advised by the physician

Thrombophlebitis

Signs and Symptoms

Superficial Thrombophlebitis

- Pain
- Local tenderness
- Inflammation
- Palpable knot or cord

Deep Vein Thrombosis

- Abrupt onset with severe leg pain worsening with activity
- Edema of affected leg
- Positive Homan's sign
- Pain with pressure
- Tenderness along length of affected area
- Palpable cord

Treatment

- Physician consultation for decisions regarding anticoagulation and antibiotics
- Elevation of the extremity
- Heat
- Elastic/surgical stockings or venodynes
- Analgesics

Table 15-1   Homan's Sign

Place one hand gently on the mother's knee.
Apply gentle pressure to keep the leg straight.
Dorsiflex the foot.
Pain is a positive Homan's sign.

Postpartum Depression

In contrast to the baby blues, which are mild and transient, true postpartum depression can develop at any point in the first months postpartum, and shares the diagnostic characteristics of major or minor depression. (See Section 4, page 91.) At the far end of the spectrum of postpartum mood disorders, the rare postpartum psychosis is characterized by suicidal or infanticidal behaviors, and delusional thinking, in addition to symptoms related to depression. Postpartum thyroiditis should be considered when evaluating postpartum depression.

Baby Blues

- Occur soon after birth
- Symptoms are relatively mild and include tearfulness, anxiety, restlessness.
- Resolve spontaneously

Predictors of Postpartum Depression

- Prenatal depression
- Child-care stress
- Life stress
- Lack of social support
- Prenatal anxiety
- Marital satisfaction
- History of previous depression
- Infant temperament
- Maternity blues
- Poor self-esteem
- Socioeconomic status
- Marital status
- Unwanted/unplanned pregnancy

Patients complete the Edinburgh Postnatal Depression Scale (EPDS), and scores for each item are then totaled. Totals of 12 or more indicate clinical depression. Borderline scores of 9-11 warrant close follow-up.

The Postpartum Office Visit

Interval History and Review of Systems

- Recollection of birth experience
- Infant feeding method and success
- Infant growth and well-being
- Appetite
- Rest and activity
- Sexual activity, contraceptive method planned or used
- Mood changes
- Support at home
- Any current physical problems or concerns

Physical Examination (Minimum)

- Breasts
- Abdomen
- Perineum, including status of repair
- Bimanual
- Speculum exam if indicated or if pap/cultures needed
- Rectal exam if any perineal lacerations, episiotomy, or trauma

Patient Teaching

Continued healing process

Beginning Contraception Postpartum

Hormonal Methods

Progestin-only methods including medroxyproges-terone acetate (Depoprovera) and progesterone-only pills may be prescribed immediately after birth for formula-feeding mothers, and at 6 weeks for breast-feeders. There is minimal breast milk transmission of progestins to the infant; no harm has been found as a result of this exposure.

Combination estrogen/progesterone methods includ-ing most oral contraceptives, Ortho Evra patch, and vaginal ring (NuvaRing) can be prescribed after birth for formula-feeding mothers, but not earlier than 2 to 3 months post-partum for breastfeeders. Ideally combined hormonal contraceptives are delayed until weaning is complete, as estrogens may reduce the supply of breast milk.

IUDs

Either the Mirena or Paraguard devices can be inserted at or after the 6-week postpartum visit. A normal Pap smear during pregnancy should be available, as well as a screen for gonorrhea and chlamydia within 1 month of insertion.

Barrier Methods

Condoms may be used at the time sexual activity is resumed. Breastfeeding mothers may find that vaginal dryness inhibits comfort. Vaginal lubricants or estrogen vaginal cream can be used to relieve discomfort.

The diaphragm and cervical cap cannot be used until the cervix has closed and returned to its nonpregnant state. Diaphragms and possibly caps will need to be refitted. Their fit can be checked at the time of the 6-week postpartum visit. However, vaginal tone may not be

SECTION 15

well enough restored for diaphragm fitting to occur at this time.

The use of contraceptive foams, creams, gels, films, etc., is not contraindicated postpartum, once all lochial bleeding has ceased. Without the use of a barrier at the same time, their effectiveness is not high.

Permanent Contraception

Tubal ligation can be performed at the time of delivery, although the risk of method failure is higher. If not done at this time, the procedure should be delayed until postpartum recovery is complete—at least 4 to 6 weeks. The insertion procedure for Essure tubal occlusion cannot be performed during postpartum recovery.

One possibility with both these methods is to provide the mother with another effective measure, such as medroxyprogesterone acetate injection, immediately after delivery to provide protection until the procedure is complete.

Natural Family Planning

Couples experienced with natural family planning can utilize this method after birth. They first need to establish a basic infertility pattern over 2 weeks of abstinence, and then can regard all days as infertile until menstrual cycles return. The lack of clear correlation with the symptoms used to identify ovulation when the mother is still hypoestrogenic may cause some increase in failures. Another difficulty may be the mother's disturbed sleep cycle in the early postpartum period that prevents evaluation of basal body temperature. Breastfeeding mothers can use the lactational amenorrhea method for several months before switching to these techniques.

Lactational Amenorrhea

Mothers who breastfeed exclusively experience ovulation suppression for 3 to 6 months postpartum unless vaginal bleeding occurs earlier. Prolactin is an effective suppressor of ovulation. During this period, no further contraception is needed. The failure rate is approximately 2%. Vaginal dryness associated with exclusive breastfeeding should be addressed with the mother, as she may wish to use a vaginal lubricant for comfort, or an estrogen vaginal cream to restore vaginal lubrication and tissue strength.

References

Varney, H., Kriebs, J. M., Gegor, C. L. (2003). *Varney's midwifery* (4th ed.). Sudbury, MA: Jones and Bartlett Publishers, Inc., 2003. Chs. 42, 44.

Cox, J. L., Holden, J. M., Sagovsky, R. (1987). Detection of postnatal depression: Development of the 10-item Edinburgh Postnatal Depression Scale. *Br J Psychiatry, 150,* 782–6.

SECTION 16

Immediate Care
of the Newborn

Physiologic Transition to Extrauterine Life

The first few moments and hours of extrauterine life are among the most dynamic of the entire life cycle. At birth, the newborn moves from complete dependence to physiological independence through the transitional period—a period that starts when the infant emerges from the mother and continues during the entire first month of life.

Respiratory Changes

Table 16-1 Normal and Abnormal Respiratory Responses

Normal	Abnormal
Average rate: 40 bpm	—
Range: 30–60 bpm	—
Diaphragmatic and abdominal breathing	Intercostal retractions, retractions of the xyphoid
Obligate nose breather	Flared nostrils
—	Grunting on expiration

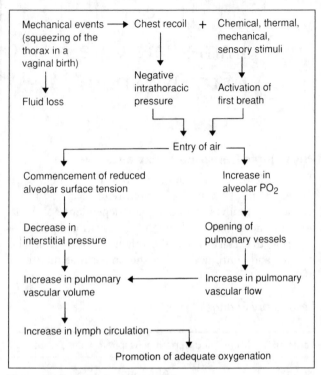

Figure 16-1   Initiation of respiration.

Source: Londong, Laedwig, Ball, and Bindler. (2002). *Maternal-newborn & child nursing: Family centered care.* Upper Saddle River, NJ: Pearson Education, Inc. Reprinted by permission.

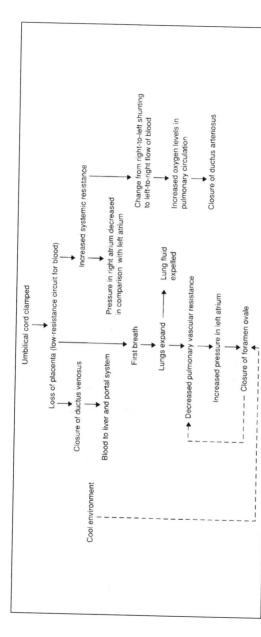

Figure 16-2 Changes from fetal to neonatal circulation.

Source: Kenner, C., Bruggemeyer, A., and Gunderson, L. (1993). *Comprehensive neonatal nursing: A physiologic perspective.* Reprinted with permission from Elsevier.

Thermoregulation

Newborns are easily stressed by changes in environmental temperature. The midwife must minimize heat loss by the wet newborn.

Contributing factors to newborn heat loss:

- Large surface area of a newborn
- Varying levels of subcutaneous fat insulation
- Degree of muscle flexion

Newborns lose heat through four mechanisms:

1. Convection
2. Conduction
3. Radiation
4. Evaporation

Methods of heat conservation:

- Prewarm blankets, hats, clothing before birth.
- Prewarm the newborn resuscitation area.
- Dry newborn immediately.
- Replace wet blankets after drying newborn.
- Set birth room temperature at 75°F.
- Do not suction newborn on wet sheets.
- Postpone newborn bath until temperature is stable for two hours.
- Place newborn care areas away from windows, outside walls, or doorways.

Hypothermia

Symptoms of hypothermia may be subtle, including tachypnea and tachycardia. Hypothermic newborn should be evaluated for hypoglycemia and hypoxia. Rewarming will take a number of hours. Rapid rewarming may lead to apnea.

Table 16-2   Methods by Which the Neonate Can Create Heat

Shivering	• Inefficient • Seen only in the most severe cold stress
Voluntary muscle activity	• Of limited benefit even in term infants with sufficient muscle strength to cry and remain in a flexed position
Nonshivering thermo-genesis—two pathways	
First pathway • Increased metabolic rate	• Norepinephrine triggers the splitting of fatty acids, which are oxidized and released into the circulation, causing a marked increase in oxygen utilization, exhausting even a healthy, term neonate.
Second pathway • Utilization of brown fat for heat production	• Amount of brown fat depends on gestational age and is decreased in growth-restricted newborns. • A nonrenewable resource of the newborn. • Use of brown fat stores does not proceed efficiently in a newborn with hypoglycemia or thyroid dysfunction.

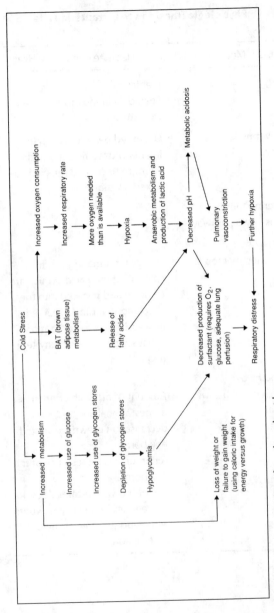

Figure 16-3 Sequelae of newborn heat loss.

Source: Blackburn, S. (2003). *Maternal, fetal, and neonatal physiology: A clinical perspective.* Philadelphia, PA: Saunders. Reproduced by permission.

Glucose Regulation

At particular risk of developing hypoglycemia are:

- Newborns with intrauterine growth restriction
- Postterm infants
- Preterm infants
- Infants experiencing fetal distress
- Infants of diabetic mothers

Hypoglycemia is:

- Defined as serum glucose <40–45 mg/dl
- Determined with heel stick and test strip
- Verified with repeat serum sample if <45 mg/dl

Symptoms of hypoglycemia:

- Jitteriness
- Cyanosis
- Apnea
- Weak cry
- Lethargy
- Limpness
- Refusal to eat

Methods of intervention:

- Utilization of breast milk/formula
  ○ Early feeding
- Utilization of glycogen stores
- Creation of glucose from other sources, especially lipids

Intervene if:

< 45 mg/dl in symptomatic infant
< 35 mg/dl in asymptomatic infant

Table 16-3   Limitations of Glucose Testing from a Heel Stick

Possible limitations of glucose testing as a result of testing a capillary sample from a heel stick include:

- Glucose oxidase reagent strips are affected by venous stasis in an unwarmed foot, leading to false high test results.
- The strips measure whole blood glucose, which is 10 to 15% lower than plasma glucose.
- Heel sticks sample venous blood, which has a lower glucose concentration than arterial blood. If a capillary sample from the foot is low (less than 45 mg/dl), or, if it is normal but the newborn is symptomatic, then a plasma glucose sample must be obtained by venipuncture.

Table 16-4   Procedure for Glucose Testing by Heel Stick

1. Gather equipment: alcohol swabs, cotton ball, sterile gauze square, lancet, glucose strips, gloves, bandage.
2. Prewarm foot with warm wet wrap for 30 seconds to decrease stasis.
3. Wash your hands, put on gloves.
4. Grasp foot firmly with hand, using some pressure to briefly occlude blood flow.
5. Prep skin with alcohol and blot dry with sterile gauze.
6. Select an area on the lateral aspect of the foot—not on the heel where a lancet stick can cause permanent damage.
7. Pierce the foot with the lancet.
8. Following instructions on the glucose test strip bottle, place the correct number of drops of blood on the reagent strip.
9. Time test accurately. Compare color on test strip with chart on bottle.
10. Wipe heel with cotton and place bandage on puncture.

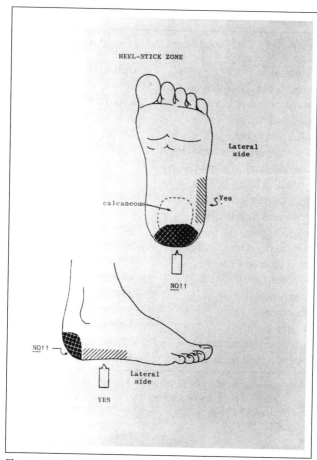

Figure 16-4   Anatomic landmarks for heel sticks.

Changes in the Blood

Table 16-5   Cord Blood Values of a Full-Term Newborn

Component	Optimal Range
Hemoglobin concentration	14.0–20.0 g/dL
Red blood cell (RBC) count	4,200,000–5,800,000/mm^3
Hematocrit	43–63%
Mean cell diameter	8.0–8.3 μm
Mean corpuscular volume (MCV)	100–120 μm^3
Mean corpuscular hemoglobin (MCH)	32–40 pg
Mean corpuscular hemoglobin concentration (MCHC)	30–34%
Reticulocyte count	3–7%
Nucleated red blood cell count	200–600/mm^3
White blood cell count	10,000–30,000/mm^3
Granulocytes	40–80%
Lymphocytes	20–40%
Monocytes	3–10%
Platelet count	150,000–350,000/mm^3
Serum iron concentration	125–225 μg/dL
Total iron-binding capacity	150–350 μg/dL

Source: Fanaroff, A., and Martin, R. (2002). *Neonatal and perinatal medicine: Diseases of the fetus and infant* (7th ed.). St. Louis, MO: Mosby. Reprinted by permission.

Fetal hemoglobin has a high affinity for oxygen. Hemoglobin values are influenced by timing of cord clamping and newborn position immediately after birth.

Advantages of delayed cord clamping:

- Can increase the blood volume by 25–40%
- Supports the natural physiological course of transition to extrauterine life

- Provides a continuing bolus of oxygenated blood during the first few breaths
- Promotes pulmonary capillary perfusion by volume expansion
- Achieves more rapid progress of adequate oxygenation leading to closure of fetal structures such as the ductus arteriosus

Disadvantages of delayed cord clamping caused by an excessive placental transfusion to the infant may be:

- Respiratory distress
- Polycythemia
- Hyperviscosity syndrome
- Hyperbilirubinemia

To support the physiologic transfusion that occurs over the first 1 to 3 minutes of life, the newborn is placed on the mother's abdomen with the cord intact. This position promotes modest amounts of blood flow to the newborn without the potential danger of a forced and large bolus of blood. By 3 minutes, most of the blood flow from the cord to the neonate is accomplished.

Care Immediately After Birth

Table 16-6 Apgar Scoring

		Score	
Sign	0	1	2
Heart rate	Absent	Slow—below 100	Above
Respiratory effort	Absent	Slow—irregular	Good crying
Muscle tone	Flaccid	Some flexion of extremities	Active motion
Reflex irritability	None	Grimace	Vigorous cry

Color	Pale blue	Body pink, extremities blue	Completely pink

Source: Apgar, V. (1966). The newborn (Apgar) scoring system: Reflections and advice. *Pediatr Clin North Am, 113,* 3, 645 (August). Reprinted by permission.

Transitional Period

The transitional period is the time when the infant stabilizes and adjusts to extrauterine independence. The activities of this period reflect sympathetic responses to the stress of birth (tachypnea, tachycardia) and parasympathetic responses (presence of mucus, vomiting, and peristalsis). See Figure 16-5.

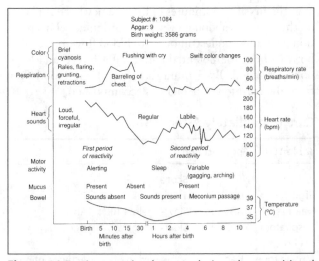

Figure 16-5 Autonomic changes during the transitional period after birth.

Source: Desmond M. M., Rudolph, A. J., and Phitaksphraiwan, P. (1966). The transitional care nursery: A mechanism for preventive medicine in the newborn. *Pediatr Clin North Am, 13,* 3, 656. Used by permission.

Table 16-7 Signs of Normal Transition

Assessment	Normal Value
Tone	Predominantly flexed
Sucking reflex	Intact
Behavior	Alertness alternating with sleep
Bowel sounds	Present after 30 minutes
Pulse	120 to 160 bpm; may vary with sleep or crying from 100 to 180 bpm
Respirations	30 to 60 rpm; diaphragmatic with abdominal wall movement
Temperature	Axillary: 36.5°–37°C (97.7°–98.6°F)
	Skin: 36°–36.5°C (96.8°–97.7°F)
Dextrostix	Greater than 45 mg %
Hematocrit	65 to 70 %

Table 16-8 The Transitional Period of the Newborn: Newborn Behaviors and Findings and Midwifery Support

First Period of Reactivity—From Birth to 30 minutes of life (approximate timing)

Behaviors/Findings

- Heart rate rapid, cord pulsation is evident
- Color shows transient cyanosis or acrocyanosis
- Respirations are rapid at the upper end of the range of normal
- Rales and rhonchi should disappear within 20 minutes
- May exhibit nasal flaring with grunting respirations and retractions
- Mucus is usually a consequence of expulsion of retained lung fluid
- Mucus is thin, clear, may have small bubbles
- Eyes are open, baby manifests alert behavior

Midwifery Support

- Maximize contact between mother and newborn
- Assist mother to hold infant to aid in the acquaintance process
- Encourage breastfeeding while the newborn is in this highly alert stage as a protection against the physiological hypoglycemia that occurs after birth
- Minimize any uncomfortable maternal procedures during this time period

- May cry, startle, or root
- Frequently has a stool immediately after birth, bowel sounds usually present by 30 minutes
- Infant focuses visually on the mother or father when they are in the appropriate field of vision
- Many will breastfeed during this period

Period of Unresponsive Sleep—30 minutes to 2 hours of age (approximate timing)

- Cardiac rate decreases during this period to less than 140 bpm
- A murmur can be heard; an indication that the ductus arteriosus has not fully closed (normal finding)
- Respiratory rate becomes more slow and even
- Deep sleep
- Bowel sounds are present but diminished

- If possible the newborn should not be disturbed for major examinations or bathing during this period.
- This first deep sleep allows the newborn to recover from the demands of birth and the immediate transition to extrauterine life.

Behaviors/Findings

Second Period of Reactivity 2 to 6 hours of age (approximate timing)

- Heart rate is labile
- Swift changes in color related to environmental stimuli
- Respiratory rate variable, related to activity, should be < 60 bpm with no rales or rhonchi
- May be interested in feeding
- May react to first feeds by spitting milk with mucus

Midwifery Support

- Early feeding
  - Helps to prevent hypoglycemia
  - Stimulates stool passage
  - Helps prevent jaundice
  - Provides bacterial colonization of the intestines
- Encourage breastfeeding
- Bottle-fed infants usually take less than an ounce per feeding.
- New mothers should be shown techniques for burping.
- Any mucus present during early feeding may interfere with adequate feeding. Large amounts of mucus may indicate a problem such as esophageal atresia. Bile-stained mucus is always a sign of illness.

Plan of Care for the First Few Days

The plan of care for the newborn includes ongoing observation, plans for physical care, feeding, assessment of elimination, blood work, screening tests, and medications. The midwife should observe for signs that the mother and other family members are ready to assume responsibility for care of the newborn. A complete physical examination and gestational age assessment must be completed. Indication of whether the infant is average for gestational age (AGA), small for gestational age (SGA), or large for gestational age (LGA) will influence the complete plan of care (Figure 16-7).

If the midwife is not providing direct care of the newborn, written orders should be provided for the nurse or birth assistant. The following is a sample of written orders:

1. Admit to well-baby nursery (in-hospital).
2. Check temperature, pulse, and respirations every 30 minutes X 4, then every hour until stable.
3. Record urination and bowel movements.
4. Weigh infant on admission and daily.
5. Administer 1 mg vitamin K intramuscularly into right anterolateral thigh.
6. Administer eye prophylaxis: erythromycin ointment 0.5% in each eye.
7. Use soap and water to care for umbilical cord. Dry and expose to air when possible.
8. Administer sponge bath to infant after temperature has been stable 1 hour.
9. May place infant in bassinet with cotton cap (in-hospital).
10. Offer breast prn or at least every 2 hours or offer bottle (name formula type) every 3 hours.
11. Administer 0.5 ml (10 mcg) hepatitis B vaccine into left anterolateral thigh.
12. Screen for PKU and hypothyroid (others as required by law) as per protocol at 48 hours of age.

Discharge Planning

Table 16-9   Criteria for Short Hospital Stay (<48 Hours)
of Term Newborns

The antepartum, intrapartum, and postpartum courses for both
mother and baby are uncomplicated.

Delivery is vaginal.

The baby is a single birth at 38 to 42 weeks' gestation and the
birth weight is AGA.

The baby's vital signs are documented as being normal and
stable for the 12 hours preceding discharge.

The baby has urinated and passed at least one stool.

The baby has completed at least two successful feedings, with
coordinated sucking, swallowing, and breathing while feeding.

Physical examination reveals no abnormalities that require
continued hospitalization.

There is no evidence of excessive bleeding at the circumcision
site for at least 2 hours.

There is no evidence of jaundice in the first 24 hours of life.

The mother has received training regarding:

1. Breastfeeding or bottle-feeding. The breastfeeding mother–
   infant dyad should be assessed by trained staff regarding
   nursing position, latch-on, adequacy of swallowing, and
   mother's knowledge of urine and stool frequency.

2. Cord, skin, and infant genital care.

3. Ability to recognize signs of illness and common infant
   problems, particularly jaundice.

4. Proper infant safety (e.g., proper use of a car seat and
   positioning for sleeping).

Support person(s), including health care providers, familiar with
newborn care, lactation and recognition of jaundice and
dehydration are available to the mother and the baby.

Laboratory data are available and reviewed, including: Maternal
syphilis and hepatitis B surface antigen status. Cord or infant
blood type and direct Coombs' test result as clinically indicated.

Screening tests are performed in accordance with state
regulations. If the test is performed before 24 hours of milk
feeding, a system for repeating the test must be assured.

Initial hepatitis B vaccine is administered or scheduled within
the first week of life.

A health care provider-directed source of medical care for both
mother and baby is identified. For discharge in less than 48
hours after delivery, an appointment has been made for the
baby to be examined within 48 hours of discharge.

Source: American Academy of Pediatrics, Committee on Fetus and the
Newborn. (1995). Hospital stay for healthy term newborns. *Pediatrics, 96,*
4, Pt. 1, 788–790. Adapted with permission.

Examination of the Newborn

See Chapter 80, *Varney's Midwifery*, 4th edition, for a
detailed review of newborn physical assessment.

Table 16-10   Medical and Perinatal Factors
and Neonatal Impact

Factors	Possible Implications for the Newborn
Maternal Medical Factors	
Cardiac disease	Chronic intrauterine hypoxia
Diabetes	Large for gestational age; trauma; hyper-bilirubinemia; stillbirth
Kidney disease	Prematurity, IUGR
Hypertension	Growth retardation; prematurity; abruptio placentae
Sexually trans-mitted diseases	Perinatal transmission
Substance abuse	Neontal withdrawal syndrome
Rh or other isoimmunization	Anemia; jaundice; hydrops fetalis
History of prior pregnancy losses	Genetic syndromes

Factors	Possible Implications for the Newborn
Prenatal Factors	
No prenatal care	Maternal substance abuse; lack of social supports
Bleeding during pregnancy	Placental defects; placenta previa
Size-dates discrepancy	Growth restriction; large newborn; trauma
Pregnancy-induced hypertension	Growth restriction; prematurity
Gestational diabetes	Macrosomia; birth trauma
Polyhydramnios	Neonatal kidney problems, inability to swallow
Oligohydramnios	Amniotic band defects; dehydration syndromes, neonatal kidney/bladder abnormalities
Infection	Perinatal transmission
Perinatal Factors	
Preterm/postterm labor	RDS; asphyxia
Prolonged labor	Neonatal trauma
Drug use in labor	Neonatal respiratory distress
Fetal distress	Asphyxia
Elevated maternal temperature	Perinatal transmission of infection
Abnormal presentation or position of fetus	Neonatal trauma
Meconium-stained fluid	Meconium aspiration pneumonia
Prolonged rupture of membranes	Perinatal transmission of infection
Excess bleeding in labor	Newborn hypovolemia; hypoxia
Prolapsed cord	Asphyxia
Maternal hypotension	Asphyxia
Fetal acidosis	Newborn acidosis

Table 16-11 Information Gathered by Observation

Gestational Age Assessment	Physical Assessment
Skin attributes	Central and peripheral body color
General maturation (female)	Muscle tone
	Characteristics of cry
Posture	Characteristics of respirations
Lanugo	Body proportions and formation of visible body parts
	Abdominal contours
	Presence of hair, fingernails, toenails
	Symmetry of eyes; movements of mouth, arms, legs
	Presence of normal external genitalia
	Straight, intact spine

Gestational Age Assessment

The NBS (Figure 16-6) can date newborns of gestational ages as low as 20 weeks. Very premature newborns should be assessed soon after birth because of rapid changes in their skin and overall condition. The NBS and other scales are accurate within a range of 2 weeks. Technical competence in performance of the NBS is critical to achieve an accurate outcome.

Table 16-12 New Ballard Scale: Neuromuscular Evaluation and Assessment of Physical Maturity

Procedure for the neuromuscular evaluation is as follows:

• Posture: with the infant supine and quiet, score as indicated on Figure 16-6.

- Square window: flex the hand at the wrist; exert pressure sufficient to get as much flexion as possible.
- Arm recoil: with the infant supine, fully flex the forearm for 5 seconds, then fully extend by pulling the hands, and release.
- Popliteal angle: with the infant supine and the pelvis flat on the examining surface, the leg is flexed on the thigh and the thigh fully flexed using one hand; with the other hand, the leg is then extended.
- Scarf sign: with the infant supine, take the infant's hand and draw it across the neck and as far across the opposite shoulder as possible; assist the elbow by lifting it across the body.
- Heel-to-ear maneuver: with the infant supine, hold the infant's foot with one hand and move it as near to the head as possible without forcing it; keep the pelvis flat on the examining surface.

Procedure for assessment of physical maturity includes the following:

- Check lanugo on the back with a direct light in order to get a clear view.
- Palpate the entire pinna of the ear for presence of cartilage.
- Palpate to accurately assess breast tissue.

Because the NBS is a standardized tool, it is important for the midwife to record findings as the assessment is made and not to rely on memory. The NBS takes approximately 2 to 3 minutes to perform and should be recorded directly on the standardized form found in most nurseries. After scores for each category of physical and neuromuscular maturity have been assigned, they are added and the aggregate score is plotted to obtain gestational age.

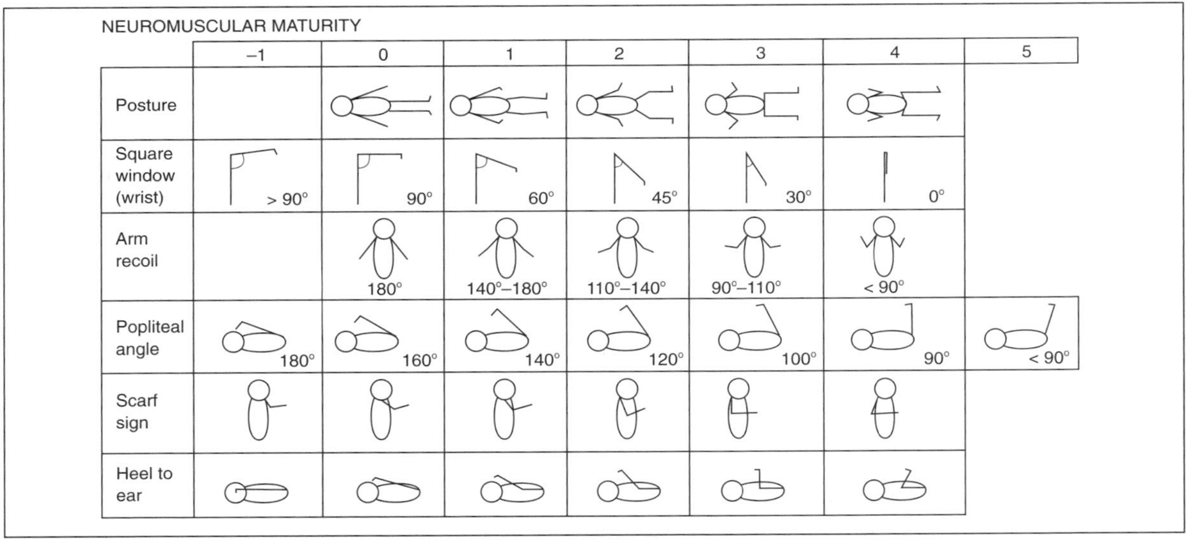

Figure 16-6 The New Ballard Scale (NBS).

Source: Ballard, J. (1991). New Ballard Scale, expanded to include extremely premature infants. *J Pediatr, 119,* 417. Reproduced by permission.

PHYSICAL MATURITY

							Leathery, cracked, wrinkled
Skin	Sticky, friable, transparent	Gelatinous, red, translucent	Smooth, pink, visible veins	Superficial peeling and/or rash, few veins	Cracking, pale areas, rare veins	Parchment, deep cracking, no vessels	Leathery, cracked, wrinkled
Lanugo	None	Sparse	Abundant	Thinning	Bald areas	Mostly bald	
Plantar surface	Heel-toe 40–50 mm: −1; < 40 mm: −2	> 50 mm, no crease	Faint red marks	Anterior transverse crease only	Creases anterior two-thirds	Creases over entire sole	
Breast	Imperceptible	Barely perceptible	Flat areola, no bud	Stippled areola, 1–2 mm bud	Raised areola, 3–4 mm bud	Full areola, 5–10 mm bud	
Eye/Ear	Lids fused loosely: −1; tightly: −2	Lids open; pinna flat, stays folded	Slightly curved pinna, soft, slow recoil	Well-curved pinna, soft but ready recoil	Pinna formed and firm, instant recoil	Thick cartilage, ear stiff	
Genitals (male)	Scrotum flat, smooth	Scrotum empty, faint rugae	Testes in upper canal, rare rugae	Testes descending, few rugae	Testes down, good rugae	Testes pendulous, deep rugae	
Genitals (female)	Clitoris prominent, labia flat	Clitoris prominent, labia minora small	Clitoris prominent, labia minora enlarged	Labia majora and minora equally prominent	Labia majora large, labia minora small	Labia majora cover clitoris and labia minora	

MATURITY RATING

Score	Weeks
−10	20
−5	22
0	24
5	26
10	28
15	30
20	32
25	34
30	36
35	38
40	40
45	42
50	44

Figure 16-6 (Continued)

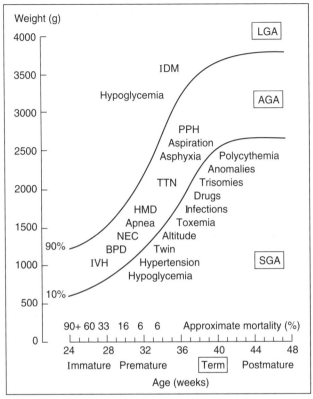

Figure 16-7 Conditions associated with birth weight/gestational age categories. Specific clinical conditions frequently encountered in the three major developmental channels: (1) large for gestational age (LGA); (2) appropriate for gestational age (AGA); (3) small for gestational age (SGA). Expected approximate overall mortality is indicated on the abscissa.

IDM, infant of a diabetic mother; IVH, intraventricular hemorrhage; BPD, bronchopulmonary dysplasia; NEC, necrotizing enterocolitis; HMD, hyaline membrane disease; TTN, transient tachypnea of the newborn; PPH, persistent pulmonary hypertension or persistent fetal circulation.

Source: Battaglia, F., and Lubchenco, L. A. (1967). Practical classification of newborn infants by weight and gestational age. *J Pediatrics, 71,* 159. Reproduced by permission.

Table 16-13 Mean Birth Weights, Lengths, and Head Circumferences of Term Newborns

Gestational Age (weeks)	Weight (g)	Length (cm)	Head Circumference (cm)
38	3050	48.3	33.6
39	3225	49.0	34.0
40	3364	49.5	34.3
41	3501	50.2	34.7
42	3598	50.5	34.9

Source: Dombrowski, M., Wolfe, H., Brans, Y., Saleh, A., and Sokol, R. (1992). Neonatal morphometry: Relation to obstetric, pediatric and menstrual estimates of gestational age. *Am J Dis Children, 146,* 852. Reprinted by permission.

Table 16-14 Common Minor Malformations of the Newborn

- Large fontanel
- Epicanthal folds
- Hair whorls
- Widow's peak
- Low posterior hair line
- Preauricular tags and pits
- Minor ear anomalies: protruding, rotated, low set
- Darwinian tubercle
- Digital anomalies: clinodactyly (curved finger); camptodactyly (bent finger); syndactyly (webbed finger); polydactyly (extra finger/s)
- Transverse palmar crease
- Shawl scrotum
- Redundant umbilicus
- Widespread nipples
- Supernumerary nipples

Table 16-15   Visual Clues that Suggest Birth Defects and Genetic Conditions

Diagnosis	Visual Clues
Mendelian Inheritance	
1. Autosomal Dominant (AD)	
Neurofibromatosis I	Cafe au lait spots
Tuberous sclerosis	Ash leaf spot
Myotonic dystrophy	Myopathic facies
Multiple epiphyseal dysplasia	Bumps at end of long bones
Waardenburg syndrome	White forelock
Peutz-Jehger syndrome	Brown lip macules
Van der Woude syndrome	Lip pits
Holt-Oram syndrome	Thumb anomaly
2. Autosomal Recessive (AR)	
Tay-Sachs disease	Cherry red spot
Galactosemia	Cataracts and neonatal jaundice
Cystic fibrosis	Meconium ileus, rectal prolapse
Congenital adrenal hyperplasia	Ambiguous genitalia
Mucopolysaccharidoses	Corneal clouding, joint contracture
Meckel-Gruber syndrome	Polydactyly, encephalocele
Rhizomelia chondrodysplasia	Short proximal limbs, cataracts
3. X-Linked Recessive (X-LR)	
Fragile-X syndrome	Large testes
Duchenne muscular dystrophy	Large calf muscle
Menke Kinky Hair syndrome	Steel-wool like hair
Usher syndrome	Retinitis pigmentosa
Lesch-Nyhan syndrome	Gravel urine, self-mutilation

Diagnosis	**Visual Clues**
4. X-Linked Fominant (X-LD)	
Incontinentia pigmenti	Pigmented skin swirls
Rett syndrome	Hand wringing
Vitamin D resistant ricketts	Bowed legs

Non-Mendelian Inheritance

1. Mitochondrial	All associated with muscle
Kearns-Sayre	weakness, ophthalmo-
Lebers disease	plegia, and recurrent
MELAS	episodes of acidosis
MERRF	
2. Uniparental Disomy	
Prader-Willi	Obesity, small hands and feet
Angelman	MR, recurrent bouts of laughter
3. Gonadal Mosaicism	
Osteogenesis Imperfecta	Blue sclera, brittle bones

Teratogen

Alcohol	Microcephaly, short palpebral fissures
Dilantin	Nail hypoplasia
Hyperpyrexia	Neural tube defects (NTD)
Tegretol	NTD
Coumadin	Flat nasal bridge
Accutane	Facial and limb anomalies

Multifactorial

Clubfoot	Same as diagnosis in each
Cleft lip/palate (CLP)	case
NTD	
Dislocated hip	
Congenital heart	
Hypospadies	

Chromosomal

Trisomy 21	Hypotonia, single palmar crease, prominent tongue
Trisomy 18	Finger and joint contracture, webbed neck
Trisomy 13	Polydactyly, CLP, scalp defects
45 XO	Short stature, webbed neck
Klinefelter	Small testes, gynecomastia
Cat-cry 5p(-)	Natal mewing

Sporadic Multiple Pattern Syndrome

Cornelia de Lange	Synophrys, phocomelia
Rubinstein-Taby	Large thumbs and great toes
Williams syndrome	Elfin facies
Sturge-Weber	Nevus flammeus
VATER ASSN	TE-fistula

Congenital Defects Minor and Major Malformations

Preauricular tags and sinus tracts	Deafness and renal disease
Nasal dermoids	Nasal sinus tract to septum and to brain in some cases
Lip pits	Cleft lip and palate
Bifid uvula	Submucous cleft
Enlarged tongue	Hypothyroidism
Two-vessel cord	Renal disease
Lumbar hair tuft	Spinal cord lesions

Source: Wardinsky, T. (1994). Visual clues to diagnosis of birth defects and genetic disease. *J Pediatr Health Care, 8,* 2, 63. Reprinted by permission.

Neurological Examination

The midwife elicits the following reflexes as part of the physical exam:

Eyes: Pupillary reflex, red reflex, doll's eye reflex, blink reflex

Upper extremities: Palmar grasp reflex
Lower extremities: Patellar reflex, plantar reflex,
                     Babinski reflex
Torso: Anal wink, tonic neck reflex

Absent, markedly diminished, or accentuated reflexes should be noted on the physical exam form; asymmetrical reflexes should also be noted. The midwife should then consult with a pediatric provider about further testing and follow-up. The Moro reflex, or embracing reflex:

- Symmetrical, disappears by 2 to 4 months
- Consists predominantly of abduction and extension of the arms with hands open and the thumb and index finger semiflexed to form the letter C
- Leg movements may occur, but they are not as uniform as the arm movements.
- With return of the arms toward the body, the infant either relaxes or cries.

The midwife must take care to elicit a Moro reflex and avoid "startles." Acceptable ways to elicit a Moro reflex include the following:

- Striking the examining table near the head of the baby
- Allowing a semisitting infant to fall backward (onto the examiner's open hand) from an angle of 30°
- Jarring the table suddenly
- Making a loud noise or handclap

Medical consultation is required if any of the following deviations is found with the Moro reflex test:

- Absence of the reflex indicates possible intracranial lesions.

- Asymmetrical response may indicate birth injury involving the brachial plexus, clavicle, or humerus.
- Abnormal persistence of embrace gesture indicates hypertonicity.
- Persistence of entire Moro reflex after 4 months indicates delay in neurological maturation.

Resuscitation at Birth

Guidelines for neonatal resuscitation are discussed in detail in *Varney's Midwifery*, 4th edition. Details of full infant resuscitation are not covered in this book.

Every midwife and birth assistant attending births should be certified in neonatal advanced life support. The training course, the Neonatal Resuscitation Program (NRP), was jointly developed by the American Heart Association and the American Academy of Pediatrics and is available nationally. Check the AAP Web site (www.aap.org/ nrp) for new developments and online review materials.

Pathophysiology of Asphyxia

The events in asphyxia include:

- Lack of oxygenation of cells
- Excess carbon dioxide retention
- Metabolic acidosis

These events cause cell damage and a biochemical environment that is incompatible with life. The goals of resuscitation are:

- Timely intervention
- Reversal of the biochemical effects of asphyxia
- Prevention of irreversible brain and organ damage

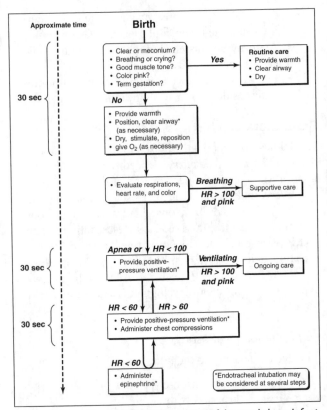

Figure 16-8 Algorithm for resuscitation of the newly born infant.

Source: Niermeyer, S., Kattwinkel, J., Van Reempts, P., et al. (2000). International guidelines for neonatal resuscitation: An excerpt from the guidelines 2000 for cardiopulmonary resuscitation and emergency cardiovascular care. International consensus on science, contributors and reviewers for the neonatal resuscitation guidelines. *Pediatrics, 106,* 3, E29. Used by permission.

Table 16-16 Procedure for Positive Pressure Ventilation

Equipment	Method	Precautions
1. Anesthesia bag with pressure gauge (manometer) or self-inflating bag with oxygen reservoir attachment	1. Suction nares and oropharynx to clear secretions.	1. Inadequate ventilation may be caused by poor seal around mask, flexed or hyperextended neck, or inadequate pressure of ventilation.
2. Infant- and premature-size face masks	2. Place infant's head in a neutral position (when hyperextended, air enters esophagus).	2. Face mask pressure near the infant's eyes can cause tissue damage.
3. Stethoscope	3. Place mask over nose and mouth, making sure seal is tight.	3. Positive pressure ventilation will cause air retention in the stomach. After bagging for a brief period of time, vent the stomach by passing a feeding tube. Any gastric contents should also be emptied. If bagging is going to continue over time (e.g., while awaiting a transport team), stop momentarily to slip a tube into the stomach to vent the stomach and prevent or reduce distention. Secure tube in place while continuing to ventilate.
4. Feeding tube	4. Pressure for first breath should be 40–50 cm H_2O.	
5. Source of humidified oxygen with flowmeter	5. Subsequent breaths need about 25 cm H_2O or the lowest pressure that will allow you to see the chest wall expanding.	
	6. Ventilate 40–50 times per minute for for 23 minutes.	
	7. Have assistant auscultate anterior upper lobes of the lungs for aeration.	
	8. Continue to provide free-flow O_2 by face mask after infant has established respirations.	

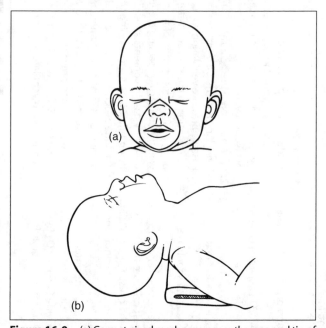

Figure 16-9   (a) Correct-sized mask covers mouth, nose, and tip of chin, but not the eyes. (b) Correct position for assisted ventilation.

Source: Kattwinkel, J. (2000). *Textbook of neonatal resuscitation* (4th ed.). Elk Grove Village, IL: American Heart Association and Academy of Pediatrics. Used with permission.

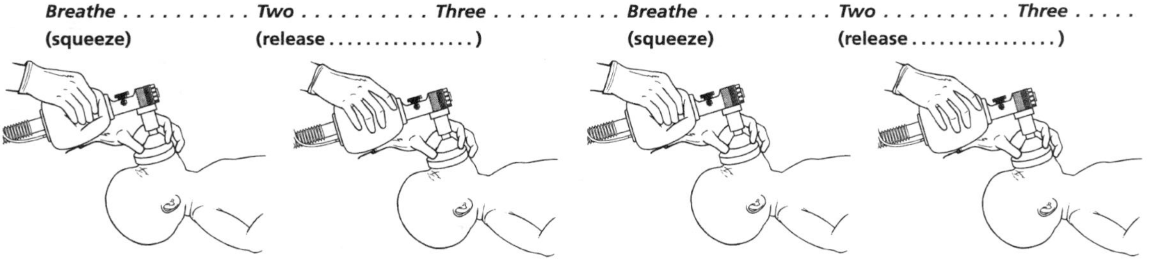

Figure 16-10 Rhythm for effective positive pressure ventilation.

Source: Kattwinkel, J. (2000). *Textbook of neonatal resuscitation* (4th ed.). Elk Grove Village, IL: American Heart Association and Academy of Pediatrics. Reproduced by permission.

Techniques of Cardiac Compression

The goal of cardiac compression is to provide the proper frequency of compression accompanied by a pressure that is effective yet avoids damage to internal organs.

Initiate if respirations <60 bpm:

- Assistance from a second trained person is needed.
- During compressions, ventilatory support must continue.
- Caregiver's fingers should give pressure downward, without splaying pressure out laterally.
- Fingers or thumbs can be positioned side-by-side in either the thumb technique or the two-finger technique (see Figure 16-11).
- Apply fingers to lower third of the sternum.
- Compress sternum to a depth of one-third of the anterior posterior diameter of the chest.
- Between compressions, do not remove the fingers from the newborn.
- Compressions should be at the rate of 90 compressions per minute.
- Intersperse with adequate ventilations in a ratio of 3:1, or three cardiac compressions to one ventilation every 2 seconds.
- After 30 seconds, pause and evaluate the heart rate for 6 seconds.
- If heart rate is >60 bpm, discontinue cardiac compressions, PPV must continue until spontaneous respirations.
- If heart rate is <60 bpm, cardiac compressions must continue.
- Newborn may need medications to strengthen and increase the heart rate so cardiac output will be adequate.
- If heart rate is >100 bpm, stop cardiac compressions and gradually decrease PPV.

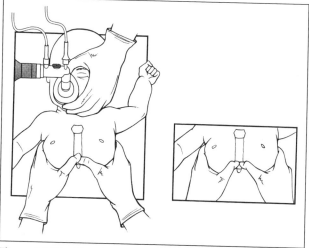

Figure 16-11   Thumb technique of chest compressions for small and large babies.

Source: Kattwinkel, J. (2000). *Textbook of neonatal resuscitation* (4th ed.). Elk Grove Village, IL: American Heart Association and Academy of Pediatrics. Used with permission.

Care of the Neonate Born in Meconium-Stained Amniotic Fluid

Prior to birth, 10% to 30% of fetuses pass meconium, which is retained in the amniotic fluid. The passage of meconium prior to birth is directly related to increasing gestational age. Theories of the etiology of meconium passage include:

- That it is a maturational event of no significance
- That it is a symptom of chronic hypoxia during the fetal period

- That it is a symptom of acute hypoxia during labor that stimulates a vagal response

The type of damage inflicted by meconium is related in part to how deeply meconium is inhaled into the lungs. Meconium can damage the newborn lungs by:

- Acting as a chemical irritant causing pneumonitis
- Causing direct blockage of the airways

The goal of care for the meconium-exposed newborn is prevention of aspiration.

- This is accomplished by deep suctioning of the baby's head as it rests on the perineum and prior to the chest recoil that occurs with the birth of the body.
- Suctioning can be done manually or with wall suction.
- The mouth and posterior pharynx are suctioned first.
- The newborn is then placed on the resuscitation surface for observation and evaluation.
- A vigorous newborn requires no special care (guidelines of AAP/AHA).
- Nonvigorous newborns require aggressive care whenever possible including:
  - Either intubation and suctioning of the cords with a meconium aspirator attached directly to the ET tube or direct suctioning with wall suction while observing the cords.
  - In a home birth, aggressive management with direct DeLee suctioning after visualization of the cords by laryngoscope.
  - Very depressed newborns should have intubation and suctioning in accordance with the standard of care in the local community or institution.

References

Gilstrap, L. Fetal acid-base balance. (1999). In Creasy R, Resnik R. eds. *Maternal Fetal Medicine* (4th ed.). Philadelphia, PA: Saunders.

Kalhan, S., & Peter-Wohl, S. (2000). Hypoglycemia: What is it for the neonate? *Am J Perintatol, 17,* 1

Mercer, J. S., & Skovgaard, R. L. (2002). Neonatal transitional physiology: A new paradigm. *J Perinat Neonat Nurs, 15,* 4, 56–75.

NACC Standards Committee. (1995). *National association of childbearing centers standards.* Perkiomenville, PA: National Association of Childbearing Centers.

Pildes, R., & Lilien, L. (1992). Carbohydrate disorders. In Fanaroff, A. A., & Martin, R. J. *Neonatal and perinatal medicine: Diseases of the fetus and infant* (5th ed.) St. Louis, MO: Mosby.

Varney, H., Kriebs, J. M., & Gegor, C. L. (2003). *Varney's Midwifery* (4th ed.). Sudbury, MA: Jones and Bartlett Publishers, Inc. Chapters 36, 37, 38, 39, 41.

Volpe, J. (1995). *Neurology of the newborn* (3rd ed.) Philadelphia, PA: Saunders.

Wiswell, T. Delivery room management of the apparently vigorous meconium-stained neonate: Results of a multicenter, international collaborative trial. *Pediatrics, 105,* 1–7.

SECTION 17

Primary Care
of the Newborn

Midwifery Role in Newborn Care

- May be minimal formal role after the birth
- May be primary care throughout the first 6 weeks of life
  - Collegial relationship with pediatric providers
  - Well-child care gradually shifts to pediatric providers

All midwives answer parents' questions about care and well-being of their newborns.

Well-Child Surveillance in the First 4 Weeks

All newborns should have at least two physical examinations before discharge from the birth center or hospital or before the midwife leaves after a home birth.

First Examinations

- Screening at birth (Section 16)
- Comprehensive exam including gestational age assessment (Section 16)

First Outpatient Visit

- Timing
  - If discharged at or before 48 hours, then see newborn again on 3rd to 5th days of life.

- If discharged after 48 hours, then the visit can be delayed until the infant is 10 to 14 days old.
- Purpose of visit
  - Reexamine the newborn.
  - Review teaching and anticipatory guidance.
  - Perform metabolic screening if not done prior to discharge (accurate PKU requires 48 hours of milk feedings).

Content of Initial Well-Child Visit

- Review maternal history, birth history, immediate neonatal course and unresolved issues regarding the birth.
- Observe parents and interview regarding family adjustment: assess well-being of parents, coping strategies, signs of depression, and for signs of parental attachment.
- Take a newborn interval history: feeding, alertness, crying, bowel, bladder, and other problems
- Measure weight, length, and head circumference.
- Perform physical exam with attention to reflexes, signs of dehydration, alertness, heart sounds, and abduction of the hips.
- Review need for metabolic screening.
- Provide teaching and anticipatory guidance.
- Schedule visit in 6 to 8 weeks for further immunization and check-up.
- Review how to reach the pediatric provider for emergencies.

Recommended Schedule for Immunizations of Infants and Children

Vaccine ▼ / Age ▶	Birth	1 mo	2 mos	4 mos	6 mos	12 mos	15 mos	18 mos	24 mos	4-6 yrs	11-12 yrs	13-18 yrs
			Range of Recommended Ages				Catch-up Vaccination				Preadolescent Assessment	
Hepatitis B[1]	HepB #1 *only if mother HBsAg(-)*	HepB #2			HepB #3						HepB Series	
Diphtheria, tetanus, pertussis[2]			DTaP	DTaP	DTaP		DTaP	DTaP		DTaP	Td	
Haemophilus influenzae Type b[3]			Hib	Hib	Hib	Hib						
Inactivated Polio[4]			IPV	IPV	IPV		IPV			IPV		
Measles, mumps, rubella[4]						MMR #1				MMR #2	MMR #2	
Varicella[5]						Varicella			Varicella		Varicella	
Pneumococcal[6]			PCV	PCV	PCV	PCV			PCV	PPV	PPV	
Hepatitis A[7]									Hepatitis A series			
Influenza[8]					Influenza (yearly)							

Vaccines below this line are for selected populations

This schedule indicates the recommended ages for routine administration of currently licensed childhood vaccines, as of December 1, 2002, for children through age 18 years. Any dose not given at the recommended age should be given at any subsequent visit when indicated and feasible. ▨ Indicates age groups that warrant special effort to administer those vaccines not previously given. Additional vaccines may be licensed and recommended during the year. Licensed combination vaccines may be used whenever any components of the combination are indicated and the vaccine's other components are not contraindicated. Providers should consult the manufacturers' package inserts for detailed recommendations.

Figure 17-1 Recommended schedule for immunizations of infants and children.

1. Hepatitis B vaccine (HepB). All infants should receive the first dose of hepatitis B vaccine soon after birth and before hospital discharge; the first dose may also be given by age 2 months if the infant's mother is HBsAg-negative. Only monovalent HepB can be used for the birth dose. Monovalent or combination vaccine containing HepB may be used to complete the series. Four doses of vaccine may be administered when a birth dose is given. The second dose should be given at least 4 weeks after the first dose, except for combination vaccines which cannot be administered before age 6 weeks. The third dose should be given at least 16 weeks after the first dose and at least 8 weeks after the second dose. The last dose in the vaccination series (third or fourth dose) should not be administered before age 6 months.

Infants born to HBsAg-positive mothers should receive HepB and 0.5 mL Hepatitis B Immune Globulin (HBIG) within 12 hours of birth at separate sites. The second dose is recommended at age 1–2 months. The last dose in the vaccination series should not be administered before age 6 months. These infants should be tested for HBsAg and anti-HBs at 9–15 months of age.

Infants born to mothers whose HBsAg status is unknown should receive the first dose of the HepB series within 12 hours of birth. Maternal blood should be drawn as soon as possible to determine the mother's HBsAg status; if the HBsAg test is positive, the infant should receive HBIG as soon as possible (no later than age 1 week). The second dose is recommended at age 1–2 months. The last dose in the vaccination series should not be administered before age 6 months.

2. Diphtheria and tetanus toxoids and acellular pertussis vaccine (DTaP). The fourth dose of DTaP may be administered as early as age 12 months, provided 6 months have elapsed since the third dose and the child is unlikely to return at age 15–18 months. **Tetanus and diphtheria toxoids (Td)** are recommended at age 11–12 years if at least 5 years have elapsed since the last dose of tetanus and diphtheria toxoid-containing vaccine. Subsequent routine Td boosters are recommended every 10 years.

3. *Haemophilus influenzae* type b (Hib) conjugate vaccine. Three Hib conjugate vaccines are licensed for infant use. If PRP-OMP (PedvaxHIB® or ComVax® [Merck]) is administered at ages 2 and 4 months, a dose at age 6 months is not required. DTaP/Hib combination products should not be used for primary immunization in infants at ages 2, 4, or 6 months, but can be used as boosters following any Hib vaccine.

4. Measles, mumps, and rubella vaccine (MMR). The second dose of MMR is recommended routinely at age 4–6 years but may be administered during any visit, provided at least 4 weeks have elapsed since the first dose and that both doses are administered beginning at or after age 12 months. Those who have not previously received the second dose should complete the schedule by the 11–12-year-old visit.

5. Varicella vaccine. Varicella vaccine is recommended at any visit at or after age 12 months for susceptible children, i.e., those who lack a reliable history of chickenpox. Susceptible persons aged ≥ 13 years should receive two doses, given at least 4 weeks apart.

6. Pneumococcal vaccine. The heptavalent **pneumococcal conjugate vaccine (PCV)** is recommended for all children age 2–23 months. It is also recommended for certain children age 24–59 months. **Pneumococcal polysaccharide vaccine (PPV)** is recommended in addition to PCV for certain high-risk groups. See MMWR 2000;49(RR-9);1–38.

(Continued)

7. Hepatitis A vaccine. Hepatitis A vaccine is recommended for children and adolescents in selected states and regions, and for certain high-risk groups; consult your local public health authority. Children and adolescents in these states, regions, and high risk groups who have not been immunized against hepatitis A can begin the hepatitis A vaccination series during any visit. The two doses in the series should be administered at least 6 months apart. See MMWR 1999;48(RR-12):1–37.

8. Influenza vaccine. Influenza vaccine is recommended annually for children age ≥ 6 months with certain risk factors (including but not limited to asthma, cardiac disease, sickle cell disease, HIV, diabetes, and household members of persons in groups at high risk; see MMWR 2002;51(RR-3);1–31), and can be administered to all others wishing to obtain immunity. In addition, healthy children age 6–23 months are encouraged to receive influenza vaccine if feasible because children in this age group are at substantially increased risk for influenza-related hospitalizations. Children aged ≤ 12 years should receive vaccine in a dosage appropriate for their age (0.25 mL if age 6–35 months or 0.5 mL if aged ≥ 3 years). Children aged ≥ 8 years who are receiving influenza vaccine for the first time should receive two doses separated by at least 4 weeks.

For additional information about vaccines, including precautions and contraindications for immunization and vaccine shortages, please visit the National Immunization Program Web site at http://www.cdc.gov/nip or call the National Immunization Information Hotline at 800-232-2522 (English) or 800-232-0233 (Spanish).

Approved by the Advisory Committee on Immunization Practices (http://www.cdc.gov/nip/acip), the American Academy of Pediatrics (http://www.aap.org), and the American Academy of Family Physicians (http://www.aafp.org).

Source: American Academy of Pediatrics. (2003). Recommended childhood and adolescent immunization schedule—United States, 2003. *Pediatrics, 111,* 1, 212. Reprinted by permission.

Common Issues in Early Physical Care
Regulation of Behavior
Each infant shows a unique ability to react to stimulation presented by the environment and its own bodily functions. Infants vary in their ability to cope with these stimuli. If parents are having trouble coping with a newborn the midwife may recommend to parents that their newborn be examined using the full Brazelton Neonatal Behavioral Assessment Scale (NBAS).

Behavioral Parts of the NBAS
The behavioral parts of the NBAS assess the infant's ability to:

- Organize behavioral states
- Decrease motor activity to cope with sensory input
- Become alert and oriented to auditory and visual stimuli
- Interact with a caregiver through cuddling
- Console self
- Habituate to repeated stimulation

The abilities to quiet down and focus, to smile and cuddle with a caregiver, and to ignore extraneous stimulation are key to coping in the world.

Bathing
Newborns need to have their heads and diaper areas sponged whenever those areas are dirty; daily full body bathing is unnecessary. Use a mild, nondeodorized soap and dry well.

Cord Care
- "Dry care" of the umbilicus is sufficient.
- The cord should dry and fall off in 2 weeks.

- Cords with a strong odor are cleaned with hydrogen peroxide.
- Call the pediatric provider if the cord oozes pus or red streaks appear on the abdomen near the umbilicus.

Skin Care in Diaper Area

- Regular diaper changes
- Thorough cleansing of the skin
- No need for routine use of powder or cream
- Barrier cream containing zinc oxide (e.g., Desitin) may stop diaper rash at the earliest stages.

Diaper Rash

Usually a reaction of the skin to the ammonia in urine and bacterial contamination from fecal material. Note the location and distribution of the problem and whether there is generalized redness, a rash, or both.

- Simple diaper rash of the irritant variety
  - Presents as flat, reddened areas without much skin fold involvement
  - Clean affected skin with mild soap and tepid water.
  - Uncomfortable when the area is cleaned
  - When possible, leave open to the air.
  - Frequent diaper changes necessary.
  - A zinc oxide barrier cream (e.g., Desitin) may prevent further skin problems.
- Fungal diaper rash caused by *Candida albicans*
  - Pronounced erythematous confluent lesions, skin fold involvement, and "satellite lesions" at some distance from the perineum and anus

- Best treated with topical antifungal preparation, e.g., topical nystatin, miconazole, or clotrimazole; fungal diaper rash will resist most other treatments.
- The baby will be in pain.
- 1% hydrocortisone cream may lessen inflammation and can be used with the fungal preparation.
- Frequent diaper changes and sponging with tepid water will also assist healing.
- A newborn must be evaluated if the parent reports peeling skin, vesicles, or an exudate.

Safety Concerns

- Falling (from a changing table or baby seat)
- Getting stuck between crib bars (should be less than 2 3/8 inches apart with a tight fitting mattress)
- Keeping mobiles out of reach
- Remove soft pillows and toys that may lead to suffocation
- Car seats—Place small infants in the backseat of the car rear facing

Prevention of Sudden Infant Death Syndrome (SIDS)

- Sleep position
  - Supine position (on the back) to minimize risk of sudden infant death syndrome (SIDS)
- Other possible contributors to SIDS include soft sleep surfaces, loose bedding, maternal smoking, bed sharing (especially with multiple family members), overheating, or preterm birth.

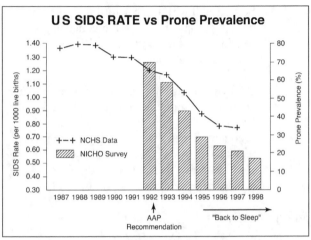

Figure 17-2   Change in incidence of SIDS since encouragement of the supine sleeping position.

Source: American Academy of Pediatrics. (2000). Changing concepts of sudden infant death syndrome: Implications for infant sleeping environment and sleep position (RE9946). *Pediatrics, 105,* 3, 650–656. Used with permission of the American Academy of Pediatrics.

Circumcision

According to the American Academy of Pediatrics:

- "Existing scientific evidence demonstrates potential medical benefits of newborn male circumcision; however, these data are not sufficient to recommend routine neonatal circumcision."
- AAP recommends that if circumcision is performed, adequate analgesia be provided via a dorsal penile nerve block or an anesthetic cream.

Nonnutritive Sucking

- Newborns use sucking as a calming activity and are better able to regulate to an alert state when they suck on a thumb or pacifier.
- There is evidence that pacifier use is associated with a lower incidence of SIDS.
- Some fetuses suck their thumb in utero and continue postnatally.

Hiccups

- Common and more annoying to the mother than to the infant
- Due to spasmodic contractions of the diaphragm from regurgitation of gastric contents
- A few swallows of water may help the contractions stop quickly.

Cradle Cap

- An adherent seborrheic exudate on the scalp
- Only of cosmetic concern
- Can be loosened by a gentle scalp massage with vegetable or olive oil and removed by shampooing and use of a very fine-tooth comb
- Usually does not return if shampooing is part of the bath

Mouth Thrush

- Caused by *Candida albicans*
  - Appears as adherent white plaque-like clumps on the tongue, gums, and hard palate
  - The baby may start to eat but then pull away from the breast or bottle while crying

○ Treated with an oral antifungal preparation or gentian violet
- Breastfeeding mothers can get a fungal infection of their nipples from an infected infant (See Section 18)

Noisy, Irregular Breathing

- Parents frequently are concerned about noises and irregularities of their infant's breathing.
  ○ The upper airways of infants are narrow; any slight nasal swelling can produce noise.
  ○ Suctioning of the nares with a bulb syringe should be discouraged, it can produce trauma and swelling, making the situation worse.
  ○ A crusted nasal discharge can be loosened with one or two drops of saline into the nares.
- Periodic breathing of the newborn must be distinguished from apnea. Direct observation of the newborn is critical to see the pattern of respiratory effort.
  ○ Periodic breathing
    - Occurs most frequently during REM sleep
    - Defined as pauses in respiratory movement for up to 20 seconds alternating with breathing
    - More prolonged pauses need evaluation, especially if accompanied by tachypnea (> 60 breaths per minute), nasal flaring, retractions, color changes, or grunting.
    - Should not be associated with a drop in heart rate.

The Fussy Baby

A frequent cause of parental desperation in the newborn's first 2 months is the fussy, inconsolable baby—often known as "high-need" or colicky babies.

History

- What are the crying and fussing patterns?
- What are the parents' expectations of the new-born's sleep-wake patterns and ability to self-comfort?
- What is the mother's mental state? Mothers who are depressed may complain about the newborn's behavior to mask their own serious depression.

Physical

- Physical examination should rule out infections, milk intolerance, and gastrointestinal blockage.
- An organic cause is rarely pinpointed.

Management

- Education of the parents in calming techniques
  - Try to feed the baby.
  - Hold the baby; try different holds that provide abdominal support.
  - Swaddle the baby.
  - Give the baby a pacifier.
  - Talk to the baby face to face using low, rhythmic sounds.
  - Reduce sensory stimulation in the room.
  - Walk the baby around the room.
  - Take the baby outside for a walk or a car ride.
- Try each technique for only 5 minutes until the baby calms.
- Urge parents to discuss their frustration and anger. A fussy baby can provoke violent responses from a sleep-deprived parent.
- Reassure parents that most fussy babies settle by the third month of life.

Feeding Patterns

- First 48 hours of life
  - Minimal interest in feeding
  - Intake may be only 1 ounce
  - Should be offered a feeding regularly
- During the first month
  - Usually hungry every 2 to 3 hours
  - Offer feeding at least every 4 hours
  - Feedings of 2 to 4 oz will become the norm.

Eating Patterns and Weight Gain

Table 17-1   Weight Gain by AGA Term Infants

In the first 3 to 5 days of life:
- Newborns may lose from 5% to 10% of their birth weight.
- Breastfed babies experience greater weight loss.
- Weight should be regained by the tenth day of life.

In the first 3 months:
- Average gain of 1 ounce per day
- Breastfed babies may gain slightly less than 1 oz per day

In the first year:
- Birth weight trebles
- Birth length doubles

History

- Birth and immediate postnatal course
- Birth weight and length
- Current age
- Interval illness or problems
- Method of feeding
- Primary caregiver

- Current family stress level
- Parental level of comfort with infant and infant feeding

Determining Need for Office Visit

- Weight check (parental reassurance)
- Any critical factor identified in Table 17-2
- If no critical indicators, a phone conversation with the parent can offer some information.

Table 17-2 Factors in Feeding History Requiring Immediate Evaluation

Regular projective vomiting

Bile-stained vomit

No stools since birth

No urination since birth

Poor muscle tone—"spread-eagle posture"

Inability to rouse infant

Inability of infant to suck

Rapid respirations over time (greater than 60 per minute)

Marked color changes during eating

Taut, swollen abdomen

More than six stools per 24 hours

Bloody or excessively watery stools

Regurgitation

- Regurgitation always needs to be distinguished from vomiting.
- Regurgitation ("spitting up") is reflux of stomach contents through the immature lower esophageal sphincter and is normal in newborns.

- The amount is usually small and the spitting up is rarely forceful.
- Overfeeding with the bottle contributes to regurgitation.
- Should not interfere with weight gain.
- Regurgitated milk will not be bile- or blood-stained.

Void/Stooling Patterns

- Babies who are being fed adequately will produce both urine and feces in a regular pattern.
- Ask parents to check the diaper prior to a feed for evidence of urine. Super absorbent disposable diapers may be hard to evaluate; a cloth diaper may be necessary.
- Six voids a day indicate adequate hydration.

Table 17-3   Types of Jaundice

Physiological Jaundice	Possible Pathological Jaundice
Not visible in first 24 hours	Visible during first 24 hours
Rises slowly and peaks at day 3 or 4 of life	May rise quickly: > 5 mg/dl/ 24 hours
Total bilirubin peaks at less than 13 mg/dl	Total bilirubin greater than 13 mg/dl
Lab tests reveal predominance of unconjugated bilirubin	Great amounts of conjugated bilirubin
Not visible after 10 days	Visible jaundice persists after one week

References

American Academy of Pediatrics Task Force on Circumcision. (1999). Circumcision policy statement (RE9850). *Pediatrics, 103*, 686–693.

American Academy of Pediatrics Provisional Committee for Quality Improvement and Subcommittee on Hyperbilirubinemia. (1994). Practice guideline: Management of hyperbilirubinemia in the healthy term newborn. *Pediatrics, 94.*

Brazelton T. B. (1984). *Neonatal behavioral assessment scale* (2nd ed.). Philadelphia, PA: Lippincott.

Ludington-Hoe S. M., Cong X., & Hashemi F. Infant crying: Nature, physiologic consequences, and select interventions. *Neonatal Network, 21*, 29–36.

Varney, H., Kriebs, J. M., & Gregor, C. L. (2004). *Varney's midwifery* (4th ed.). Sudbury, MA: Jones and Bartlett Publishers, Inc. Chs. 36–41.

Infant Feeding

Breastfeeding

Nutritional supplementation with solid foods for exclusively breastfed infants should not be needed until 4–6 months of age.

Breast milk is low in iron, calcium, and zinc, all of which are readily bioavailable. Exclusively breastfed infants do not need iron supplement until 4-6 months of age.

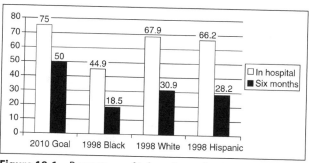

Figure 18-1 Percentage of infants breastfeeding.

Source: Ross Products Division, Abbott Laboratories, Ross Mothers' Survey.

Table 18-1 Ten Steps to Successful Breastfeeding

Every facility providing maternity services and care for newborn infants should:

1. Have a written breastfeeding policy that is routinely communicated to all health care staff.
2. Train all health care staff in skills necessary to implement this policy.
3. Inform all pregnant women about the benefits and management of breastfeeding.
4. Help all mothers initiate breastfeeding within one hour of birth.
5. Show mothers how to breastfeed and how to maintain lactation even if they should be separated from their infants.
6. Give newborn infants no food or drink other than breast milk, unless *medically* indicated.
7. Practice rooming-in to allow mothers and infants to remain together 24 hours a day.
8. Encourage breastfeeding on demand.
9. Give no artificial teats or pacifiers.
10. Foster the establishment of breastfeeding support groups and refer mothers to them on discharge from the hospital or clinic.

Source: World Health Organization/UNICEF. Accessed online at http://www.unicef.org. Used by permission.

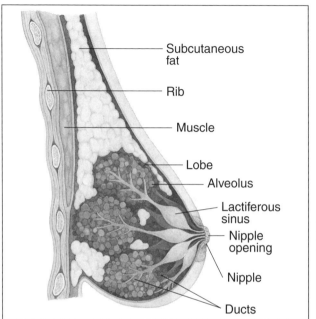

Figure 18-2 Lactating breast.

Source: Walker, M. L. (2002). *Core curriculum for lactation consultant practice.* Sudbury, MA: Jones and Bartlett Publishers, Inc.

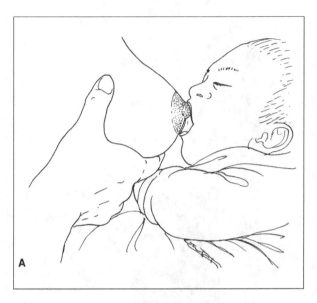

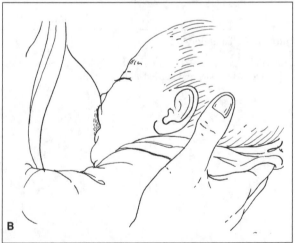

Figure 18-3 Latch on: (a) mouth gaped open; (b) grasping breast.

Nipple Pain

Can be caused by improper latch or position, blisters, cracking or fissures, candidiasis, eczema

Treat with:

- Warm compresses
- Hydrogel dressings
- Pain medication—usually NSAIDs
- Manage each diagnosis as indicated

Nipple pain associated with fissures can be a precursor to mastitis. Culture before treating with penicillinase-resistant antibiotic (such as dicloxacillin) for ten days.

Mastitis

Inflammatory process which, unrelieved, can progress to infection and abscess. Initial symptoms: mild breast pain, redness, flulike syndrome.

Diagnostic Signs

- Rapid temperature rise, often above 101°F
- Tachycardia
- Chills
- Malaise
- Tender, painful, hot, swollen, well-localized area
- Acute pain
- Hard enlarged milk glands, usually one-sided

Breast Abscess

Firm fluctuant mass, reddened, with purulent nipple discharge (sometimes), and acute pain

Common Organisms

S. aureus, Streptococci species, *H. parainfluenzae, E. coli*

Medications

Dicloxacillin (Dynapen) 500 mg po q 6 hours for
10–14 days

Cloxacillin (Cloxapen) 250–500 mg po q 6 hours
for 10–14 days

Oxacillin (Prostaphin) 500–1000 mg po or IM q
4–6 hours for 10–14 days

Cephalexin (Keflex) 250–500 mg po q 6 hours for
10–14 days

Cephaclor (Ceclor) 250–500 mg po q 6 hours for
10–14 days

Patient Teaching

- Hand washing
- Correct latch and breastfeeding technique
- Feed frequently, from both breasts unless nipple
  discharge is purulent.
- Warm compresses to area, ice if mother prefers
- Breast massage, milk expression from affected
  lobe
- Increase po fluids.
- Give pain medication as indicated.

Follow-up: 2-4 days after beginning therapy, culture
if no improvement.

Yeast Mastitis

Associated with nipple injury, thrush, maternal yeast.
Symptoms include acute onset of sharp, stabbing pain at
the nipple when the infant nurses, reddened or cracked
nipples that do not heal.

Medications
Topical

- Clotrimazole 10%, nystatin 100,000 u/g, keto-conazole, or miconazole, applied to nipple and areola after each feeding for 14 days, plus 1 ml nystatin suspension in the infant's mouth after each feeding.

Oral

- Fluconazole 200 mg qd for 14–28 days if resistant to topicals

Patient Teaching

- Frequent thorough hand washing
- Careful breast care that avoids touching both nipples without washing hands between
- Frequent changes of breast pads
- Arrange for infant treatment at the same time as the mother.

Medication Use in Breastfeeding Mothers

Many medications are believed to be contraindicated during breastfeeding, when they are in fact safe. However, not all medications safe in pregnancy are safe for nursing infants. Before any medication is prescribed, or breastfeeding cessation recommended, a reliable source should be used to determine the safety of the medication and its concentration in breast milk. Medications that have been studied or observed in infants are preferable to those that have not.

Table 18-2   Guidelines for Breastfeeding and Medication Use

- Reserve the use of pharmaceuticals for situations where they are necessary.
- Delay the use of pharmaceuticals as long as possible since maturation of the infant includes ability to better metabolize agents.
- Use the lowest dose for the shortest time that is therapeutic.
- Whenever possible, choose an agent that:
    Is used in pediatrics
    Has a short half-life
    Has a milk plasma ratio of 1 or less
    Is not sustained release
- Manipulate timing so that the lowest amount is in the milk—usually immediately after a feeding or before the baby has a long sleep period.
- Observe the baby for any changes, including behavior or physical signs like a rash.
- Teach a woman about manual expression or use of a breast pump if the only drug available is contraindicated for the baby.
- Encourage the woman to continue to breastfeed and not see use of medications as a reason she must wean her baby.

Source: Adapted from Riordan, J., and Auerbach, K. (1999). *Breastfeeding and human lactation* (2nd ed.). Sudbury, MA: Jones and Bartlett.

See also Section 3, for a scheme to classify categories of medications during lactation.

Increasing Milk Supply

- Oxytocin nasal spray, 1 spray each nostril 2–3 minutes before nursing or pumping
- Metclopromide (Reglan), 10 mg po tid for 7 days, bid for 7 days, qd for 7 days

- Fenugreek, 2–3 capsules tid, can be recommended as safe to mothers wishing to use an herbal remedy.

Medical Reasons for Supplementation
Infant Reasons

- VLBW infants
- Severe dehydration with inadequate milk supply for rehydration
- Galactosemia
- Phenylketonuria (may partially breastfeed)
- Lactase deficiency

Maternal Reasons

- Acute, severe illness (e.g., eclampsia)
- Maternal medications that are contraindicated in breastfeeding
- HIV infection when an acceptable substitute is available (including women at high documented risk)
- Untreated tuberculosis
- Herpes simplex lesion of the breast
- Drug or alcohol abuse (does not include moderate tobacco use)
  - Nicotine patch safe for use during lactation

Table 18-3 Comparison of Human Milk, Cow's Milk, and Formula

Nutrient (Unit)[2]	Minimum Level Recommended[1]	Mature Human Milk	Typical Commercial Formula	Cow's Milk (Mean)
Protein (g)[2]	1.8	1.3–1.6	2.3	5.1
Fat (g)[3]	3.3	5	5.3	5.7
Carbohydrate (g)	—	10.3	10.8	7.3
Linoleic acid (mg)	300	560	2300	125
Vitamin A (IU)	250	250	300	216
Vitamin D (IU)	40	3	63	3
Vitamin E (IU)	0.3 FT 0.7 LBW 1 g linoleic	0.3	2	0.1
Vitamin K (µg)	4	2	9	5
Vitamin C (mg)	8	7.8	8.1	2.3
Thiamin (µg)	40	25	80	59

Riboflavin (µg)	60	60	100	252
Niacin (µg)	250	250	1200	131
Vitamin B$_6$ (µg)	15 µg/g protein	15	63	66
Folic acid (µg)	4	4	10	8
Pantothenic acid (µg)	300	300	450	489
Vitamin B$_{12}$ (µg)	0.15	0.15	0.25	0.56
Biotin (µg)	1.5	1	2.5	3.1
Inositol (mg)	4	20	5.5	20
Choline (mg)	7	13	10	23
Calcium (mg)	5	50	75	186
Phosphorus (mg)	25	25	65	145
Magnesium (mg)	6	6	8	20
Iron (mg)	1	0.1	1.5 in fortified	0.08
Iodine (µg)	5	4–9	10	7

Nutrient (Unit)	Minimum Level Recommended[1]	Mature Human Milk	Typical Commercial Formula	Cow's Milk (Mean)
Copper (μg)	60	25–60	80	20
Zinc (mg)	0.5	0.1–.05	0.65	0.6
Manganese (μg)	5	1.5	5–160	3
Sodium (meq)	0.9	1	1.7	3.3
Potassium (meq)	2.1	2.1	2.7	6
Chloride (meq)	1.6	1.6	2.3	4.6
Osmolarity (mosm)	—	11.3	16–18.4	40

[1]Committe on Nutrition, American Academy of Pediatrics.

[2]Protein of nutritional quality equal to casein.

[3]Includes 300 mg essential fatty acids.

Source: Hambridge, K., and Krebs, N. (1995). Normal childhood nutrition and its disorders. In Hay, W., et al. *Current pediatric diagnosis and treatment* (12th ed.). Norwalk, CT: Appleton and Lange. Reprinted by permission.

Most commercial formulas are based on heat-treated, nonfat cow's milk, to which vitamins, minerals, fats, and sugars are added. Others are based on soy products. The choice of an initial formula is generally made by the pediatrician.

References

Riordan, J., & Auerbach, K. G. (2005). *Breastfeeding and human lactation* (3rd ed.). Sudbury, MA: Jones and Bartlett Publishers.

Varney, H., Kriebs, J. M., & Gegor, C. L. (2004). *Varney's midwifery* (4th ed.). Sudbury, MA: Jones and Bartlett Publishers. Chs. 10, 40, 43.

Walker, M. L. (2002). *Core curriculum for lactation consultant practice*. Sudbury, MA: Jones and Bartlett Publishers.

World Health Organization. Accessed online at http://www. who.org.

Appendix A

Table of Normal Laboratory Values for Nonpregnant
and Pregnant Women

Laboratory Test	Nonpregnant	Pregnant
Hematology		
Hematocrit	37%–47%	33%–44%
Hemoglobin	12–16 g/dL	11–14 g/dL
Erythrocyte count	$4.8 \times 10^6/mm^3$	$4.0 \times 10^6/mm^3$
Leukocyte count	$6.0\ (4.5–11) \times 10^3/mm^3$	$9.2\ (6–16) \times 10^3/mm^3$
Neutrophils	$4.4\ (1.8–7.7) \times 10^3/mm^3$	$(3.8–10) \times 10^3/mm^3$
Lymphocytes	$2.5\ (1–4.8) \times 10^3/mm^3$	$(1.3–5.2) \times 10^3/mm^3$
Monocytes	$0.30\ (0–0.8) \times 10^3/mm^3$	No change
Eosinophils	$0.20\ (0–0.45) \times 10^3/mm^3$	No change
Platelet count	130,000–400,000/mL	Slight decrease
Fibrinogen	200–450 ng/dL	400–650 ng/dL
Folate		
Red blood cell	150–450 ng/mL cells	100–400 ng/mL cells
Ferritin	25–200 ng/mL	15–150 ng/mL
Iron	135 µg/dL	90 µg/dL
Iron-binding capacity	250–460 µg/dL	300–600 µg/dL
Coagulation studies		
Bleeding time (Duke)	<4 min	No change
Partial thrombo-plastin time	24–36 sec	No change
Prothrombin time	12–14 sec	No change
Thrombin time	12–18 sec	No change

Laboratory Test	Nonpregnant	Pregnant
Factors		
VIII	60%–100%	120%–200%
X, IX	60%–100%	90%–120%
VII, XII	60%–100%	No change
II, V, XI	60%–100%	No change
V	60%–100%	No change

Renal

BUN	10–20 mg/dL	5–12 mg/dL
Creatinine	<1.5 mg/dL	<0.8 mg/dL
Magnesium	2–3 mg/dL	1.6–2.1 mg/dL
Osmolality	285–295 mOsm/kg H_2O	275–280 mOsm/kg H_2O
Sodium	136–145 mEq/L	130–140 mEq/L
Potassium	3.5–5 mEq/L	3.3–4.1 mEq/L
Carbon dioxide content	21–30 mEq/L	18–25 mEq/L
Chloride	98–106 mEq/L	93–100 mEq/L
Uric acid	1.5–6 mg/dL	1.2–4.5 mg/dL
Urinary protein	<150 mg/day	<250–300 mg/day
Creatinine clearance	91–130 mL/min	120–160 mL/min
Complement (total)	150–250 CH50	200–400 CH50
C3	55–120 mg/dL	100–180 mg/dL

Endocrine

Glucose, fasting (plasma)	75–115 mg/dL	60–105 mg/dL
ACTH	20–100 pg/mL	No change
Aldosterone (plasma)	<8 ng/dL	<20 ng/dL
Aldosterone (urinary)	8–20 µg/24 hr	15–40 µg/24 hr
Cortisol (plasma)	5–25 µg/dL	15–35 µg/dL
Growth hormone, fasting	<5 ng/mL	No change
Insulin, fasting	6–26 µU/mL	8–30 µU/mL
Parathyroid hormone (Bio–intact)	20–30 pg/mL	10–20 pg/mL
Prolactin	2–15 ng/mL	50–400 ng/mL
Renin activity (plasma)	0.9–3.3 ng/mL/hr	3–8 ng/mL/hr
Thyroxine (T_4), total	5–12 µg/dL	10–17 µg/dL
Triiodothyronine (T_3)	70–190 ng/dL	100–220 ng/dL

Free T$_4$	1–2 ng/dL	No change
T$_3$ resin uptake	25%–35%	15%–25%
Free thyroxine index	1.75–4.95	No change
TSH	4–5 μU/mL	No change
Calcium		
Total	9.0–10.5 mg/dL	8.1–9.5 mg/dL
Ionized (serum)	4.5–5.6 mg/dL	4–5 mg/dL
Inorganic phosphorus	3.0–4.5 mg/dL	No change

Hepatic and Enzymes

Bilirubin (total)	0.3–1 mg/dL	No change
Cholesterol	120–180 mg/dL	180–280 mg/dL
Triglyceride	<160 mg/dL	<260 mg/dL
Amylase	60–180 U/L	90–350 U/L
Creatine phosphokinase	10–70 U/L	5–40 U/L
Lactic dehydrogenase (LDH)	200–450 U/mL	No change
Lipase	4–24 IU/dL	2–12 IU/dL
Alkaline phosphatase	30–95 mU/mL	60–200 mU/mL
Alanine amino transaminase	0–35 U/L	No change
Aspartate amino transaminase	0–35 U/L	No change
γ–Glutamyl transpeptidase	1–45 IU/L	No change
Ceruloplasmin	27–37 mg/dL	40–60 mg/dL
Copper	70–140 ng/dL	120–200 ng/dL
Protein (total)	5.5–8 g/dL	4.5–7 g/dL
Albumin	3.5–5.5 g/dL	2.5–4.5 g/dL
IgA	90–325 mg/dL	No change
IgM	45–150 mg/dL	No change
IgG	800–1500 mg/dL	700–1400 mg/dL

The exact values depend on the individual laboratory.

ACTH, adrenocorticotropic hormone; BUN, blood urea nitrogen; IgA, IgG, and IgM, immunoglobulins A, G, and M; TSH, thyroid-stimulating hormone.

Source: Burrow, G.N., Duffy, T.P., & Copel, J.A. (2004). *Medical complications during pregnancy* (6th ed.). Philadelphia: Elsevier Saunders. Used by permission.

APPENDIX B

A Timeline of Modern 20th Century Midwifery

by Helen Varney Burst

At the beginning of the 1900s, midwifery was neither an organized nor a well-respected profession in the United States, although European and African midwives had practiced since their first arrival on the continent, and the presence of Native American midwifery is documented in drawings created during the western expansion of European Americans.

This timeline briefly represents the changes that began occurring in midwifery and in women and infant health care at about the same time. For a detailed discussion of these issues, the reader is referred to the first chapter of *Varney's Midwifery*, 4th edition.

1903	—Federal Children's Bureau is proposed by Lillian Wald; established in 1912; promoted prenatal care
1911	—Bellevue School of Midwifery in NYC is established to educate indigenous midwives (closed 1935)
1918	—Maternity Center Association (MCA) is established in New York City with Hazel Corbin, RN, as executive director; promoted family-centered maternity care, developed childbirth education materials,

	demonstrated specialized maternity care with Henry Street Visiting Nurses Association
1921–1929	—Shepherd-Towner Act facilitates education, licensure, and supervision of African American and immigrant midwives; mandated provision of maternity care for all women
1923	—Preston Retreat Hospital, Philadelphia, opens a course in midwifery for practical nurses, and later, registered nurses (closed 1960)
1925	—Frontier Nursing Service (FNS), originally known as the Kentucky Committee for Mothers and Babies, is founded by Mary Breckinridge
	—Manhattan Midwifery School opens, the first school specifically established to educate graduate nurses as midwives
1929	—Kentucky State Association of Midwives is founded for nurse-midwives associated with FNS; later becomes the American Association of Nurse-Midwives
1931	—Lobenstine Midwifery Clinic is incorporated in New York City, organized by the Association for the Promotion and Standardization of Midwifery (closed 1958)
1932	—Lobenstine Midwifery School opens; Hattie Hemschemeyer, director of the clinic and the school, is a graduate of the first class; the school becomes the Maternity Center Association School of Nurse-Midwifery in 1934
1939	—FNS opens the Frontier Graduate School of Midwifery in Hyden, Kentucky

1941	—Tuskegee School of Nurse-Midwifery opens in Tuskegee, Alabama (closed 1946)
1942	—Flint-Goodrich School of Nurse-Midwifery opens in New Orleans, Louisiana (closed 1943)
1944	—National Organization of Public Health Nurses (NOPHN) adds a nurse-midwifery section
	—Catholic Maternity Institute (CMI) founded in Santa Fe, New Mexico; provides clinical services at home and in a birthing center (La Casita) (closed 1969)
1945	—CMI School of Nurse-Midwifery opens with Sister Theophane Shoemaker as director of both the school and the service (closed 1968)
1947	—Catholic University of America, Washington, DC, in affiliation with CMI, opens the first master's degree program for nurse-midwives (closed 1968)
1949	—The Nurse-Midwifery section within the NOPHN publishes the first national descriptive data gathered about nurse-midwives
1952	—The NOPHN is dissolved and absorbed into the American Nurses Association and the National League for Nursing; neither of these organizations make any provision for a recognizable entity of nurse-midwives
1954	—The Committee on Organization is formed with Sister Theophane Shoemaker as chair

1955 —The American College of Nurse-Midwifery is incorporated; Hattie Hemschemeyer is the first president, Sister Theophane Shoemaker is president-elect, the *Bulletin of the American College of Nurse-Midwifery* is designated the official publication of the ACNM

1956 —The ACNM is accepted into the International Confederation of Midwives (ICM)

1960s —The Madera County Project, with Armentia Jarrett as the principal nurse-midwife, demonstrates effectiveness and safety of nurse-midwifery care in a rural California community

1967 —ACNM Foundation incorporates; initially conceived and implemented by Ruth and Bill Lubic

1968 —Maternal-Infant Care (MIC) program is established in New York City with Dorothea Lang as director

1969 —A nurse-midwife (Ingeborg Rathke) first practices in the Indian Health Service
—The American College of Nurse-Midwifery and the American Association of Nurse-Midwives merge to become the American College of Nurse-Midwives

1970s —Nurse-midwives enter private practice in the United States

1971 —Official recognition by organized obstetrics; first joint statement by the American College of Obstetricians and Gynecologists, the Nurses Association of the American College of Obstetricians and Gynecologists, and the American College of Nurse-Midwives

1972	—ICM-US: ACNM is host for triennial meeting of ICM; Lucille Woodville, ACNM past-president is ICM president
1973	—The *Bulletin of the American College of Nurse-Midwifery* becomes the *Journal of Nurse-Midwifery*
1974	—The ACNM board recommends that separate statutory recognition be the basis for nurse-midwifery practice
1977	—ACNM archives are gifted to the National Library of Medicine
	—The ACNM Division of Examiners is a founding member of the National Commission of Health Certifying Agencies
	—First national meeting of lay midwives occurs in El Paso, Texas
1978	—CHAMPUS legislation passed by Congress includes the first national mandate for direct reimbursement of nurse-midwives
1980	—*Nurse-Midwifery* by Helen Varney (Burst) is the first nurse-midwifery textbook published in the western hemisphere; name is changed to *Varney's Midwifery* with third edition in 1997
1981	—ACNM receives its first international grant, targeted for training traditional birth attendants, which leads to the development of the Special Projects Section, later known as the Department of Global Outreach; first directed by Bonnie Pederson
1982	—The ACNM Division of Accreditation (DOA) is first recognized by the U.S. Department of Education as an accrediting

agency for nurse-midwifery education programs

—Midwives Alliance of North America (MANA) is founded

1986 —The North American Registry of Midwives (NARM) evolves from MANA and is separately incorporated

1990 —The Division of Competency Assessment (formerly the Division of Examiners) separates from ACNM and is incorporated as the ACNM Certification Council, Inc. (ACC)

1991 —Midwifery Education and Accreditation Council (MEAC) evolves from MANA

1993 —ACNM establishes a Department of Professional Services, with Deanne Williams as the first director

1994 —The ACNM Fellowship is established under the leadership of Mary Ann Shah

—*An Administrative Manual for Nurse-Midwifery Service Directors* is first written and published as a project of the Service Directors Network

1996 —The Midwifery Business Institute is developed at the University of Michigan

—The first program preaccredited by the ACNM DOA for the education of direct entry midwives opens at the State University of New York Downstate Medical Center in Brooklyn in affiliation with North Central Bronx Hospital

2001 —ACNM Division of Accreditation is recognized by the U.S. Department of Education to accredit direct entry midwifery education programs, whose graduates are certified as Certified Midwives (CMs) by the ACC upon passage of the same certification examination as CNMs

—MEAC is recognized by the U.S. Department of Education to accredit education programs for direct entry midwives. Graduates of these programs take the NARM examination to become Certified Professional Midwives (CPM)

—National Association of Certified Professional Midwives is formed

—*The Journal of Nurse-Midwifery* becomes the *Journal of Midwifery and Women's Health*

Index